To Eric Engleman MD
Best wishes for a successful and
rewarding future in Urology
Allan H. Haward MD

DIAGNOSTIC AND THERAPEUTIC AIDS IN UROLOGY

DIAGNOSTIC AND

THERAPEUTIC

AIDS IN UROLOGY

By **HENRY BODNER, M.D.**

Associate Clinical Professor
Department of Surgery (Urology)
Loma Linda University School of Medicine
White Memorial Hospital Division
Los Angeles, California

In Collaboration with

JOHN S. ARCONTI, JR., M.D.
Formerly Clinical Instructor
Department of Surgery (Urology)
University of California Center for the Health Sciences
Los Angeles, California

ALLAN H. HOWARD, M.D.
Associate Clinical Professor
Department of Surgery (Urology)
University of California Medical Center
Irvine, California

ROBERT O. PEARMAN, M.D.
Associate Professor
Department of Surgery (Urology)
University of California Center for the Health Sciences
Los Angeles, California

Illustrated by

JOHN S. ARCONTI, JR., M.D.

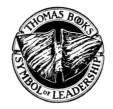

CHARLES C THOMAS • PUBLISHER
Springfield, Illinois

Published and Distributed Throughout the World by

CHARLES C THOMAS · PUBLISHER

Bannerstone House

301-327 East Lawrence Avenue, Springfield, Illinois, U.S.A.

© *1974, by* CHARLES C THOMAS · PUBLISHER

ISBN 0-398-02969-5

Library of Congress Catalog Card Number: 73-12745

*With THOMAS BOOKS careful attention is given to all details of
manufacturing and design. It is the Publisher's desire to present books
that are satisfactory as to their physical qualities and artistic possibilities
and appropriate for their particular use. THOMAS BOOKS will be true
to those laws of quality that assure a good name and good will.*

Printed in the United States of America

PP-22

Library of Congress Cataloging in Publication Data

Bodner, Henry, 1910–
    Diagnostic and therapeutic aids in urology.

    1. Urology. I. Title. [DNLM: 1. Urologic
diseases—Diagnosis. 2. Urologic diseases—Therapy.
3. Urology—Instrumentation. WJ100 B663d 1973]
RC871.B63   616.6   73-12745
ISBN 0-398-02969-5

To Dorothy, for her unfailing
patience, forbearance, and understanding during the many
months expended in the preparation of this volume.   H.B.

PREFACE

"I expect to pass through this world but once. Any good therefore that I can do, or any kindness that I can show to any fellow creature, let me do it now. Let me not defer or neglect it, for I shall not pass this way again."

Attributed to Stephen Grellet

THE PRACTICAL "TRICKS of the trade," gadgets, and shortcuts in diagnostic, surgical, and therapeutic applications in all phases of medicine are usually passed down from physician to physician, though not necessarily recorded in standard textbooks. On approaching the post-residency period, the neophyte urologist frequently finds himself faced with many unanswered questions. These may include uncertainty as to future type of practice (university, salary, administrative, or private practice), location, special and general equipment needs, layout and size of offices, treatment rooms, etc. There are questions as to what procedures should be done in one's office, when to hospitalize, types or means of anesthesia, etc. There are doubts in the urologist's mind as to the value of specific techniques, the use of one modality vs. another, in addition to the ubiquitous practical problems of recordkeeping, bookkeeping, and myriad administrative details which obviously are omitted from medical textbooks.

To fill the need for guidance in some of the areas mentioned above, the authors have combined their years of urologic experience to point out some applicable aids in the practice of urology. Obviously one can in a short volume present only a *limited number* of such concepts. We feel, nonetheless, that this book should be helpful to general practitioners and to specialists in many branches of medicine, as well as to our fellow urologists —residents, in particular. The practical tricks of the trade, gadgets, and shortcuts in diagnostic, surgical, and therapeutic applications may possibly be of value even to men of long experience who have themselves amassed a "bag of tricks."

Initially presented are needs encountered in setting up office or clinic urological practice. Useful instruments and equipment, and methods for their practical use, are included. Suggestions are made for treatment rooms, X-ray and laboratory setups. Emergency equipment, anesthesia, and amnesic agents are considered.

A chapter on the urine is included. Related factors deal with varied effects on urinary tract symptomatology of drugs and other agents. Urine collection methods, residual urine, and urinary flowrates are appraised.

A few aids in urological roentgenology are presented. The various parts of the urinary tract are also dealt with, beginning with the kidney.

It is manifest that changing techniques, equipment, and therapy modes will make obsolete many of the ideas contained herein almost before they are written. Therefore, this book presents its subjects in short, precise form, devoid of long discussion and controversy, and with the idea of periodic revision. The usual and customary techniques appearing in standard textbooks on urology are for the most part avoided in this work. However, when variations on standard diagnostic and therapeutic techniques are recognized, they are presented.

The authors expect that this publication will motivate others to produce similar types of guidebooks in other specialties.

ACKNOWLEDGMENTS

In the evolution of this volume, it has been my privilege to have the collaboration of fellow urologists of wide clinical and teaching experience. My longtime partner in practice, Dr. Allan H. Howard, wrote Chapters Five and Nine, while Dr. Robert O. Pearman contributed Chapter Six. Dr. John S. Arconti, Jr., shared his artistic gifts by his illustration of the entire book. In addition, he spent many weeks in critical evaluation of the manuscript, to which he added many ideas of his own. All of the authors collaborated on the entire contents.

Since 1957, I have been publishing a regular edition of the "Weekly Urological Clinical Letter" (W.U.C.L.). Once a year, each of approximately 150 urologists in this Letter group, on request, contributes a one-page article relative to ideas on treatment, new devices, gadgets, or innovative uses for various equipment in the field of urology. These articles are edited, typed, reproduced, and sent to members of the Letter group throughout the nation and to many urologists in foreign countries. We have in this book included a great many of these contributed ideas, in order to share widely the thoughts of the member urologists, who are men in private practice as well as members of the faculties of university medical centers. Though many of the ideas submitted had been known and used by us previously, the authors wish to thank all the members of the W.U.C.L. group and most gratefully acknowledge their contributions.

The large number of contributing W.U.C.L. members (past and present) precludes mention of individual names and titles with each specific subject. In addition, the multiplicity of ideas and the diversity of their exact origins renders impractical the conferral of credit for each line, sentence, and paragraph. Therefore, the names of the contributing member urologists are listed as an appendix—we trust that we may be forgiven the task of referencing each bit of information, in the interest of disseminating that information while it is still topical.

We are grateful to Virginia Reed Hansen for her untiring efforts in editing, rewriting, and typing the manuscript throughout the long period of the book's preparation, and for her valued advice concerning literary form. Much credit is also due my faithful secretary, Marjorie Cooper, whose innumerable hours of work served to enable the project to be completed.

Our most sincere thanks are extended to Mr. Payne Thomas and the publishing house of Charles C Thomas for their continuing, patient encouragement and many kindnesses.

HENRY BODNER

FIGURES

xi

TABLES

DIAGNOSTIC AND THERAPEUTIC AIDS IN UROLOGY

Chapter One

ARMAMENTARIUM

GENERAL FACILITIES AND EQUIPMENT

A FTER RESIDENCY TRAINING, the neophyte urologist must very often choose his office location and equipment without prior experience except that gained by visiting other urologists in the area where he intends to practice. A professional planning service from an equipment manufacturer, or an interior decorator, may be helpful in providing room and equipment layout. The general planning and choice of color scheme and furnishings should befit the convenience and reflect the taste of the individual physician. University clinic facilities should receive the same careful consideration.

Facilities

Waiting Room

Since the patient receives the first impression of his physician by the appearance of the reception area, the waiting room should be cheerful and attractive, and as spacious as necessary to provide comfortable seating room for the expected number of patients and accompanying family members or friends. The size and number of seating places required is governed by individual needs. Small sofas—for two or three persons—or individual chairs are more practical than long sofas on which patients tend to spread themselves out at the ends, thereby discouraging the seating of new arrivals between them.

Comfort and relaxation for the waiting patient, simplicity of design, sturdy construction, and upholstery that is easy to care for should be considered in choosing the furniture.

Receptionist's Office

The office of the receptionist should be readily accessible from the waiting room. In most instances a sliding glass window and wall separate the receptionist from the waiting room. She should, however, be visible to the patients, lest they feel neglected. The receptionist's area will doubtless adjoin the business office area which will be equipped with the usual office desks, counters, filing cabinets, bookkeeping machines, intercommunications units, etc.

Consultation Room

The consultation room should be large enough to accommodate the patient and possibly two members of the family, a minimum of nine feet by eleven feet in size. This room, too, should be attractive to the patient, for it is here that he develops his possible lasting impression of his physician.

Treatment and Cystoscopy Rooms

Most one-physician offices require only two to three treatment rooms, since it is not possible for one physician to treat more than three patients at one time. A fourth such room may be justified by the occasional patient who must spend an unusually long period of time for recovery following a minor surgical procedure or other treatment in the office.

Treatment rooms should be so planned that when a patient is on the examining table, his head is toward the door. When the door of a treatment room is open the patient should be behind the door if at all possible.

The treatment room size should preferably be a minimum of seven by ten feet. A cystoscopy room should be a minimum of nine by twelve feet, whereas an operating cystoscopy room should preferably be the size of a standard operating room. Ideally, a one-physician facility should have one cystoscopy room to two treatment rooms.

Recovery Room

In some parts of the United States, retrograde pyelography is done in the physician's office. The performance of such a procedure makes necessary the provision of a recovery room. In other parts of the country, such examinations are done in the hospital, the physician's treatment room being reserved for simple cystoscopic observations, dilations, intravenous pyelography, and other procedures which require only local anesthetics or anesthesia to the amnesia level.

Other Facilities

A *bathroom* (toilet and lavatory) within the suite (4 feet by 4 feet, minimum) is a basic necessity for the urological office.

Provision of *laboratory facilities* will, of course, be at the option of the physician. Plans for a small clinical laboratory are available from biological supply companies. The ease of performing urine cultures and sensitivity testing with present-day culture media warrants these procedures being done by the urologist.

X-ray facilities provided in the office minimize hospital time or may even obviate hospitalization. The physician may therefore elect to include these in his office plans.

Sinks in treatment rooms, whether built in with cabinets around them, or standing as a single unit, need be no larger than 12 by 12 inches * and should preferably be at 28- or 29-inch level. This height facilitates the collection of urine specimens by male patients in a treatment room. The patient may, for example, in catching urine in three bottles, switch from bottle to bottle. With the sink at this height, spillage will be into the sink and not onto the floor. Avoidance of a wide border around the sink at the periphery also enables the patient to more conveniently void into the container.

For male patients on whom one is to do prostatic massage (on an empty bladder), utilization of the sink in the treatment room is more convenient than having the patient proceed back and forth from a bathroom to void.

Floor drains should be preplanned and provided in treatment rooms for use with the urological examining and cystoscopic tables. The collection of bladder irrigating fluids in buckets is thereby eliminated.

Provision for *adequate lighting* is essential and should be thoroughly preplanned. This also applies to *telephone and intercommunication systems.* It is practical to have an extension telephone and "intercom" unit within each treatment room and in easy reach, so that the physician while treating a patient may answer telephone calls in a treatment room without having to make frequent trips back to a consultation room. The treatment room telephones should not have outside dialing facilities—patients while waiting in treatment rooms have been known to make long-distance calls.

Additional standard equipment such as cabinets, lavatories, waste and laundry receptacles, etc., will obviously be needed. These should be designed for the convenience of the individual physician. Deep pullout bins lined with large plastic disposal bags are convenient and out-of-sight means of collecting waste and soiled laundry items. A discard hole cut directly over the bin in the counter top makes unnecessary the pulling out of the bin each time a disposal is made. Sink enclosure cabinets may be purchased as prefabricated units or may be custom-made.

A wallboard mounted over the treatment room sink area is a convenient location for dispensers of paper towels, liquid soap, tissues, adhesive tapes, gloves, clear plastic wrap (such as Saran Wrap ®), etc.

A built-in shelf, 12 inches wide and 30 inches long, on the wall next to a cystoscopy or treatment table very conveniently will hold the trays of cold sterilizing solution in which cystoscopes, sounds, etc., are immersed. The irrigating tubing and the cords for the battery operated or fiber optic power unit lie immersed in the solution ready for instant use. The same shelf holds the power units, as well as lubricating jelly, etc.

In treatment rooms, cabinet drawers may be partitioned either transversely or lengthwise to hold cystoscopic instruments, sounds, bougies,

---

* One standard-size sink (either in the laboratory or other work area) should be provided to enable nurses to adequately clean equipment and instruments.

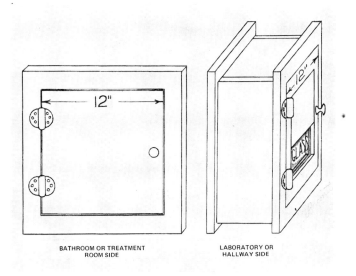

BATHROOM OR TREATMENT
ROOM SIDE   LABORATORY OR
                                                 HALLWAY SIDE

1. Pass-through for urine specimens

catheters and other items. Most urological instruments will fit into drawers at least 3 inches high and 18 inches long (inside dimensions). This drawer partitioning makes it easier to put instruments away in their proper places and permits instant availability of the desired instruments.

For the efficient operation of a urological office and the rapid collection of urine specimens, a *pass-through for urine specimens* is recommended. The patient may void into a plastic disposable urine specimen glass, open the door of the pass-through box and place the glass in the wall cubicle. The specimen should be visible to the nurse (through a one-way-view glass strip) from the hallway or laboratory, and available to her through a similar door. The patient's privacy is maintained and urine can be collected with no loss of time or embarrassment to either patient or nurse. Hinged doors with magnetic latches are suggested (see Fig. 1).

Equipment

Basic Equipment List

For a physician beginning the practice of urology a basic equipment list is here suggested. Obviously, one is necessarily guided by the funds available for the purchase of such equipment. In some areas of the country, hospitals supply a limited amount of equipment. In others, the urologist must supply his own. Only that equipment used in the office and not provided for hospital use need be purchased.

Equipment needed for the completely furnished urologic office follows:

SUGGESTED BASIC UROLOGIC EQUIPMENT LIST

1 ea.	Portable fiber optic power source
2 ea.	Instrument bundles or fiber optic light cord
1 ea.	Miniature cystoscope
1 ea.	Foroblique telescope
1 ea.	Visual lithotrite
1 ea.	Cystourethroscope, 22 French
1 ea.	Retrospective telescope
1 ea.	Right-angle telescope
1 ea.	Infant resectoscope (seldom used)
1 ea.	Resectoscope with long- or short-beak fiberglass sheaths and extra working element
1 ea.	Flexible scissor forceps with handle, 7 French
1 ea.	Flexible rongeur forceps without handle, 7 French
1 ea.	Flexible foreign body forceps without handle, 7 French
1 ea.	Lowsley grasping forceps
1 ea.	Kollmann dilator, curved, with handle
1 ea.	Kollmann dilator, pediatric model
1 ea.	Otis urethrotome
2 ea.	McCrea or Van Buren stainless steel sounds, 8-30 French, even numbers
1 doz.	Olive tip filiforms, 1/56 thread, sizes 3, 4, 5, and 6 French
1 doz.	Spiral filiforms, 1/56 thread, sizes 3, 4, 5, and 6 French
1 doz.	Coudé filiforms, 1/56 thread, sizes 3, 4, 5, and 6 French
6 ea.	Cutting loops, yellow, 0.012 inch
6 ea.	Cutting loops, grey, 0.015 inch
1 doz.	Cutting loops, blue, 0.015 inch
2 ea.	Knife electrode, yellow
1 ea.	Knife electrode, grey
1 ea.	Knife electrode, blue
2 ea.	Dormia ureteral stone dislodger
1 ea.	Portable electrosurgical unit
plus	Cystoscopic X-ray table with complete 200-ma rotating anode tube and accessories, developing tank, complete darkroom equipment, film as selected ⎫ optional
plus	Laboratory setup: centrifuge, microscope, testing chemicals as selected, sink, counters, cabinets, emergency setup (complete)
plus	Examining and treatment tables, sinks, counters, cabinets, stools, lights, cystoscopic equipment for treatment rooms
plus	Office equipment: desks, chairs, typewriter, adding machine, photocopy unit, files, stationery items
plus	Furnishings for reception room
plus	Furnishings for consultation room

NOTE: Assorted catheters (ureteral and urethral) are not here included. See *Urological Instruments for the General Practitioner* in this chapter; also *Catheter* category in INDEX.

Light Sources

Battery operated or fiber optic light sources are necessary. Two 1-½-volt dry-cell batteries in series (3 volts) serve well to illuminate any cystoscopic light bulb. Maximum safe illumination is obtained at 3 volts. The bulbs will usually burn out at 3.2 volts plus. In all probability, bulb-type cystoscopes will be replaced entirely by fiber optic equipment within the next few years.

It is suggested that one inspect and consider the fiber optic equipment manufactured by several American and foreign firms. Lenses which may be interchanged with equipment of multiple manufacturers are most desirable. (See *Adapters for Use of Various Fiber Optic Lenses* near end of this chapter.)

Equipment for Cystoscopic Irrigation

A practical system for office cystoscopic irrigation apparatus requires preplanning for proper installation. One may depend on the prepared plastic bag solutions or bottles of distilled water put out by the various pharmaceutical houses, with component sterilized plastic tubing for direct connection to the cystoscope, or one may employ a Valentine irrigating jar utilizing weak antiseptic solutions. Deionized water is utilized by some urologists while boiled, sterilized tap water is used by others.

Distilled water must be used if fulguration of a small lesion such as a bladder tumor is performed in the office, as the electrolytes in tap water disturb cutting and coagulation. Built-in irrigation systems are available.

Suggested Cystoscopic Irrigation System

This system, designed for a urological group or a cystoscopic suite in a hospital, provides sterile distilled water automatically with a minimum of maintenance. The essential parts of the system are a deionizer to pretreat the water, a still for further purification and sterilization, and a recirculating system to deliver the water to the point of use. The size of the water still is dependent on the water volume required per hour.

The heart of the system is a master control that senses water pressure in the incoming line and water level in the storage sump. This control opens and closes the supply of water and starts and stops the still as required to maintain the water supply. The delivery system has a pump to move the water to the use points and return the unused water to the storage sump. The system (storage sump) also has an ozone generator and a 0.45μ filter to maintain sterility in this part of the system. For protection of the system there is a pressure switch in the incoming line to shut down the still should the building water supply fail, and a low-level switch in the storage sump to shut off the pump before the water level in the storage sump drops so low as to permit the pump to run dry.

The system operates with a minimum of attention. The deionizer must be exchanged upon exhaustion (every two to three months), which requires only a telephone call to the water deionizer distributor. The still pot should be flushed according to the manufacturer's recommendations. As a safety precaution, scheduled cultures should be run on samples taken from the point of use to assure that the system remains sterile.

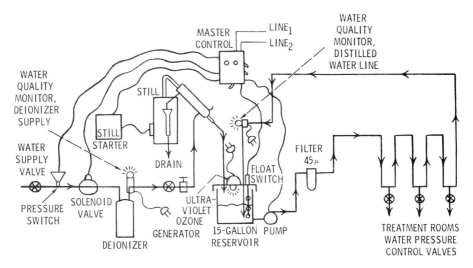

WATER
QUALITY
MONITOR,
DISTILLED
WATER LINE

MASTER
CONTROL
LINE₁
LINE₂

WATER
QUALITY
MONITOR,
DEIONIZER
SUPPLY

STILL

STILL
STARTER

WATER
SUPPLY
VALVE

DRAIN

FILTER
45 μ

FLOAT
SWITCH

PRESSURE
SWITCH

SOLENOID
VALVE

ULTRA-
VIOLET
OZONE
GENERATOR

15-GALLON
RESERVOIR

PUMP

DEIONIZER

TREATMENT ROOMS
WATER PRESSURE
CONTROL VALVES

2. Flow chart of sterile water irrigation system

Between cystoscopic procedures, the water connector and about two feet of plastic tubing lie continuously in the pan of cold sterilizing solution used to sterilize cystoscopes. Aqueous activated dealdehyde (Cidex)* or equivalent solution is recommended. It is important to remember, however, that *cutting loops should be gas-sterilized* (see succeeding section on *Electrosurgical Units*).

It is recommended that plastic tubing only be used for cystoscopic irrigation systems, and that the system be equipped with Luer-lock adapter valves.

Figure 2 is a flow chart of the described cystoscopic irrigation system.

X-Ray Equipment

A 200-milliampere (minimum) X-ray machine is most desirable for office or outpatient clinic use. This machine should have a rotating anode. Because of exposure time, the 100-ma X-ray unit is not too satisfactory for use with the heavier patient or with children. Intravenous pyelography and cystography are best done with the larger unit.

The volume of X-ray work done by most urologists probably does not warrant the use of an automatic developing unit like the X-OMAT® by Kodak. Group practice urologic offices and outpatient clinics, however, have sufficient volume to consider this type of developing equipment. Much time and effort is conserved by its use. A busy clinic or university urology depart-

---

* Important Note: Throughout this volume, when drug names are not marked with the customary ®, we have followed the generic name with the trademarked name in parentheses. The first letter of the trademarked name is capitalized; generic names are not so indicated.

ment may utilize the portable image amplifier with television monitor for visualization of renal pelvis filling, etc.

Electrosurgical Units

A small electrosurgical unit is a necessary part of the office or outpatient department. Many excellent units are available. With this unit one may fulgurate tiny bleeding surfaces or tumors in the bladder or in the urethra under sodium methohexital (Brevital) amnesia without the necessity for hospitalizing the patient.

A small self-contained, battery-operated electrosurgical unit developed for use in ophthalmology works exceedingly well for meticulous hemostasis in such procedures as hypospadias repair; these units (OPTEMP®) are inexpensive and disposable.

SAFEGUARDS IN USE OF ELECTROSURGICAL UNITS. Operating room personnel as well as urologists must learn to use an ohmmeter to check power cords, loops, and working elements of all electrosurgical units to be certain there is no shorting-out of current in the system. The testing cords and clips of the ohmmeter may be cold-sterilized, as are the power cords and the working elements. *Cutting loops*, however, *should be gas-sterilized* and preferably packaged in pairs.

One may also use a battery-operated electrical circuit tester. This simple instrument is so made that if there is any electrical continuity, an indicator light will go on. Therefore, when there is any shorting-out, there will be evidence of electrical continuity where there should not be.

It is essential that operating room personnel, under the supervision of the urologist, realize that the patient grounding plate surface area required by most electrosurgical units demands limitation of 1.5 watts to a square centimeter of indifferent electrode contact. *It is therefore critical that the plate be placed entirely under the patient, where complete contact is made, so that there will not be any exceeding of 9.675 watts per square inch of body surface. It is also essential that not even a small portion of the sheet or towel slip between the plate and the patient's body.*

Now available on the market are electrosurgical units which automatically are inactivated when not properly grounded. This transistorized equipment is a marked improvement over previous units.

USE OF CUTTING CURRENT OF ELECTROSURGICAL UNIT INSTEAD OF COAGULATING CURRENT FOR HEMOSTASIS. In the performance of open surgery, many surgeons utilize the cutting current of the unit rather than the fulgurating current for hemostasis. The current, obviously, is set at a lower level than that ordinarily used for cutting. One merely slaps or touches the electrode for a fraction of a second against the hemostat to obtain the same coagulating effect as that obtained by holding the electrode against the hemostat for a period of a number of seconds when using the fulgurating current.

This use of the cutting current is a great timesaver. At times, however, bleeding is not controlled by fulguration, or by a combination of fulguration and compression of the bleeding site with a sponge for a number of minutes. In such cases, a Penrose drain may be held against the oozing area. The combination of fulguration and pressure with this non-adhering surface will often effect hemostasis.

Electrocoagulation Forceps

There is available an insulated bayonet-type forceps with coagulation current which may be activated by closure of the forceps. This instrument may be adapted to various electrosurgical units. Insulation to the tip prevents inadvertent coagulation of tissue. Enclosure contact obviates the necessity for a foot switch.

This is a very useful and timesaving instrument for the hemostasis of minor vessels. The Turner-Warwick insulated electrosurgical thumb forceps, hemostatic forceps, and hemostatic scissors are also helpful instruments for use with the electrosurgical unit.

Cystoscopic and Examining Tables

It has been difficult to decide upon a universally acceptable table for use in urologic procedures. Some popular tables are the Hamilton ® (as modified for urologic use), the Ritter Model 75 Universal®, the Utilex®, and Hydradjust ® tables (the last two made by Liebel-Flarsheim). Over the past few years these and other very satisfactory units have been on the market. It would behoove the urologist to look around well before making a decision as to which specific tables to use in his office or hospital urologic suite.

LABORATORY FACILITIES

Additional Reasons for Laboratory Facilities in the Office

Provision for urinalysis in the urologist's office is obviously required. In addition, equipment for culture and sensitivity testing will prove to be of extreme value. Many variations of systems and media are available from commercial sources.

The incubator serves well for gonococcus culture on Difco ® media. Female patients may be subjected to cervical and urethral cultures without disclosing the reasons for the cultures. Should a culture be positive, the patient must be so informed. Most patients under such circumstances are most cooperative. This testing, together with the proper reporting required by law but all too often ignored, will help to disclose and eradicate the female reservoir of gonococci which presently amounts to an epidemic.

Sterilizing Equipment

Steam Sterilization

An autoclave should be available for steam sterilization of dressings and sounds and other instruments which may be sterilized under steam pressure.

Cold Sterilization

Large plastic trays, inert with the chemical solutions to be contained therein,* may be purchased in any photographic supply shop. These trays are usually employed in photo developing. Approximate dimensions for trays which are adequate to hold most urological instruments (including cystoscopes) are 12 by 16 by 3-½ inches.

Cold-Sterilizing Solutions. Because of damage to lens cement, it is universally accepted that resectoscopes, etc., are best sterilized by cold-sterilizing solutions or gas sterilization. The cutting loops of resectoscopes are now known to be damaged by cold-sterilizing solutions. These must be gas-sterilized.

Numerous sterilizing solutions are available on the market. In the past oxycyanide of mercury was a favorite until it was shown that many varieties of organisms were able to grow within the substance. Aqueous benzyl (dodecyl-carbamyl methyl) dimethyl ammonium chloride (Urolocide) is an excellent cold-sterilizing solution. A quartian ammonium (or benzalkonium chloride) solution sold under the trade name Zephiran ® may also be used as a cold-sterilizing solution. Zephiran does, however, tend to damage cystoscopes, especially when used without anti-rust tablets.

A preferred solution for cold sterilization is aqueous activated glutaraldehyde (2% solution supplied under the trade name Cidex). This is a quick acting and highly effective disinfectant with bactericidal, sporicidal, fungicidal, tuberculocidal, and viricidal properties. A contact time of 10 minutes is recommended for the destruction of vegetative bacterial and fungal cells, Mycobacterium tuberculosis, and viruses. Ten hours of contact time is recommended to totally destroy more resistant spores.

Cidex is of low toxicity for the user and the patient. It has no reported deleterious effects upon plastic or rubber goods or upon lensed instruments or their metal and metal-thread components. It has a short sterilization time, but is effective for an interval of at least two weeks and can be reused during this period. Its low-protein coagulability is advantageous. It has a mild odor, low volatility, and is noninflammable.

Cidex is bactericidal, tuberculocidal, pseudomonicidal, and viricidal within ten minutes; it is sporicidal within three hours. The agent must be

---

* Plastic trays are utilized with cold-sterilization solutions since the use of stainless steel pans may result in electrolysis of the chome- and nickel-plated instruments, causing them severe damage. The trays should be kept covered, if possible.

activated with sodium bicarbonate before it becomes effective, and recommended contact times should be closely followed (see also cautions below).

SOME DANGERS OF COLD-STERILIZING SOLUTIONS. In addition to the cystoscope damage previously mentioned with reference to Zephiran, the following cautions should be added regarding the use of Cidex.

Since aqueous activated glutaraldehyde is an irritant to bladder and ureteral mucosa, instruments must be carefully washed in sterile distilled water after being soaked in Cidex. The agent collects inside the rubber stoppers of the cystoscope and may not be rinsed out when instruments are placed in sterile water.

To properly wash out the rubber stoppers, they must be removed from the cystoscope and first soaked and then squeezed (milked) several times in the distilled water to force out Cidex held on the inner surface by negative or capillary pressure. When Cidex remains in the rubber stoppers, a ureteral catheter passing through the ureter may deposit concentrated solution within the channel.

All stop cocks on instruments should be opened during sterilization with Cidex, as well as during and after rinsing to ensure washing out of the concentrated solution.

Cases of oliguria have been reported which were apparently due to edema of ureteral orifices following catheterization with Cidex-soaked ureteral catheters which had not been properly rinsed after sterilization. Prompt recovery from creatinine levels of 5.0 mg percent occurred following 72 hours of further ureteral catheter drainage in two of the author's cases.

Gas Sterilization

Most hospitals now use gas sterilization in their operating suites. This has certain advantages over steam sterilization. With gas, the maximum temperature needed for sterilization is 130 degrees C, for a 3½-hour exposure time (though each 30° increase in temperature over 130° allows an exposure time rate decrease of 50% for bacterial kill). This compares with 240 degrees C temperature needed for steam sterilization for a 30- to 45-minute load; 275 degrees C temperature is needed for 3-minute "flashings." With gas, the pressure used within the chamber is 7.3 pounds per square inch. The cost per load for sterilization is minimal.

There is no condensation in the cystoscopic lenses or tubes when gas sterilization is used. The cement now used by the American Cystoscope Makers, Inc. and other cystoscope manufacturers is nonreactive to the inert gas used.

Sterilized instruments should not be put in use for several hours after sterilization, so that gas trapped within catheters and cystoscopes is allowed to escape.

All types of urological instruments may be sterilized by this means: ureteral catheters, cystoscopes, resectoscopes, balloon-type catheters, waxed filiforms and followers. There is no deterioration of catheters and dilators by use of this method. The cutting loops of the resectoscopes are safely sterilized *only* by this type of sterilization.

Small units for gas sterilization in the urological office are manufactured in either tray or canister form. The tray container should be approximately 16 inches long, 10 inches wide, and 4 inches deep. The canister should be about 8 inches in diameter and 10 inches deep. In both, rubber goods and metal equipment are wrapped separately and placed in the container. A sensitized color tape is placed within each envelope to ensure adequate sterilization. A special envelope containing the gas ampule is then placed within the container and crushed. The lid is locked in place by means of clamps.

An added advantage of gas sterilization is that a complete set of needed cystoscopic instruments may be stored in a regular cabinet and kept ready for use at any time.

Ethylene oxide is the gas used in some of this equipment.

Other Laboratory Equipment

Thought should also be given to choice of microscope, centrifuge, small refrigerator, culture and sensitivity testing equipment, locked storage for narcotics, etc.

EMERGENCY EQUIPMENT

Introduction

At all times emergency equipment should be available in physicians' offices. Such equipment is demanded not only by common sense but by medical-legal requirements.

Most important of all are the rebreather mask and oxygen. Simple rebreather masks (in adult and child sizes) are available at surgical supply houses. Oxygen tanks, with their various valve attachments, etc., may be rented from a medical oxygen supply house. Intracath should be available. Mouth-to-mouth resuscitation equipment is necessary. It is desirable that the urologist be familiar with cardiopulmonary resuscitation.

It is advantageous to have on hand a No. 10 or 12 gauge short-beveled needle which may on rare occasions be useful in penetrating the cricoid cartilage instead of performing a tracheotomy.

Emergency Medications

The following medications may be considered for inclusion with the urologist's emergency equipment:

Adrenalin Chloride ® (1:1000 Adrenalin—epinephrine inj. U.S.P.)

Aminophylline

Anectine ® (succinylcholine chloride)

Aramine ® (metaraminol as bitartrate)

Aromatic spirits of ammonia

Atropine sulfate

Benadryl ® (diphenhydramine hydrochloride)

Caffeine and sodium benzoate

Calcium chloride in ampule for intravenous use

Dextrose (5% in distilled water)—in 500-ml or 1000-ml flasks

Distilled water (for injection)

Emivan ® (ethamivan-vanilic acid diethylamide in 5% aqueous solution of diethanolamine)

Isuprel ® (isoproterenol hydrochloride, U.S.P.)

Novocain ®, 1 percent (procaine hydrochloride)

Sodium bicarbonate (5%)

Sodium chloride

Solu-Cortef ® (hydrocortisone sodium succinate)

Trilafon ® (perphenazine)

Vasoxyl ® (methoxamine hydrochloride)

Other Emergency Equipment

Additional suggested equipment for emergencies includes:

Disposable and nondisposable syringes in sizes from 2½ to 50 cc

Disposable and nondisposable needles

Intravenous infusion sets, small and large, with injection sites for adding medication

Suction machine and aspirator

Scissors

Penrose tubing (sterile pack)

Cut-down tray (sterile pack)

Sterile blades for scalpels

Sterile sutures, absorbable and nonabsorbable

ANESTHESIA AND AMNESIC AGENTS

Introduction

A medical office or hospital outpatient department is no place for general anesthesia, as a rule. Nonetheless, some physicians do such procedures as retrograde pyelograms in their offices. Office procedures should be done under local anesthesia or anesthetic agents used to the *amnesia level only.*

Among the local anesthetic agents currently in use are lidocaine hydrochloride and dyclonine. The Duke University Trilene ® (trichloroethylene) inhalation mask is still popular with some urologists. Others prefer the use of hypnosis, a modality which is not too popular because of the amount of time it requires. At the time of this writing, acupuncture is under study as an amnesic medium. Its merits are as yet not completely determined.

Recommended Amnesic Agents

Sodium Methohexital (Brevital) for Urologic Procedures

At one time pentothal sodium administration to the amnesia level, as done by the psychiatrists, served as a valuable office procedure for performing cystoscopic or urethral instrumentation. Meperidine (Demerol) later came into favor for this purpose, succeeded now by sodium methohexital (Brevital) which has proven still more useful. Though about three times as potent as pentothal sodium, methohexital is only about one-half as long in action.

Our experience with this short-acting oxybarbiturate over a period of approximately ten years, for a total of nearly 50,000 injections, has been so successful and so much appreciated by grateful patients that it warrants describing in considerable detail.

Sodium methohexital, used in the dosage of 6 to 10 ml of one-half percent (or 30 to 50 mg) intravenously, has proved remarkably safe for use with outpatients subjected to urethral instrumentation such as dilation, simple cystoscopy, bladder dilation for interstitial cystitis, fulguration of small recurrent bladder tumors, needle biopsy of the prostate, or any other short procedure. In an occasional *rare* situation when the patient is fully awake, a second injection has been used to complete a procedure.

Patients should be first questioned as to sensitivity to any medications, including the barbiturates. Should they be allergic, the medication is not used. They are questioned, too, as to any other medication taken that day. Tranquilizing drugs potentiate the effect of barbiturates, and therefore smaller dosage is warranted.

The medication is not used in the very young or the very old. It is not used on patients in shock, with severe anemia or uremia, with advanced cardiorespiratory diseases, with myasthenias, with hepatic or adrenal dysfunction or insufficiency, with obstructive respiratory disease or debilitative state, or in patients who have been treated with hypotensive agents or steroids.

Appropriate equipment for the treatment of anesthetic emergencies should be available, even though an amnesic effect only is the application of the drug recommended; the use of this equipment has not been necessary in our large series of injections.

Methohexital causes no impairment of hepatic or renal function. There is no blood hemolysis and a true fall in blood pressure is a rarity. There is relatively no venous irritation. There is minimal effect on blood pressure; thus the drug may be used with safety in cardiac patients. Hiccoughing occurs in a very small percentage of cases. Infrequently a patient may develop hyperactive laryngeal reflex.

One may ignore the above incidents, however, since sodium methohexital in the recommended dosage is metabolized rapidly. The patient is completely awake before one could initiate therapeutic procedures for any complication. *Therein lies the safety of this drug in the recommended dosage schedule.* A dosage schedule above this amount is contraindicated as an office (or hospital outpatient) procedure since one is then placing the patient at an *anesthetic* level.

The necessary urological procedure must be completed within one or two minutes; thus instruments must be ready to use and the patient washed and draped for treatment prior to administration of the drug. The urologist must move rapidly in his performance of the necessary urologic procedure. From 6 to 10 ml (30 to 50 mg) of one-half percent sodium methohexital is injected rapidly intravenously. The dosage is dependent on the patient's weight and age, on an estimate-only basis.

This difference in dosage is not critical. No specific end point is utilized. There is a wide margin of safety in the dosage recommended, as 30 to 50 mg is the usual test dose administered by most anesthesiologists when sodium methohexital is used for anesthesia in hospital surgical procedures. *It is imperative*, however, *that the physician not exceed the recommended one-injection dosage* even though the patient may thrash about, cry out, or scream. Complete amnesia for these events is assured.

Patients often awaken after the completion of the treatment with the remark, "Don't begin yet, I'm still awake." Though patients are completely awake and able to proceed to their homes five to seven minutes after administration of the drug, they should not be allowed to leave for about thirty minutes for added safety reasons.

Though the additional use of preanesthetic agents or larger doses of medication would allow for longer procedures, it is again emphasized that anesthesia has no place in the office or in the outpatient department of a hospital. Sodium methohexital in the dosage herein recommended serves as an amnesic agent which is remarkably safe under office circumstances. The ease of its administration, its rapidity of effect, freedom from complications, and the extreme thankfulness of the patient, warrant the use of sodium methohexital by other physicians for short, painful urologic procedures.

Use of Diazepam (Valium)

Intravenous diazepam (Valium) in 5- to 10-mg intravenous dosage, has also become popular for short instrumentation procedures in recent years. This has been used, as well, by some physicians as premedication before the injection of sodium methohexital. It does prolong the effect of the medication. Side effects, however have been ascribed to the use of premedication and to combined usage of the two drugs, and we therefore recommend that sodium methohexital be used alone. For longer procedures, hospitalization, with the use of anesthesia and anesthesiologist, is urged.

OTHER EQUIPMENT USEFUL IN UROLOGIC PRACTICE

Devices, Gadgets, and Supplies

The Computer in the Future of Urology

In addition to the widening use of computer programs in hospitals and teaching institutions, in large medical groups and medical insurance coverage programs, there are currently in effect pilot programs to research the use of the computer in individual private practice.

Use of this space-age tool in tabulating the incidence of disease, frequency of procedures and operations, progress of patients, and in cost analysis, automatic patient recall, billing, insurance, etc., can be expected to increase vastly and to make an immense contribution to the evaluation of patients and to the accumulation of meaningful statistical research data for urologists and all others engaged in the practice of medicine.

Informed Consent: Use of Audiovisual Aids

In the present era of medical-legal awareness, informed consent has become mandatory before the performance of surgical procedures. Patients should have explained to them as thoroughly as possible the procedures contemplated. Many physicians utilize diagrams to enhance their explanations. Others use models of one type or another.

Presently available are audiovisual aids of wide variety. These may be used to great advantage in acquainting patients with the procedures to which they are to be subjected. Audiovisual machines of the type manufactured by Bell and Howell, and Fairchild, utilizing taped cassettes, are easily operated and can be employed to demonstrate with live action and animation the particular *modus operandi* which will answer the patients' questions and help them to understand their problem and its contemplated solution.

It is a simple matter, then, to ask a patient to sign his name to a record book stating that he has seen this particular film. This is a timesaver for the urologist and for other physicians.

Urological Instruments for the General Practitioner

Office instruments needed by general practitioners who are called upon to perform limited urological procedures should include woven nylon filiforms and woven (e.g., Phillips) or metal (e.g., Le Fort) followers.

A catheter which is of utmost value to the general practitioner is the rubber Coudé-tip (or Tiemann) catheter. Very often, in patients in retention due to prostatic hyperplasia, a physician will find it impossible to pass an ordinary red rubber rounded-tip Robinson catheter but will find to his amazement that a Coudé-tip Tiemann catheter will readily pass. The Phillips urethral catheter is a particularly useful instrument for patients with stricture.

Choice of Sheets, Drapes, Gowns, etc.

The economics of medical practice require laborsaving, timesaving, and moneysaving ideas. Disposable paper sheets, drapes, and gowns may prove more practical and more hygienic than those made of cloth.

Disposable paper gowns for patients' office use also make excellent and inexpensive drapes for the patient in the lithotomy position for pelvic examinations, cystoscopy, etc. The gown, designed to slip over the head of the patient poncho style, is opened, turned, and applied sideways. The lower limbs are covered. The opening in the middle of the gown adequately exposes the genitalia and pelvic area. Cellulose pads, some of which are polyethylene-backed (e.g., the TIDI POLYTOWL ®), are also most helpful and inexpensive table protectors for treatment room use.

Plastic Protective Sheet for Older Patients

Elderly male patients often have difficulty getting undressed due to long underwear or high-laced shoes and will occupy a dressing or treatment room for a lengthy period of time. Therefore, patients in whom one plans either to instill medication, pass sounds, or check residual urine, are simply asked to get on the treatment table, slip down their trousers, and open their underwear. A heavy plastic sheet with a central opening in it is placed over the perineum and abdomen. The penis is passed through the opening of this sheet. Absorbable paper or like material can be placed on the lower portion so that any leakage is absorbed.

All treatment rooms may be supplied with these sheets which can be washed and used again and again. A great deal of wasted time for the doctor and needless effort for the patient are thus eliminated.

Shields for Radiation Protection

Where urologists perform retrograde pyelography in their offices, a shield for protection against scatter irradiation during this procedure should be available. A length of lead-glass fabric may be suspended from the tube stand of a cystoscopy table in such a way that the shield hangs between the patient's thighs, leaving the genitalia exposed. The shield should be so placed on the tube stand that when not in use the screen may be swung upward, where it rests on the support.

One may use a leaded apron which may be draped over the X-ray tube

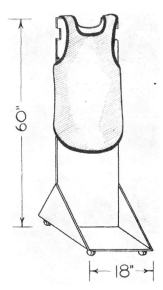

3. Movable stand for radiation shield apron

stand and in between the patient's thighs. Tapes may be used to tie this around the tube stand so that the apron serves as a portable X-ray shield which may be moved from room to room.

A screen made of ½-inch plywood may be affixed to a stand mounted on large ball-bearing casters. Over the screen may be draped the standard leaded apron. This device is also easily transported from room to room. The screen serves as a support to hang the apron so that there is no cracking or bending of the lead within the garment. The screen is wide enough to give adequate protection (reducing body exposure by approximately 80%), yet narrow enough to permit freedom of movement in performance of retrograde pyelography. See Figure 3.

Glasses for Endoscopic Work

Urologists who must wear bifocal lenses find these very awkward for endoscopic work. "Half-eye glasses" (see Fig. 4) are quite helpful for this purpose. They should be made with rigid frames. The glasses may be mounted on the frame in such a manner that the upper half of the frame is utilized for the glasses instead of the usual customary lower half. By raising one's head, one is looking below the glasses when performing cystoscopy or transurethral surgery. One must then lower one's head to look through the bifocal aspect of the lenses.

The lenses may preferably be made with the convexity of the lower limit of the lens curving upward, so that one can more readily look into the lensed cystoscopic instrument. Any competent optician can make these glasses to order.

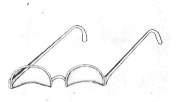

4. "Half-eye glasses" for endoscopic work

Magnifying Loupe for Use in Minute and Precision Surgery

Urologists should have the use of a magnifying loupe to be employed in fine surgery such as small vessel anastomosis or vas reanastomosis or other plastic procedures. Usually the 2.5X to 4X magnification is most satisfactory.

These loupes may be obtained through the optician of one's choice or through surgical supply houses.

Magnification Lenses in Ureteral Repair

The anastomosis of a ureter is greatly facilitated by the use of a Keeler loupe for magnification of the operating field. Such a loupe is also valuable in performing a cutaneous uretero-ileostomy. The use of these glasses, with a focal length of approximately 13.5 inches, enables one to place sutures with great accuracy in anastomosing small structures. The use of 6-0 chromic suture with a ventral cutting-edge type of needle is also advantageous for this type of surgical repair.

Improvising a Fine-Tip Fulgurating Electrode

Occasionally one has need of an electrode to use through a cystoscope or panendoscope, and none is available. A ureteral catheter stylet may be placed into a whistle-tip (preferably No. 4 French) ureteral catheter. The metal stylet passes through the catheter for 2-3 mm beyond the whistle tip of the catheter. The distal end may then be bent over so that the position in the catheter will not change. The distal bent-over end of the stylet and the male end of the electrosurgical cord are laid on each other and gripped thusly with a hemostat. Adhesive tape may be wound snugly around the connection point before applying the hemostat.

A rubber glove is then placed over the hemostat and connection point so that danger of short-circuiting and burn is eliminated. The rubber glove is taped on to the connection area, as illustrated in Figure 5A.

The stylet may be held against the electrosurgical unit cord by adhesive tape so as to eliminate the hemostat (Fig. 5B). This, however, often leads to poor connection and poor function of the hastily made substitute electrode.

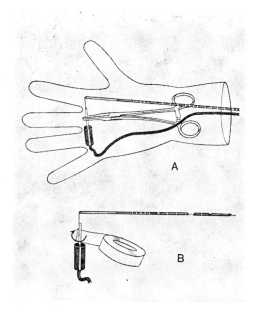

5. Improvised electrodes
    A. With rubber-glove insulation
    B. Without hemostat and rubber glove

The electrosurgical unit should be set at the lower aspect of its usual cutting and fulgurating range to minimize the possibility of burning out the whistle-tip end of the wire.

Meatotomy Ureteral Electrode

One may be faced with the necessity of doing a ureteral meatotomy in a child, or fulgurating posterior urethral valves, etc. The need of passing an electrode through a small-caliber instrument arises. The instrument described above may be employed, using a No. 3 or 4 French ureteral catheter.

Use of Crochet Hook to Remove Buried Nonabsorbable Suture

In most instances where one may have a chronic draining sinus, due in all probability to a nonabsorbable suture, one may probe this sinus with a sterilized crochet hook. By moving and rotating the hook, one may encounter the buried suture, grasp it and remove it from the depths of the wound.

This instrument may also be useful in probing for and elevating an inadvertently buried nonabsorbable skin suture.

Devices for Holding Cystoscopy Cords, Tubing, etc.

Numerous devices have been designed to allow the operator freedom of movement with the resectoscope or cystoscope, and to avoid the entanglement of the plastic irrigating tubing, light cord, and electrosurgical unit cord

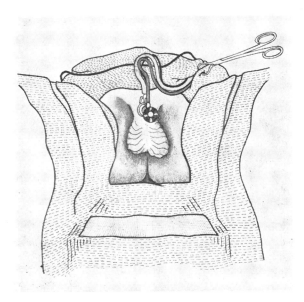

6. Practical arrangement of equipment for transurethral surgery and instrumentation

with each other. These pieces of paraphernalia should be draped in from the right side of the cystoscope or resectoscope (from the left side of the patient's body). Several means of holding these in place are suggested:

1) The tubing and cords may be placed in the region of the patient's groin and a towel clip fastened over the draperies so that all conduits may slide easily in and out under the towel clip (Fig. 6).

2) A coil-spring metallic device designed to attach on to an ironing board and to prevent entanglement of the ironing cord, may instead be attached to the X-ray support. The electrosurgical cord, light cord, and water tubing are wedged into the spring. There is sufficient elasticity in the contrivance to permit easy movement of the resectoscope with all of its attachments without any of these conduits becoming entangled in each other.

3) A metal stand with several hooks on it may be attached to the X-ray tube stand. The conduits are held by the various hooks.

4) Several long elastic bands may be attached to each other and to the complex of conduits and then attached to the X-ray tube stand. The bands must be of sufficient length to keep all of these structures just above the working aspect of the resectoscope.

5) A heavy S-shaped plastic gadget used for shower curtains serves well to hook over the arm of the X-ray tube to hold irrigating tubing and light cords. Coat-hanger wire bent into the same shape may be substituted. The upper arm of the S hangs over the arm of the X-ray stand; the lower arm holds the conduits.

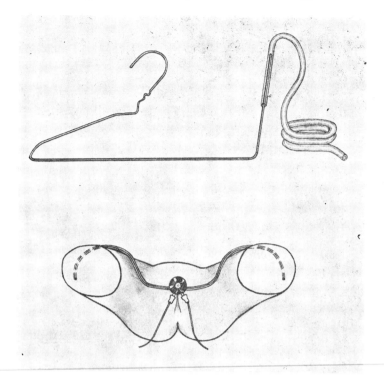

7. Simple cystoscope holder

Large Test Tube to Hold Plastic Tubing

A large test tube, containing cold-sterilizing solution such as aqueous activated glutaraldehyde (Cidex) may be attached on the arm of the X-ray tube stand. The end of the tubing used in cystoscopy, with its connecting irrigating tip, may be placed in the test tube between cystoscopic procedures—sterility is all the more assured.

Cystoscope Holder

Following the introduction of ureteral catheters some urologists will allow the cystoscope to remain in the bladder. To hold the cystoscope in place a simple holder may be made by using a wire about the strength and size of a clothes-hanger wire, and passing this through a small-size rubber or plastic tubing of the same length. The wire should be about 24 to 30 inches long and bent into the shape of a capital U, with the upper arms of the U bent so as to rest over the patient's thighs.

This is especially handy in female patients while collecting ureteral specimens or awaiting X-rays. Figure 7 illustrates this easily fashioned device.

Identification of Instruments

One may identify various cystoscopes, etc., by color-coding with varied-color tapes. For example, when several cystoscopes are in a cold-sterilization pan and one wishes to pick up a specific instrument, the color-coding makes it easily and quickly identifiable.

Identification of Medications and Solutions

It is extremely valuable to color-code all solutions and medications for instant identification. Local anesthetic may be colored with vegetable coloring dye so that when one sees in an Asepto ® syringe, for example, a pink or red solution, one automatically knows that this is local anesthetic if this is the selected color code for such an agent. Intravenous substances may be identified by placing on the syringe a sticker of whatever color or shape one wishes to use for code identification. Contrast material such as Hypaque ® or Renografin ® may be identified in the syringe by a blue triangle or blue circle sticker. ·

Solutions for Bladder Instillation

Following instrumentation we invariably will instill into the bladder a local anesthetic in addition to an antiseptic solution. On sucking up into an Asepto syringe some furantoin solution (yellow), plus lidocaine viscous, the solution takes the pink color of the latter substance. Lidocaine viscous is utilized for bladder instillations in our offices because it is low in cost, is already color-coded, and may be autoclaved without any change of the substance.

Usefulness of Indigotindisulfonate Sodium (Indigo Carmine) or Tetramethylthionine Chloride (Methylene Blue)

In transurethral resection, perineal or retropubic surgery, and ureteral lithotomy: Approximately one hour before planned transurethral surgery, an intravenous is started using two ampules of indigo carmine per 1000 ml of fluid. Promotion of this early hydration process on the patient makes it possible to see the blue spurts from the ureteral orifices during transurethral prostatectomy. Given in this manner, the dye excretion lasts much longer than when one ampule is administered intravenously at the time of surgery.

This facilitates the identification of ureteral orifices during transurethral resection of a median bar or bladder tumor lying close to the ureteral orifice. It is particularly useful in operations on patients who have had a prior ureteroneocystostomy. It is also valuable for the identification of the orifices in performing perineal or retropubic radical prostatectomies.

When one is doing a ureteral lithotomy, use of the dye helps to identify the lumen of the ureter. This is of value when trying to use a hooked blade to enter the lumen of the ureter at some distance above a stone.

In identification of ureteral or vesicovaginal fistulae: Milk may be instilled in the urinary bladder, a tampon inserted in the vagina, and indigo carmine may be given intravenously. If a heavy blue concentration is noted on the tampon, the source is a ureteral fistula.

In ileal conduit surgery: At the time of surgery, after making the ileo-ureteral anastomosis, a solution of indigo carmine may be instilled into the ileal conduit to check for leaks at the ileoureteral anastomotic sites.

In identifying the course of the ileal conduit during reexploration: In patients with dense adhesions around the ileal conduit which prevent the passage of a catheter, 10 ml of methylene blue may be injected into a balloon-type catheter inserted through the ileal stoma into the conduit to a site just below the peritoneal attachment. The balloon then may be inflated to prevent dye leakage. The ileal conduit is distinguishable by a light blue, dusky discoloration which sets it apart from adjacent loops of small bowel.

In postsurgical drainage: Methylene blue or indigo carmine may be placed in the balloon of a balloon-type urethral catheter. If at any time in the post-operative course the urinary drainage turns blue, one can determine that the balloon is leaking and that the catheter may soon be slipping out. This is particularly helpful to assure one of nonleakage of a balloon-type catheter used as a nephrostomy tube.

Lubricating Jelly

Some urologists prepare their own lubricating jelly or ask their local pharmacist to make it up for them. The lubricant made from the following formula serves exceedingly well for rectal lubrication in prostate palpation and massage, etc. The jelly may be contained in two-ounce cold cream jars into which the physician merely inserts his gloved finger to obtain the lubricant.

The formula for the *rectal lubricant* is as follows:

1000 ml distilled water

7 oz glycerine

3 oz tragacanth

4 drops lavender oil

4 drops phenol

vegetable coloring (as desired)

It is prepared by placing glycerine, tragacanth, lavender oil and phenol into a blender with a small quantity of the distilled water which has been heated. Blend slowly at first, adding the balance of the warm distilled water a bit at a time. When thoroughly blended, add vegetable coloring to the desired tint. The lavender oil is added merely for fragrance, and the phenol serves to inhibit bacterial growth.

To concoct a *lubricant for urethral instrumentation,* 4 drops of Zephiran concentrate may be substituted for the phenol. The mixture is prepared in the previously described manner.

The vegetable coloring used in either case preferably should not be red or pink since patients on drying themselves may interpret this as rectal or urethral bleeding.

Cleaning Laboratory Equipment

Alconax ® powder (one tablespoon per gallon of warm water) is very effective for cleaning glass, porcelain, metal and plastic laboratory equipment. The solution remains stable for as long as one week. It is available through most wholesale drug supply companies. A 1:1 solution of 0.75 percent hexachlorophene solution such as Septisol ® answers the same purpose, as does Pine-sol ®, a phenolic compound available at drug stores and supermarkets. Slides, cover slips, used sounds and other instruments may also be effectively cleaned with these solutions.

Cleaning Lumen of Instruments

Female dilators such as the Walther dilator are readily sterilized by autoclaving or cold sterilization. However, physical cleansing of the lumen, after use, may be difficult in smaller sizes. Ordinary pipe cleaners have been found satisfactory for cleaning these dilators prior to sterilization. Longer pipe cleaners may be used for longer hollow instruments. Kollmann dilators may be cleaned by extremely cautious use of applicator sticks.

Cystoscopes must also be cleaned with extreme care. They are ordinarily supplied with long metal rods to which one applies cotton for use in cleaning.

Maintaining Surface Finish on Stainless Steel Instruments

Vaginal specula, sounds, and other stainless steel instruments develop a dull film after long use. These instruments can be made to look like new by the following method: Fill sterilizer one-half to two-thirds full of water. Place stainless steel instruments in sterilizer. Empty one four-ounce packet of Pel-Toner ® into water and boil for thirty minutes. Rinse sterilizer and instruments. When dry, brush off any remaining tarnish and apply silver polish. (Pel-Toner is available from surgical supply houses.)

Useful Method for Measurement

A simple means of measurement is to use relationship to one's own anatomy. When one wishes to estimate with fair accuracy the size, for example, of a calculus or specific structure, one can use the width of one's fingernail (of the thumb or little finger, etc.) as a guideline for estimating the size. The measurement from one knuckle to another may be used as a means of comparison to which one may relate, or the length of the terminal phalanx may be employed as a gauge of measurement.

The same indices should be used at all times so that one becomes accustomed to using these same units for specific measurements.

Improvised Cover Slips

Slides containing prostatic secretions taken by a urologist during a hospital visit often become dried out before reaching the laboratory. If cover slips are not readily available on the hospital ward, a piece of cellophane or plastic cut to size will serve as a cover slip to preserve the specimen for examination.

Incontinence Devices for Emergency Use by Male Patients

The following devices are suggested as readily available incontinence aids, to be employed on a temporary basis only:

—A rubber or plastic examining glove (in which the thumb side has about two inches cut out of the wrist section) may be pinned to the underwear or suspended from the waist by a heavy piece of string. The penis hangs free inside the glove.

—A "Baggie ®" (plastic bag) may be suspended from the waist to contain the penis and scrotum.

—A condom may be unrolled and affixed to the penis with adhesive tape.

—A hole may be cut in an athletic supporter and a condom or a plastic bag or glove may be attached to the inside aspect of the hole.

—A large abdominal pad may be held in place over the perineum by a tight athletic supporter.

—A wide abdominal band may be held in place with a tight athletic supporter, holding the penis upward on the abdomen.

—Cunningham clamps or "bent to fit" hair curling clips may be used.

—Firm wrapping with Kling ® dressing may control leakage.

Medications employed to control incontinence include testosterone preparations, propantheline bromide (Pro-Banthine), chlorpheniramine maleatephenylpropanolamine hydrochloride-isopropamide compound (Ornade) and imipramine hydrochloride (Tofranil). These are further discussed in the chapter on The Bladder. (Incontinence devices for females are also treated in the latter chapter.)

Convenient Carrying Case for Urological Instruments

A compact lightweight unit for carrying the resectoscope, cystoscope, and allied equipment may be made from an oversized attaché case. The case used by the authors measures 17¾ inches long by 13 inches wide by 6½ inches in depth. Ethafoam ®, Wilshire P-2 ® foam, or other suitable plastic material (approximately 1⅝ inches thick) is purchased and cut into three panels to fit inside the case.

The urological instruments are placed on this material and traced around with soft lead pencil. Using a sharp razor or the tip of an electrically heated soldering iron, one then may cut out the spaces in the plastic for the respective instruments.

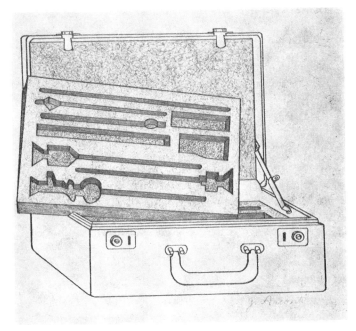

8. Instrument carrying case
   A. Attaché case modified for urologic equipment

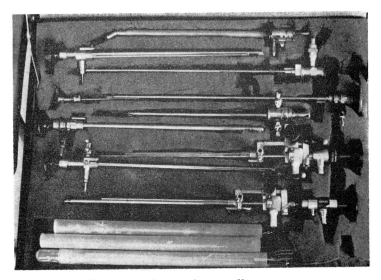

B. Plastic panel shaped to cradle instruments

In an attaché case of the described size it is simple to enclose several resectoscopes, a number of cystoscopes (including an infant cystoscope), cystoscopic handles and rongeurs, urethrotomes, lithotrites, Kollmann dilators, and all types of accessory lenses (Figs. 8A, 8B).

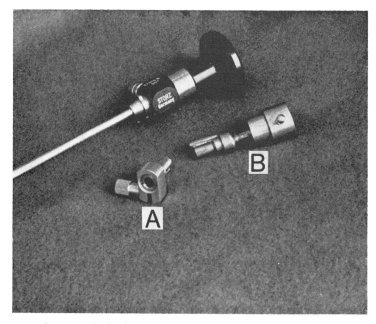

9. Adapters which allow various lenses to be used with the ACMI
resectoscope working element
A. Adapter for Fairfield lens
B. Adapter for Storz lens

Adapters for Use of Some Fiber Optic Lenses

The presently available Storz lens, Fairfield lens, Wolf lens, and the
MICROLENS® telescope (68M) made by the American Cystoscope
Makers, Inc. (ACMI)—all forward-vision lenses—may all be utilized with
the ACMI resectoscope working element by the use of specific adapters.

Available with the Fairfield lens is an adapter (Fig. 9A) which allows this
lens to be used with the ACMI resectoscope working element. In view of
the need to change the resectoscope sheath and working element when
using the Storz unit, the Storz lens has also been adapted (by H.B.) to the
ACMI working element (Fig. 9B). It is now simple to use the various lenses
desired with relatively little difficulty, interchanging them in a single operation for purposes of comparison and use.

The following conclusions have been reached as a result of experience in
using these various lenses, each of which has advantages and disadvantages. The ACMI 68A incandescent telescope lens has a smaller field than
do the Fairfield or Storz lenses, and is therefore not completely satisfactory.
The Storz lens has the largest field of the three just named. The fields of
vision with the ACMI 68M MICROLENS telescope, Wolf, and Fairfield
lenses closely approximate each other. However, the depth of focus of the
ACMI 68M MICROLENS telescope and Wolf lenses seems better than that

of the Fairfield or Storz lenses. The magnification with the ACMI MICRO-LENS telescope is greater.

At the outset, in performing a prostatectomy, a wide-angle view with the Storz lens is desirable, so that a wide field may be used to set the landmarks of the resection. However, after the beginning stages of the resection, it is difficult to continue with the Storz lens because of the feeling that one is attempting to "work in a small corner of a ballroom when one has to contend with the entire ballroom in his field of vision."

Perhaps this is the peculiarity of this operator (H.B.), who has used other lenses for a number of years, or perhaps this is the peculiarity of the particular lens. In contrast with the above, the Fairfield lens seems to allow less forward vision and more right-angle vision, so that it is more difficult to localize bleeding points.

The ACMI 68M MICROLENS telescope gives a wider angle than the ACMI incandescent telescope (68A) lens, and the depth of focus and magnification seem to be improved over that of the lenses of other manufacturers. Since the ACMI MICROLENS telescope gives a larger field than does the 68A incandescent telescope lens, one seems to adapt more easily to this increased field, which is not so large as to be distracting. The depth of focus is such that one seems closer to the tissue to be resected, with a closer range of view.

Obviously, various operators will have various reactions to the different lenses and one's technique will have been developed with the lens that one is accustomed to using. Therefore, it is suggested that urologists who have been trained with American-made instruments, and who are switching to various fiber optic equipment, should so modify the equipment that they may be interchanged and various lenses may be used during the performance of a prostatectomy. Thus, one may "get the feel" of the particular lens that best suits one's own purpose.

It is expected that a urologist utilizing a specific instrument with its particular angle will not easily adjust to a new lens with a different angle of view.

Convenient Dilators for Patient Self-Use

Some of the plastic containers for disposable needles may serve as urethral meatal dilators. Alternatively, one may give to the patient for use after each voiding a urethral catheter plug, golf tee, or any other similarly shaped plastic device of 24 to 28 French size (see Fig. 10) to retain patency of the urethral meatus during the healing phase.

Catheter Hints

BALLOON CATHETER CLIPPERS. When the urologist, on making hospital rounds, wishes to remove a balloon catheter, he may utilize an ordinary

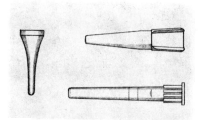

10. Urethral dilators for use by patients

fingernail clippers (usually carried by physicians) to cut the filling arm of the balloon. Should he carry a pocket knife or small pair of scissors (or a combination of same), he may use one of the two to cut the filling arm after putting it on stretch. The fluid may be collected in a bedside kidney basin, paper cup, or facial tissue.

BUILT-IN PLUG FOR RETENTION CATHETERS. A patient on continuous balloon catheter drainage, on disconnecting his catheter from the drainage tube or leg urinal, may simply insert the inflation tube end of the catheter into the drainage lumen of the catheter. This end of the catheter will not slip or leak even when the patient is ambulant. Caution in sterilizing the end of this catheter must, of course, be exercised.

BALLOON CATHETER PLUGS. The drainage lumen of the balloon catheter may be easily plugged when the patient is to be ambulatory by using one of the plastic containers for disposable needles such as Yale®, B-D®, Jelco®, or

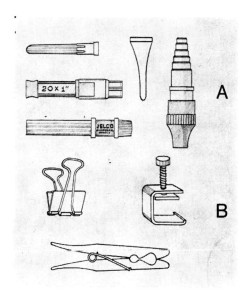

11. Balloon catheter aids
   A. Plugs
   B. Clamps

Monoject® needles. A golf tee or a patented valve such as the Gatnos® valve may be employed (see Fig. 11A). All of these devices may be cold-sterilized before use as plugs.

On occasion, a balloon catheter stopper may be improvised by using an ordinary cocktail stirring rod with a small ball on one end. This fits very adequately into the outlet of the catheter and can be easily handled by the elderly patient.

CATHETER CLAMPS. Numerous devices may be utilized to clamp a urethral catheter. The end of a retention catheter may be folded over on itself and held in the clamped-off position by use of an ordinary rubber band. Other contrivances used for clamping include small plastic spring-type clothes pins, screw clamps, or spring clips of the I.D.L.® binder* type (see Fig. 11B).

One must bear in mind that some senile patients are unable to manipulate certain devices.

Variation in Catheter Outflow Rates

The scientifically precise labeling of rate of flow from a catheter is of great importance to the urologist. A recent comparative evaluation of the outflow rate of catheters made by various manufacturers (dependent, obviously, on inside diameter) gives the results shown in Table I.

The catheters tested include a small representation only of the various brands available, and the values given are typical of only a small number of samples of each type and manufacture. They are not to be construed as large-scale authoritative test results. They do, however, serve to demonstrate effectively the wide variance in flowrates obtainable with catheters of differing materials, even those of the same manufacturer.

Measurements of outflow rate were made using a 4-inch head of distilled water at room temperature. The stated French size and the actual French size of the outside of the catheter, the inside dimensions, the area in square inches, and the flow rate in milliliters per minute and milliliters per second were recorded. It is obvious that in some instances the nominal and actual sizes on the French scale do not agree, and that the outflow rate of some of the catheters evaluated is far superior to that of others.

It may be postulated that the outflow rate of a catheter in itself may have some bearing on the possible establishment of bacteria in the bladder. Where one is concerned about the best possible outflow from the bladder, these findings may be of value.

(See also additional suggestions for catheter use, included in chapters covering the various parts of the urinary tract.)

---

* Available in all stationery stores.

TABLE I

COMPARISON OF VARIOUS BALLOON-TYPE CATHETERS
AS TO FLOWRATES AND RELATED FACTORS

	French Size		Inside Dimensions Maximum (inch)	Inside Dimensions Minimum (inch)	Area $(inch^2)$	Flow Rate (ml/min)	Flow Rate (ml/sec)
Manufacturer	Nominal	Actual					
A	16	16	0.10	0.10	0.137	245	4
	18	18	0.12	0.09	0.165	345	5.7
	24	25-26	0.17	0.15	0.396	438	7.3
Teflon	24	26	0.17	0.16	0.421	364	6
Plastic	24-26	24-28	0.19	0.16	0.514	492	8.2
B	16	18	0.13	0.08	0.176	290	4.8
	24	25	0.17	0.13	0.380	341	5.6
C	16	16	0.11	0.08	0.148	310	5.1
	18	18	0.13	0.09	0.172	489	8.1
	24	25	0.17	0.12	0.379	715	11.9
Plastic {	16	16	0.13	0.09	0.199	350	5.8
	18	18	0.15	0.11	0.286	570	9.5
	24	24	0.19	0.18	0.534	1040	17.3
D Plastic	16-18	18	0.15	0.11	0.265	525	8.8
E	24	25	0.19	0.18	0.578	1080	18
F	18	18	0.12	0.11	0.17	454	7.6
G {	18	20	0.11	0.07	0.15	320	5.3
Oval-shaped {	16	18	0.10	0.07	0.12	250	4.2

Coding:

Manufacturer

A Bard   E Travenol
B Dow-Corning   F Rusch
C Pharmaseal   G Curity
D Cutter (Resiflex®)

Note: Catheters are rubber unless otherwise noted.

Chapter Two

THE URINE AND RELATED FACTORS

URINE AND SYMPTOMATOLOGY

THE CHAPTER WHICH follows is devoted to some observations relative to the urine. The many effects of drugs and other agents on urinary tract symptomatology are recorded. Urine testing, study of urinary flow-rates, modes of specimen collection, and factors relating to residual urine are included in this section.

Office bacteriology only is presented. Though this serves a practical purpose, complete bacteriological studies, colony counts, identification of bacteria, etc., have been adequately recorded elsewhere.

Urinary Chromatology

The reaction of many agents leads to abnormal coloring of the urine. Red urine may be due to the patient's having ingested beets or red-colored candies, or to a reaction with hypochlorite used in cleaning toilet bowls. Sulfonamide therapy may cause red-colored urine. Blood may be ejaculated into the vagina by the husband, erroneously suggesting pathology in the wife.

The red color of urine due to blood may vary from pink due to bleeding in the lower urinary tract to coffee-ground appearance due to old blood from the upper urinary tract. Hematoporphyrin may color the urine to a port-wine appearance. Bile may cause a yellow or yellow-brown color.

Furantoin and some vitamin preparations containing flavones will give a greenish-yellow color (fluorescent if due to flavones). Methylene blue changes the urine to various shades of blue and greenish blue. Melanin produces a brown urine which may become black on standing. Table II shows other agents which may cause change in urine color.

Pharmacological Agents and Urinary Tract Pathology

Drugs and categories of drugs implicated in conditions and with symptoms found in urological practice are listed in Table III. This listing was compiled from a recent American Medical Association drug evaluation.

Etiology of Dysuria

Many medications are causal factors in dysuria. Numerous other causes in addition to the usual organic pathological lesions are related to painful or

TABLE II

VARIATIONS IN COLOR OF URINE

Color	Source	Common Cause
Colorless	Dilute urine	Excessive fluid intake, chronic renal disease, diabetes insipidus
Yellow to amber with pink sediment	Acid urine with excess urates	Hyperuricemia and gout (may be normal, too); bile; Pyridium, furantoin; vitamins and flavones; indandione
Yellow to amber with white sediment	Alkaline urine and excess phosphates;	Normal variation
	WBC in urine	Numerous causes
Milky	Lymph in urine	Parasitic disease; lymphatic obstruction
Orange-red to red	Gross blood	Innumerable pathologic lesions
	Hemoglobin breakdown	Injury, malaria, various hemoglobinurias
	Porphyrins	Porphyria
	Medications	Levodopa, selenium, certain sulfonamides, P.S.P. in alkaline urine, senna, cascara
	Foods	Beets, strawberries, vegetable dyes
Deep orange to mahogany	Bile in urine;	Jaundice
	Certain cathartics and chemicals	Cascara, rhubarb, senna, P.S.P. in acid urine
Green-blue to brown; black from dark brown, brown to black	Methylene blue, melanin, alkapton bodies in urine	Levodopa, urine exposed to air; melanoma, Pyridium on occasion

difficult urination. Some of these causes are the use of certain soaps, powders, deodorants, scented or alkaline douching agents, scented or tinted toilet tissue, bubble bath, pessaries, tampons, sanitary napkins, synthetic underwear, laundry detergents, etc.

Poor hygiene or defective laundering methods may play a part in causing dysuria. Allergic manifestations may also be a factor. For example, in some persons the ingestion of chocolate, coffee, tea, cola drinks, or use of anovulatory drugs contribute to urinary frequency, urgency, and dysuria. Localized instrumentation, accidental or purposeful, must also be considered in seeking the cause of urinary tract symptomatology.

URINALYSIS

Points of Emphasis

Repetitive urine testing continues to remain of utmost importance in urology. Proper collection of urine obviously is necessary to obtain significant

TABLE III
DRUGS AND DRUG CATEGORIES IMPLICATED
IN URINARY TRACT SYMPTOMATOLOGY

Albuminuria
  antimony potassium
    tartrate
  kanamycin sulfate
    (Kantrex)
  lithium carbonate
  mercurial compounds
  phenindione (Danilone,
    Eridione)
  suramin sodium
  viomycin sulfate
    (Vinactane Sulfate,
    Viocin Sulfate)

Anuria
  chlorprothixene
    (Taractan)
  colchicine
  dextrose, subcutaneous
  phenylbutazone
    (Butazolidin)
  sulfonamides

Azotemia
  calcium carbonate
  ethacrynic acid (Edecrin)
  furosemide (Lasix)
  melphalan (Alkeran)
  mercurial compounds
  radiopaque media,
    intravascular
  sodium bicarbonate
  triamterene (Dyrenium)

Bladder, Atony
  ganglionic blocking
    agents
  Lomotil (M)

Blood creatinine, increased
  arginine glutamate
    (Modumate)
  arginine hydrochloride
    (R-gene)
  colistimethate sodium
    (Coly-Mycin M
    Intramuscular)
  colistin sulfate (Coly-
    Mycin S Oral
    Suspension)
  mithramycin (Mithracin)
  polymyxin B sulfate
    (Aerosporin)

Blood urea nitrogen,
    increased
  amphotericin B, injection
    (Fungizone)
  arginine glutamate
    (Modumate)
  arginine hydrochloride
    (R-gene)
  colistimethate sodium
    (Coly-Mycin M
    Intramuscular)
  colistin sulfate (Coly-
    Mycin S Oral
    Suspension)
  diuretics, thiazides
  levodopa (Dopar,
    Larodopa)
  methoxyflurane
    (Penthrane)
  mithramycin
    (Mithracin)
  polymyxin B sulfate
    (Aerosporin)
  triamterene (Dyrenium)

Crystalluria
  acetazolamide (Diamox)
  sulfonamides

Cylindruria
  kanamycin sulfate
    (Kantrex)
  suramin sodium
  viomycin sulfate
    (Vinactane Sulfate,
    Viocin Sulfate)

Dysuria
  anticholinergics
  antispasmodics
  atropine
  belladonna
  ethionamide (Trecator)
  hyoscyamine
  iopanoic acid (Telepaque)
  ipodate calcium, sodium
    (Oragrafin)
  methenamine hippurate
    (Hiprex)
  methysergide maleate
    (Sansert)
  pyrazinamide

Hematuria
  amphotericin B, injection
    (Fungizone)
  chloroguanide
    hydrochloride
    (Paludrine)
  levodopa (Dopar,
    Larodopa)
  phenylbutazone
    (Butazolidin)
  sulfonamides
  suramin sodium
  viomycin sulfate
    (Vinactane Sulfate,
    Viocin Sulfate)

Hyperuricemia
  antineoplastic agents
  diuretics, oral
  diuretics, thiazides
  ethacrynic acid
    (Edecrin)
  furosemide (Lasix)
  niacin
  pyrazinamide

Hypervolemia
  citrated whole human
    blood
  dextran 40
  dextran 75 (Gentran 75,
    Macrodex)
  mannitol (Osmitrol)
  normal human plasma
  normal human serum
    albumin
  plasma protein fraction
    (Plasmanate,
    Protenate)
  urea (Ureaphil,
    Urevert)

Hypocalcemia
  disodium edetate
    (Endrate)
  mithramycin (Mithracin)
  polystyrene sulfonate,
    sodium (Kayexalate)
  viomycin sulfate
    (Vinactane Sulfate,
    Viocin Sulfate)

TABLE III
(Continued)

Hypochloremia
  diuretics, mercurial
  diuretics, thiazides
  ethacrynic acid
    (Edecrin)

Hypokalemia
  acetazolamide (Diamox)
  adrenal corticosteroids
  aminosalicylates
  ammonium chloride
  amphotericin B, injection
    (Fungizone)
  dichlorphenamide
    (Daranide, Oratrol)
  digitalis glycosides
  disodium edetate
    (Endrate)
  diuretics, mercurial
  diuretics, oral
  diuretics, thiazides
  ethacrynic acid
    (Edecrin)
  ethoxzolamide
    (Cardrase, Ethamide)
  laxatives, irritant
  laxatives, saline cathartics
  methazolamide
    (Neptazane)
  mithramycin
    (Mithracin)
  sodium sulfate
  urea (Ureaphil, Urevert)
  viomycin sulfate
    (Vinactane Sulfate,
    Viocin Sulfate)

Hypomagnesemia
  sodium sulfate

Hyponatremia
  ammonium chloride
  diuretics, mercurial
  diuretics, thiazides
  ethacrynic acid
    (Edecrin)
  mannitol (Osmitrol)
  posterior pituitary
    preparations
  urea (Ureaphil, Urevert)

Impotence
  desipramine hydrochloride
    (Norpramin, Pertofrane)
  disulfiram (Antabuse)
  ethionamide (Trecator)
  ganglionic blocking
    agents
  haloperidol (Haldol)
  methyldopa (Aldomet)
  nortriptyline
    hydrochloride
    (Aventyl
      Hydrochloride)
  phenelzine sulfate
    (Nardil)
  protiptyline
    hydrochloride
    (Vivactil
      Hydrochloride)
  quaternary ammonium
    compounds
  thiothixene (Navane)
  tranylcypromine sulfate
    (Parnate Sulfate)

Kidney, calculus
  acetazolamide (Diamox)
  allopurinol (Zyloprim)

Kidney, constriction
  angiotensin amide
    (Hypertensin)

Kidney damage, unspecified
  amphotericin B, injection
    (Fungizone)
  anticonvulsants
  antineoplastic agents
  APC (M)
  cephaloridine
    (Loridine)
  chloroform
  colistimethate sodium
    (Coly-Mycin M
    Intramuscular)
  colistin sulfate (Coly-
    Mycin S Oral
    Suspension)
  Cremomycin (M)
  diatrizoate sodium,
    meglumine
  dimercaprol (BAL)
  disodium edetate (Endrate)

Donnagel with Neomycin
    (M)
  edetates
  ergocalciferol
    (vitamin D₂)
  gentamicin sulfate,
    injection (Garamycin)
  iothalamate sodium,
    meglumine
  kanamycin sulfate
    injection (Kantrex)
  Kaomycin (M)
  methoxyflurane
    (Penthrane)
  neomycin sulfate, injection
  paromomycin sulfate
    (Humatin)
  phenindione (Danilone,
    Eridione)
  polymyxin B sulfate
    (Aerosporin)
  streptomycin sulfate
  suramin sodium
  vinyl ether (Vinethene)

Kidney failure
  antineoplastic agents
  fibrinolysin (human)
    (Thrombolysin)
  iopanoic acid (Telepaque)
  ipodate calcium, sodium
    (Oragrafin)
  mercurial compounds
  phenazopyridine
    hydrochloride
    (Pyridium)
  phosphates, infusion
  radiopaque media,
    intravascular

Oliguria
  colistimethate sodium
    (Coly-Mycin M
    Intramuscular)
  colistin sulfate (Coly-
    Mycin S Oral
    Suspension)
  dextrose, subcutaneous
  halothane (Fluothane)
  lithium carbonate
  mercurial compounds
  polymyxin B sulfate
    (Aerosporin)
  sulfonamides

Polyuria
carbarsone

Proteinuria
aurothioglucose
(Solganal)
gold sodium thiomalate
(Myochrysine)
mithramycin (Mithracin)
radiopaque media,
intravascular

Spermatogenesis, depressed
furazolidone

Uremia
cephaloridine (Loridine)
vancomycin hydrochloride
(Vancocin
Hydrochloride)

Ureter, calculus
acetazolamide (Diamox)
dichlorphenamide
(Daranide, Oratrol)
ethoxzolamide (Cardrase,
Ethamide)
methazolamide
(Neptazane)

Urinary incontinence
acetophenazine maleate
(Tindal)
hydroxystilbamidine
isethionate, intravenous
levodopa (Dopar,
Larodopa)
neostigmine (Prostigmin)
physostigmine

Urinary tract obstruction
methysergide maleate
(Sansert)

Urine, casts
amphotericin B, injection
(Fungizone)
chloroguanide
hydrochloride
(Paludrine)
melarsoprol
suramin sodium

Urine, protein, false-positive
iopanoic acid (Telepaque)
ipodate calcium, sodium
(Oragrafin)

Urine retention
amphotericin B,
intrathecal
(Fungizone)
anticholinergics
antihistamines
antipsychotic agents
atropine sulfate
ephedrine
fluphenazine
hydrochloride
(Permitil,
Prolixin)
isocarboxazid (Marplan)
levodopa (Dopar,
Larodopa)
methixene hydrochloride
(Trest)
protriptyline
hydrochloride
(Vivactil
Hydrochloride)
tricyclic compounds

interpretation. Hematuria, pyuria, albuminuria, and bacteriuria may all, for example, be present in contaminated specimens to suggest erroneous information.

Though modern tape and dipstick tests of urine have remarkably shortened and simplified urine testing, many points of emphasis bear repetition:

1) Chemicals impregnated in the dipstick may be dissolved out if dipsticks are kept too long in the urine.

2) When more than one chemical reaction is arranged on a single stick, e.g., pH, protein, and glucose, the chemical reagents for each are separated from each other by a water-impermeable barrier. Too long a soaking in urine may also break down this barrier.

3) Since dipsticks are activated by moisture, the bottle containing the sticks should be kept dry and stoppered.

4) Since the first morning urine is the most concentrated and most apt to show positive findings, this is the most desirable specimen for collection.

5) For routine urinalysis, a "prepped" midstream specimen in the male and female is preferable.

6) For initial examination of male patients, no other preparation need be done. The usual three-glass test pattern of collection should be instituted. The patient is instructed to pass the first 2 to 3 ounces of urine in glass #1 and with

a continuous stream collects most of the remaining urine in glass #2. Then when he feels that he is nearing termination of urination, the last 2 to 3 ounces should be collected in glass #3. Totally unsuspected anterior urethritis is often discovered by the cloudy urine and shreds in glass #1 after acidification. In the event glass #2 and #3 both show evidence of pyuria, one must also suspect upper urinary tract involvement in addition to prostatitis and cystitis.

7) Urine may have a low specific gravity due to dilution. Under these circumstances microscopic findings are not as significant. Twenty-four hour urine specimens collected for measurement of total urine protein, creatinine, electrolytes, etc., should be refrigerated during collection. Several drops of an appropriate preservative such as toluene may also be added to the specimen to prevent bacterial growth, chemical changes, etc.

8) If a random specimen of urine has a specific gravity exceeding 1.020, it is usually unnecessary to do a specific gravity concentration test.

9) Contrast material for pyelography may increase urine specific gravity for as long as twenty-four hours after injection of the medium.

10) If the urine quantity is too small to measure with the urinometer, one may dilute the specimen with an amount of water equal to or double that of the urine and then multiply the results by two or three. If the quantity is still too small to measure with the urinometer, thus diluted, one may utilize the refractometer. In some specific situations one may determine the osmolality and obtain the freezing point depression. A modern laboratory should not return a report of specific gravity as "q.n.s." (quantity not sufficient).

11) A simple clinical test of concentrating ability is the Fishberg modification of the Mosenthal test. The patient eats or drinks nothing after 6 p.m. Urine specimens are collected at three successive hours such as 6, 7, and 8 a.m. of the following morning. The specific gravity of each urine should be above 1.020, with the 8 a.m. specimen slightly more concentrated than the 6 a.m. one.

12) Tests for urinary concentration should not be done during induced diuresis.

13) High-molecular-weight solutes in urine will result in higher specific gravity and may obscure results of concentration tests. For example, each gram of glucose per 100 ml of urine will increase specific gravity by 0.003.

14) ·Specific gravity of 1.010 or less may occur in:
    a) acute renal failure.
    b) intrinsic tubular defects such as Fanconi syndrome with hypokalemia.
    c) renal parenchymal disease such as chronic pyelonephritis, polycystic kidney disease, hydronephrosis, etc.
    d) severe potassium deficiency (colitis, bowel fistula, diuretics, pyelonephritis).
    e) hypercalcemia (sarcoidosis, bone disease, multiple myeloma, vitamin D intoxication, hyperparathyroidism).

15) The pH must be measured in fresh urine. Breakdown of urea to ammonia results in an alkaline pH.

16) Persistently alkaline urine occurs in some infections, metabolic disorders, and due to use of certain drugs.

17) Persistently acid urine occurs in a variety of metabolic diseases.

18) Urinary pH is important in the management of conditions treated with certain antibiotics or chemotherapeutic agents.

19) Less than 30 mg protein per 100 ml of urine is usually insignificant; therefore, 24-hour determination should be done for greater accuracy.

20) Proteinuria may be transient and associated with fever. It may be due to cardiac disease, central nervous system lesions, thyroid disorders, blood disorders, or use of certain drugs.

21) Proteinuria may be caused by systemic disorders such as collagen disease, diabetes, subacute bacterial endocarditis, septicemia, multiple myeloma, amyloidosis, parasitic infections, and disorders associated with the use of drugs and certain chemicals.

22) Proteinuria may be due to eclampsia and also to primary renal diseases.

23) Proteinuria may erroneously be due to vaginal discharge, prostatitis, and cystitis.

24) Casts frequently are dissolved by alkaline urine. This must be considered in 12-hour or 24-hour urine collections for Addis counts.

Bacteriuria Test

Extremely helpful in office practice are such diagnostic kits as the UTI-tect ® Bacteriuria Diagnostic Test Kit (available from local medical supply houses). With this kit one can in a one-step workup identify, screen, and quantitate the common gram-negative organisms which cause 80 to 90 percent of urinary tract infections.

The test kit contains four culture media in one compact package. A simple "dip and streak" procedure inoculates them. After a single incubation bacteriuria can readily be detected and any of the pathogens identified. The test also gives clues as to the identity of other bacteria involved.

Transfer to a blood agar plate for sensitivity studies is an easy matter. No equipment need be sterilized and the test is disposable. Results are easily readable with the flow sheet provided with the kit.

Office Bacteriology with the Unibac ® System

Identification of common urinary tract pathogens in twenty-four hours with the Unibac ® one-step kit is simply done by means of visual comparison.

The antibiotic of choice is indicated. Patients are saved a three- to four-day wait for laboratory results. A unique procedure for colony counts (with automatic pipette and disposable sterile tips) is incorporated into the system, which is available from local medical supply houses.

It must be remembered that the comparison with conventional colony count methods varies from 60 to 90 percent in accuracy. It is granted that these levels of confidence are disappointing.

Many other bacteriologic kits such as the above-described system are available. Mention of a particular kit does not constitute an endorsement of that system, but is made simply to demonstrate that the urologist can readily provide such laboratory services with timesaving and costsaving advantages to himself and his patients.

URINE FLOWRATE DETERMINATION

Value of Uroflowmetry

A qualitative measurement of a patient's urine flowrate should be part of every physical examination. Nonetheless, most physicians, including urologists, do not own, let alone use, a uroflowmeter. Sophisticated equipment is necessary for complete evaluation of the true hydrodynamics of bladder and urethral outflow. However, a simple measurement of flowrate alone will provide enough information to appraise the need of further investigation.

Should the urine flowrate be abnormally low, then the usual routine methods of endoscopy, bougie-à-boule, urethrography, cystography, etc., should be used. Ultrasound study is now being utilized to estimate residual urine in neurogenic bladders, obviating catheterization.

Most patients are not aware of the relative size of their own stream. The flow may have decreased over a long period of time, so that patients are unaware of the diminution. An occasional male patient may note the difference in his urinary stream by accidental observation of a neighbor in a public toilet or by chance comparison with his own son. A female patient may become aware of a difference in her stream by the sound of another female in a public toilet.

Techniques and Aids in Flowrate Determination

Types of Flowmeters

Several brands of flowmeters are available from medical supply houses. They present a very reliable, accurate, and graphic way of showing doctor and patient alike the impedance of urinary flow, and thus help to determine the necessity for future therapy.

The Scott Uroflowmeter, recently improved, is a fine instrument which affords excellent patient uroflow studies. It is a valuable research tool for hospital use. The Kaufman Uroflometer ® has been used by the authors over the years with reliable results. Other newer units have been reported in the recent urological literature.

Stopwatch Technique for Flowrate Determination

An ordinary stopwatch may be used for a fairly accurate determination of urine flow. The patient is asked to press the stopwatch after his urinary flow is started and he begins to void into a container. When he begins to note a decrease in the size of his stream near the end of micturition, he again presses the stopwatch and ceases to void into the container, finishing the evacuation into the toilet bowl. Thus, the full strength of his urinary flowrate is the force measured.

One needs only divide the time in seconds into the volume in milliliters to obtain the urinary flowrate in number of milliliters per second.

Bodner Cup Uroflowmeter

Recently used by us for uroflowmetry are plastic cups (obtainable at all drug stores for a nominal amount) which are modified by drilling a hole $7/32$ inch in diameter in the bottom of the cup. This allows an outflow of 16 ml per second. The patient may void into the cup in his own bathroom or in the office. If the cup remains empty on voiding into it, the flowrate is poor. If urine accumulates in the cup, the flow is more than 16 ml per second. If the "cup runneth over," the patient has a most adequate flow.

Women may use the cup by sitting on the toilet seat backwards. The cup, being plastic, may be washed for reuse. Patients with urethral stricture may use the cup as a guide as to when to return for further dilation. Women with urethrostenosis may use the cup in the same way. The uroflow cup may be used as a measure of postoperative prostatectomy results, etc.

Nine-ounce cups are used for adults, four-ounce cups with smaller holes in the cup and slower flowrates are used for small children. Hole diameters for varied flowrates are as follows (note that tests were done at 2-inch head of water input):

Hole Size (inch)	Flowrate (ml/sec)
1/4	18
15/64	17
7/32	16
3/16	15
13/64	13
3/32	5

Figure 12 illustrates the simplicity of the cup uroflowmeter device, shown with a wall-type dispenser unit. A small sign underneath the wall dispenser cautions that "these cups are not for drinking purposes."

Alternatively, a soft plastic receptacle about 5 cm wide and 15 cm long, open at the top narrow end, and with a hole of appropriate size at its lower end, may be used in the previously described manner.

Privacy for the Patient

It is of utmost importance that the patient be asked to lock either a bathroom or treatment room door when testing his urine flowrate in a physician's office. Only in this way can he void with a feeling of safety from interruption, and only thus can a true flowrate be obtained.

Simple Uroflowmetry Seat for the Female Patient

For obtaining precise flowrate determination in women and children

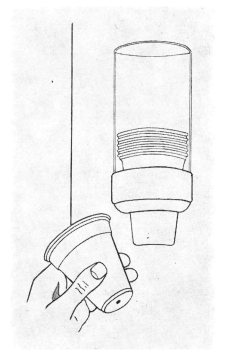

12. Simple cup uroflowmeter

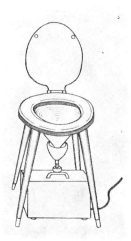

13. Uroflowmetry seat for the female patient

there is a need for a commode type of seat which may be used with one of the commercially available flowmeters. Manufactured units are designed specifically for this use, or one may very simply construct an inexpensive seat for use with the uroflowmeter as follows.

A toilet seat and cover may be purchased at any hardware store. A piece of ¾-inch plywood is outlined to the contour of the toilet seat. This is done also for the inner aspect or opening through the plywood, except that the plywood opening is cut ¼ to ½ inch larger than the toilet seat itself to avoid moistening of the wood during the act of micturition.

Four metal or wooden legs, approximately 19 to 20 inches long, may be attached to the plywood. This is a comfortable height for most women as well as being the necessary height under which most uroflowmeters will fit. The flowmeter may then be equipped with a large plastic funnel which fits against the inside of the toilet seat unit (Fig. 13).

The total cost of construction for a unit such as this should not exceed $20.

SPECIMEN COLLECTION

Non-Contaminated Specimens

Obtaining Clean-Catch Urine Specimens on Female Patients

A female patient may be instructed or shown how to wash in between the labia minora with one single downward stroke of a cotton pledget soaked with liquid soap or 0.75 percent hexachlorophene solution. This should be done with the patient sitting backwards on the toilet seat facing the water tank, or facing the wide part of a bedpan. By virtue of straddling the toilet seat or the bedpan, the patient's labia are spread apart.

After three or four pledgets are utilized to wash downward in between the labia, a glass of warm, preferably sterile, water is poured down between the separated labia. When the specimen is obtained in the home of the patient, boiled, but cooled, water may be used.

With the labia still spread apart with one hand, the patient then empties the bladder, catching a midstream specimen into a sterile vessel.

A clean-catch specimen *when negative* is of value. When a clean-catch specimen is positive, a catheterized specimen should be taken.

New Collection Device to Avoid Urethral Contamination

A device currently under clinical trial holds a good deal of promise in eliminating the possibility of contamination from the distal one-third of the urethra.

The device unrolls a film of sterile plastic material over the urethra as a catheter passes on the inside of this plastic film with no contact whatsoever with the urethra. The plastic material unrolls as the sterile catheter attached to the material is pushed slowly and gently on into the bladder. The urine specimen is thus obtained purely from the bladder.

Other Means of Sterile Specimen Collection

Suprapubic needle puncture or catheterization under aseptic technique still remain the best means of collecting sterile urine specimens in the female at this time.

Obtaining Urine Specimens from Infants

There are on the market plastic materials with a sealing edge to apply around the penis and scrotum of infant boys and around the genitalia of infant girls to collect urine specimens.

However, should these not be readily available, a satisfactory urine-collecting device may very easily be made. One may utilize a finger cot, the end of which has been cut to fit over a sterile test tube. The finger cot is applied to the penis of a male infant and held there with a narrow piece of adhesive plaster or transparent tape. The end of the finger cot may be cut along its superior and inferior border, or along its lateral borders, and by "fishmouthing" the proximal end and sticking this to the female patient with transparent tape, a voided specimen may be obtained.

A rubber or plastic glove may also be used, or a commercial plastic bag of any type may be employed in the same manner. The specimen may then be poured into any suitable container.

Collection of Urine Specimens on a Cystoscopy Table

One often attempts to get the patient to void on a cystoscopy table in order to perform a voiding cystourethrogram or to obtain a urine specimen and measure the residual urine. It is important to elevate the table so that any urine draining will flow into a drain pan rather than onto the cystoscopy table and up on the patient's back.

To keep the legs of the patient from moving together, the stirrups are maintained in position. However, at times it may be necessary to have the patient sit up almost vertically. By placing the stirrups so that the crossbar is in the transverse position, a ridge is formed upon which the patient may sit. In most tables, this involves exchanging the right stirrup to the left side and vice versa. In this way, the patient's legs are locked in and will not be spread more widely apart.

RESIDUAL URINE DETERMINATION

Mechanical Techniques

Catheter Technique for Residual Urine Determination

The patient may be asked to void and immediately after voiding have a catheter passed and residual urine obtained and measured. Should one have a catheter already in the patient and wish to determine residual urine, one may then fill the bladder to a stated amount in milliliters until such time as the patient feels his bladder to be at capacity. The catheter is then removed and the patient asked to void into a container. The difference between the amount placed in the bladder and the amount obtained on urination is the residual urine.

Use of a Sound to Estimate Residual Urine

A rough estimate of the amount of residual urine in patients with known vesical atonia can be made by passing a sound and feeling the inside of the bladder with the tip of the sound. This is particularly helpful in post-operative patients in whom one might be passing a sound in any case. This method is highly inaccurate and impracticable. If one is to instrument, then a *catheter* may be passed.

Percussion Method of Residual Urine Estimation

One may have the patient void and then percuss over his abdomen. Should he have a residual urine over 250 ml, then one may be able to percuss the bladder; residual urine below 250 ml is usually not percussible. Many factors make this method of residual urine estimation variable: the thickness of the bladder wall, adiposity and body conformation of the patient, ana-tomical depth of the pelvis, presence of adhesions due to previous inflam-mation or surgery, etc.

Chemical and Radiographic Techniques

Indirect Test of Residual Urine (Phenolsulfonphthalein Test)

A good laboratory test for measuring residual urine is the phenolsul-fonphthalein (P.S.P.) test first described by Dr. Donald Smith of the Uni-versity of California many years ago.

The patient's morning urine specimen is examined, including specific gravity. A specific gravity of less than 1.020 is suggestive of upper urinary tract disease. The patient is given 600 ml of water and 30 minutes later one milliliter of phenolsulfonphthalein is injected intravenously (6 mg/ml). In 30 minutes the patient is asked to void completely.

The percent of P.S.P. recovered, using color standards, is computed. If the patient excretes 50 percent of the P.S.P. in the first 30 minutes, one can be assured that the patient has good renal function and no appreciable re-sidual urine.

Should the P.S.P. excretion fall below 50 percent, another specimen is collected 30 minutes later and the percentage of P.S.P. again determined. A greater percent of P.S.P. in the second specimen than in the first suggests an appreciable residual urine or bilateral renal damage.

Modified Phenolsulfonphthalein Test for Children

The above-described test may be modified for children. All of the urine voided in the first three hours after the injection of the dye is collected. Another specimen is collected of the total amount of urine excreted for the following 12 hours. Under usual circumstances, the first three-hour specimen will contain 87 to 97 percent of the dye and the second specimen will be free of the dye. Urinary retention is suspected if there is any trace of P.S.P. present at the end of 12 hours.

For infants one may save the wet diapers collected for the 3 hours following injection and place them in a graduate partly filled with a liter of water. If 50 percent of the contrast material or more is collected at the end of 3 hours, in all probability this infant has no residual urine.

Iodized Oil (Lipiodol) Test for Residual Urine

One may inject Lipiodol®, or any other oil-based contrast material which is most apt to float on top of urine, into the patient's bladder. Twenty-four hours later a flat film is taken. If the Lipiodol is still present in the patient's bladder, it is evidence that there is residual urine and that this may not be drained out of the bladder at any time.

Residual urine above 10 to 15 ml in the adult or 9 to 10 ml in the child is conducive to bacterial growth.

(See also *Pyelographic Determination of Residual Urine,* and *Ultrasound for Bladder Residual,* in Chapter Three.)

ROENTGENOLOGY OF THE URINARY TRACT

FACILITIES AND TECHNICAL AIDS

NEWER AND MORE sophisticated diagnostic modalities such as ultra-sonography, cineradiography, aortography, radioisotope renography, percutaneous antegrade pyelography, renal photoscanning, etc., are used increasingly in urologic study. Nonetheless, the routine diagnostic X-ray methods are still indispensable in evaluation. Therefore, aids in techniques and administrative aspects of standard radiological procedures in urologic departments or offices are still of utmost importance.

Facilities for Pyelography and Cystoscopy

In many parts of the United States pyelography is done in the offices of the urologist. In some medical centers pyelography is performed in the urology outpatient department rather than in the department of radiology. The cystoscopy room, though part of the urologic outpatient department, should be immediately adjacent to the radiology department.

Image Fluoroscopy, Image Amplification, Television Monitoring, and Video-Tape Recording as Adjuncts to Cystoscopy Units

A room in a urologic office equipped with X-ray should also serve as a cystoscopy room. The hospital outpatient cystoscopy unit should also have image fluoroscopy with television monitoring capabilities. The *image amp-lifier, with T.V. monitoring and video-tape recording for later review,* is most helpful for many purposes:

1) *Passage of ureteral catheters.* Adequate visualization of the entire upper and middle urinary tract enables this procedure to be performed with accuracy and dispatch.

2) *Extraction of ureteral calculi.* Visualization with image amplification is most helpful in attempted extraction of a ureteral calculus. The usual precautions and complications involved with attempting to extract a calculus from the lower ureter are not as a rule modified by virtue of the vastly improved visualization.

3) *Evaluation of ureteropelvic and ureterovesical junctures.* Preoperative and postoperative assessment of these areas is improved immeasurably by use of the image amplifier.

4) *Positioning or changing of nephrostomy tubes.* The accurate placement of these tubes is facilitated by image amplification.

5) *Adequate cystography and voiding cystourethrography.* Often vesicoure-

teral reflux is demonstrated by this method whereas it may have been missed with usual radiologic technique.

6) *Adequate seminovesiculography, vasography, and epidymography.* These delicate procedures may be more accurately performed with image amplification.

7) *Translumbar and percutaneous femoral aortography and inferior venacavography.* These techniques are most handily done with the aid of the image amplifier.

8) *Renal cyst visualization.* With the aid of the image amplifier a needle may be more easily passed to a renal cyst and aspiration of fluid done. The injection of contrast material and visualization thereafter may be done most efficiently with image amplification.

Radionuclide Cystography, an Improvement over X-Ray Cystography

Recent clinical study employing radionuclide cystography to detect vesicoureteral reflux in children has proven this to be superior to roentgenographic cystography. There is also a marked reduction in radiation dose to the patient. Reflux into the renal pelvis that is missed on X-ray examination is picked up when the radionuclide cystography method is used.

For the radionuclide study, 1 mc of ^{99m}technetium pertechnetate is instilled into the bladder through a catheter, along with saline, until the bladder is filled. Polaroid ® film is used to record the images. The scintillation camera is positioned to observe the dome of the bladder and the upper urinary tracts. Superior posterior and posterior oblique views (right and left) are recorded. A final postvoiding posterior image of the urinary tracts is then recorded to document reflux occurring only during voiding. The total dose to the bladder is usually about 30 millirads per 30 minutes.

When contrasted with comparable X-ray technique, radionuclide cystography affords at least a 50- to 100-fold reduction in radiation dose.

Helpful Guidelines in Urologic Radiology

Avoidance of Unnecessary X-Ray Exposures

In many instances the urologist may minimize the number of X-ray exposures so that the patient need not be unnecessarily exposed to a complete series of X-rays.

This is especially true, for example, in patients with prostatic hyperplasia in whom one is anxious to determine the status and function of the upper urinary tract. A patient passing a ureteral calculus in whom previous recent pyelography has been done may need only a follow-up flat plate to determine the progress of a small calculus. Intravenous contrast material may be injected and one or two X-ray exposures only may be necessary to follow the progress of a passing calculus causing minimal hydronephrosis or ureterectasis.

One should in these' cases give specific instructions to the radiology department. The choice of exposures in many institutions is at the discretion of an X-ray technician, who subjects the patient to a routine series as dictated by a radiologist. No assessment of specific needs in a particular instance may be made—this may be known only to the urologist.

Often there are instances in which the urologist may require delayed emptying films over prolonged intervals. One must be specific in giving instructions to the X-ray technician in such cases.

In the special case of pregnant women, two exposures should be sufficient for diagnosis in most conditions.

Caution in Intravenous Injection in Iodine-Sensitive Patients

A test dose of the contrast material is always administered intravenously to a patient about to be subjected to intravenous urography. Testing with small doses is not a reliable indicator of possible severe reactions. Some physicians have dropped into the patient's eye a drop of contrast material, while others have resorted to the subcutaneous injection of a small quantity of contrast material. These, too, are unreliable tests.

For the most part, an injection of one minim to a milliliter of contrast material should be given intravenously. One should then wait five to fifteen minutes before proceeding with the remainder of the injection. Should the patient demonstrate edema of the eyelids or complain of generalized itching, "a tightness in the throat" or slight difficulty in inspiration and expiration, one should proceed immediately with anti-allergic therapy. This consists of the use of intravenous Adrenalin and/or an intravenous antihistamine. In some instances of more severe reactions one may have recourse to the use of intravenous steroid therapy.

Reactions occur most frequently in patients with a history of allergies. The history should be most complete in this respect, the patient being questioned very closely and specifically. Reactions may or may not increase with the rapidity of injection and increase of dosage.

Intravenous urography should not be attempted unless the physician is prepared to deal with all of the necessary emergency procedures involved in reversing a severe reaction to the contrast medium. One must first of all be familiar with cardiopulmonary resuscitation techniques. There should be oxygen available, with rebreather masks. Equipment must be on hand for endotracheal intubation and tracheotomy may be necessary on some occasions. Suction apparatus should be on hand. All of the usual emergency medications should be immediately available.

The medico-legal importance of the necessary available equipment, medication, and application of these cannot be emphasized enough. (See *Emergency Equipment* in Chapter I, Armamentarium.)

X-Ray Visualization on Minimal Dosage

Should the patient have a mild allergic manifestation while being sub-jected to intravenous pyelography, the injection procedure should be stopped. One should not forget, however, to proceed with taking X-rays. With as little as one milliliter of contrast material, it is surprising that one may get, on occasion, an acceptable pyelogram.

Contrast Media, Iodine Concentration, and Grams of Iodine per Dose

The most commonly used media for intravenous urography, cystography, and urethrography are those shown in Table IV. The amount of iodine present in the contrast media used in urography and the number of grams the patient receives determine the density of these substances on the X-ray film.

TABLE IV

IODINATED CONTRAST MATERIALS FOR INTRAVASCULAR USE

Product	Composition	Bound Iodine (%)	How Supplied (ml)	Iodine/Dose (gm)
Conray®	Meglumine iothalamate 60%	28.2	20 30 50	5.6 8.4 14.1
Conray®-400	Sodium iothalamate 66.8%	40	25 50	10 20
Cysto-CONRAY® (not for IV administration)	Meglumine iothalamate 43%	20.2	50 100 ✳	 10.1 20.2
CYSTOKON®	Sodium acetrizoate 30%	20	†	—
VASCORAY™	Meglumine iothalamate 52% and sodium iothalamate 26%	40	25 50	10 20
Renografin®-60	Meglumine diatrizoate 52% and sodium diatrizoate 8%	29	30 50	8.7 14.5

Renografin®-76	Meglumine diatrizoate 66% and sodium diatrizoate 10%	37	20 50	7.4 18.5
Reno-M-60™	Meglumine diatrizoate 60%	28.2	30 50	8.4 14
Reno-M-Dip®	Meglumine diatrizoate 30%	14	300	42
Hypaque® Sodium 25%	Sodium diatrizoate	15	300	45
Hypaque® Sodium 50%	Sodium diatrizoate	30	20 30 50	6.0 9.0 15.0
Hypaque® Meglumine 60%	Meglumine diatrizoate	28.2	20 30 50	5.6 8.4 14.1
Hypaque®-M 75%	Sodium and meglumine diatrizoates	38.5	20 50	7.7 19.2
Hypaque®-M 90%	Sodium and meglumine	46.2	20 50	9.2 23.1

* Also available in single-dose bottles of 250 ml and in 250-ml and 500-ml dilution-unit bottles containing 100 ml and 250 ml respectively of Cysto-CONRAY. For cystography and cysto-urethrography, adults usually require a volume of 200-400 ml of Cysto-CONRAY. Children require a volume in proportion to body size, usual dose 30 to 300 ml. For retrograde pyelo-ureterography: ordinarily 20 ml for bilateral and 10 ml for unilateral pyeloureterograms. Children require volume reduced in proportion to body size.
† CYSTOKON available in 100- and 250-ml single dose bottles, and in 250- and 500-ml dilution-unit bottles.

No attempt is made here to evaluate one product over another.

Many urologists continue to use sodium iodide as a contrast material for cystography. Others object to its use as a contrast medium for the bladder because of its reputed irritability.

Instruction Sheets for Patients Prior to Intravenous Urography

Sheets of instructions for patients preparing for genitourinary tract X-rays are printed and distributed by various manufacturers of contrast materials or drug products specified in preparation of the patient for X-ray. These instruction sheets are frequently made available by the manufacturer, gratis. Figure 14 illustrates such a form.

```
┌─────────────────────────────────────────────────────┐
│              PREPARATION FOR KIDNEY X-RAYS            │
│                                                       │
│  (NIGHT BEFORE X-RAYS)                                │
│  1.  One hour before evening meal, take two table-    │
│      spoonfuls Phospho-Soda® (Fleet) in a glass of    │
│      water, and follow with one-half glass of water.  │
│  2.  No liquids after 11 p.m.                         │
│  (DAY OF X-RAYS)                                      │
│  3.  No liquids the following morning.                │
│  4.  Further instructions:                            │
│           For Breakfast:  2 soft-boiled eggs          │
│                              toast and jelly           │
│                                                       │
│           In brushing teeth, do not swallow water.    │
│           If thirsty, chew gum.                       │
│  5.  Report to office:                                │
│                                                       │
│           Name (of urologist)_____ │
│           Address _____ │
│                       _____  │
└─────────────────────────────────────────────────────┘
```

14. Sample instruction sheet for kidney X-ray preparation

Intravenous Pyelography in the Afternoon

Patients receiving intravenous pyelography in the afternoon do not require dehydration from the evening of the preceding day. Under such circumstances it may be perfectly permissible to allow the patient to have a "light breakfast." However, no liquids should preferably be allowed for a period of eight to ten hours before the scheduled time for radiography.

Pills, Capsules, and Suppositories of Radiopaque Nature

Rectal and vaginal suppositories often contain radiopaque substances which may be mistaken for calculi or other foreign bodies when the patient is subjected to radiography. The heavy metals in tablet or capsule form also are radiopaque. Should these lie over the renal pelvis area, one may confuse them with renal calculi. It is therefore very important to determine the recent medication history of the patient, especially when there are opacities overlying the urinary tract.

The following[*] preparations, listed together with the substance which could possibly cause artifacts, should be considered suspect when X-ray examination demonstrates opacities overlying the urinary tract:

---

[*] There may be other preparations which have been inadvertently omitted.

A & D ®	(bismuth subgallate)	
Anugesic ®	(bismuth subgallate, bismuth resorcin compound)	
Anusol-HC ®	(bismuth subgallate, bismuth resorcin compound, bismuth subiodide)	
Desitin Calmol 4 ®	(bismuth subgallate)	Rectal Suppositories
Desitin HC ®	(bismuth subgallate)	
Medicone-HC ®	(oxyquinoline sulfate)	
P N S ®	(bismuth subcarbonate)	
Wyanoids HC ®	(bismuth oxyiodide, bismuth subcarbonate)	
Xylocaine ®	(bismuth subgallate)	
Baculin ® Tablets	(diiodohydroxyquinoline)	
Floraquin ® Tablets	(diiodohydroxyquin)	
Gynben ® Inserts	(diiodohydroxyquin)	Vaginal Preparations
Lycinate ® Tablets	(diiodohydroxyquin)	
Quinette ® Inserts	(diiodohydroxyquin)	
Vioform ® Inserts	(iodochlorhydroxyquin)	

Storage of X-Ray Film

The lack of storage facilities makes it impractical to retain all old X-rays for long periods of time. Several methods of film storage may be utilized:

1) A photographic miniature of the X-ray most representative of a patient's pyelogram may be made by a professional minifilm company. The miniatures (usually 3 by 3½ cm) are then labeled and kept on file. All films showing pathology may be kept on file indefinitely, but only representative films of a series may be kept.

2) One may select one or two films representative of a specific pyelogram and in the office make photocopies of these films. A Polaroid camera with portrait lens may be so fixed to a wall bracket that distance, focus, etc., are unchanged in relation to a fixed view-box. Thus personnel untrained in photography may film pyelograms for size reduction. These small photos may then be filed in patients' charts so that the films are always readily available.

3) One may select one or two films most representative of a patient's pyelogram and file these in numerical order in one X-ray folder. Each folder holds about 50 films. The range of the X-ray identification numbers is recorded on the outside of the film envelope. Some 90 percent of the storage space previously required for complete sets or series of films with respective envelopes is thereby eliminated.

Quick Drying of X-Ray Film

With the X-ray film in a hanger, both sides of the wet film may be sponged, utilizing long straight strokes. The rapid absorption of excess fluid in this manner allows the film to dry much more rapidly than it would otherwise.

Flat Film of Abdomen for Bladder Size

Urinary retention may be suspected in a patient in whom catheterization is contraindicated. A plane film of the abdomen may be taken over the bladder area. If the bladder shadow does not appear on the first film, a second film with different X-ray penetration may be done. Usually with a full bladder the X-ray will very adequately demonstrate bladder volume; tomography will more accurately demonstrate residual urine.

Pyelographic Determination of Residual Urine

One may determine the quantity of residual urine by first performing the usual intravenous pyelogram. The patient, after completion of the usual upper tract study, is then asked to void following the 25-minute post-injection films. Immediately during voiding and immediately after the patient's bladder is said to be emptied, X-ray exposures are made directly over the bladder and urethral areas. One thus has a visual picture of the voiding urethrogram and of the patient's residual urine.

The X-ray department should be requested to always obtain a postvoid film over the bladder area to determine residual urine on all patients.

A simple means of approximating the amount of the residual is to measure the breadth of the contrast material in milliliters in the transverse diameter and then add to this diameter the breadth of the contrast material from a superior-inferior basis. One then takes the sum of these two figures and divides this by two to obtain an average. This average figure is multiplied by a factor of ten. The result is a rough approximation of the residual urine in the bladder.

Additional Gains from Postvoiding Film for Residual Urine

In addition to determining the amount of residual urine in the bladder with the postvoiding film, one also often obtains an excellent outline of a bladder diverticulum or visual demonstration of vesicoureteral reflux, since reflux causes increase of the contrast material in the ureter and renal pelvis. This is not, however, too reliable a method of demonstrating ureteral reflux.

Bladder tumors of small size, or nonopaque calculi, may at times visualize only on the postvoid film.

Ultrasound for Bladder Residual

As previously mentioned, ultrasound, "echogram," or "sonogram" techniques may be utilized for residual urine evaluation in the bladder. This is particularly helpful in the case of a patient with a neurogenic bladder where it is preferable to avoid catheterization.

(See also *Iodized Oil (Lipiodol) Test for Residual Urine,* in Chapter Two.)

Diuretic as an Aid in the Diagnosis of Intermittent Hydronephrosis

Intermittent hydronephrosis may be an elusive entity. The taking of a diuretic prior to pyelography is a valuable aid in establishing the presence of "polyhydration nephrosis." Some of the rapid-acting diuretics such as furosemide (Lasix) are most suitable for this application.

Avoidance of Compression During Intravenous Urography

When mass lesions are suspected or known to exist, compression must be avoided in the performance of urography. Extravasation of contrast material caused by compression may lead to unfortunate complications in subsequent surgery.

UROGRAPHIC TECHNIQUES

Radiologic Aids in the Study of Male Infertility

The male partner is the primary cause of sterility in almost 40 percent of sterile marriages. Following semen analysis and the diagnosis of azoospermia, testicular biopsy with vasography, epididymograms, and seminovesiculograms are in order. The continuity of the seminal tract may be demonstrated with these studies.

Catheterization of the ejaculatory duct with radiography often fails to demonstrate satisfactorily the vas deferens. Bilateral vas exposure, however, with a tiny transverse or vertical incision to expose the lumen of the vas, insertion of a cannular-tip 23-gauge needle, and then filling with 2 to 3 ml of contrast material demonstrates beautifully the vas deferens and the seminal vesicles. One may reverse the direction of the needle and also obtain an epididymogram. One or two 5-0 chromic sutures are used to repair the small incision made in the vas.

When an epididymogram is done, approximately 0.5 ml of contrast material (Hypaque or Renografin) is injected towards the epididymis. When 2 to 3 ml of radiopaque material is injected towards the seminal vesicle, some of the fluid should escape into the urethra and bladder, showing patency of the ejaculatory duct.

Inferior Venacavography

Most patients with suspected carcinoma of the kidney should have venacavography before definitive surgical therapy is undertaken. Unsuspected tumor metastases in the renal vein or vena cava are visualized much more often with this procedure than one would suspect.

Aortography and Arteriography

Though transfemoral aortography is the procedure of choice for arteriography of the kidney, there are circumstances in which one must still consider the possibility of translumbar aortography. This is especially true in the older arteriosclerotic patient.

Angiography and Visualization of Testicular Tumor and Varicocele

In instances of suspected testicular tumors, one may do a testicular angiogram by exposing the spermatic artery in the spermatic cord and cannulating the artery. The rapid injection of 5 ml of contrast material, with rapid X-ray exposure, demonstrates the testicular arterial tree.

In this same manner one may do X-rays of the veins in the scrotum, especially in those instances where a varicocele exists.

Renal Scans in Patients with Reflux

In a patient with ureteral reflux on whom one wishes to do a renal scan for one reason or another, it is important to keep the bladder empty by means of an indwelling catheter on continuous drainage. The radioisotope department should be forewarned. Reflux may confuse the picture from the standpoint of isotope densities in the kidney.

Ureteral Reflux and Cystography

Cystograms, up to recent years, had been done primarily on children. Increasing recognition of ureteral reflux in adults with recurrent urinary tract infection has resulted in the more frequent performance of cystography. It is recommended that all patients subjected to cystoscopic evaluation (in addition to upper urinary tract evaluation) have as part of their study cystography and voiding cystourethrograms. If there is a high degree of suspicion of reflux in an adult patient, but this is not demonstrated on cystography, it *may* be demonstrated on voiding cinecystography.

Cystourethrography vs Cineradiography in Children

Cineradiography in younger children is a difficult procedure to perform. It is best done under general anesthesia. Many urologists voice objections to the technique because they feel that the emptying of a bladder by a patient under complete anesthesia is not a physiological type of bladder emptying. A patient's bladder, however, may be filled under anesthesia, after which the patient is awakened. One may then do a voiding cinecystourethrogram of the patient in the awakened state.

The above technique may prove to be laborious since the child often will not cooperate in voiding on command, and a good deal of patience and time must be devoted to the patient by the X-ray technician. This is not always feasible, and therefore cine study of bladder emptying has become a less popular procedure.

Cineradiography, however, will prove to be a very profitable and informative procedure, should one be able to execute the examination. Frequently when one strongly suspects reflux not demonstrated by the usual cystourethrogram, motion picture X-ray emptying of the bladder shows the suspected reflux.

Voiding Cystourethrogram Techniques

Controversy exists among urologists as to the proper technique for obtaining a voiding cystourethrogram on the pediatric patient. Several routines are employed:

Method 1. Under anesthesia the patient's bladder is filled (by gravity), using a catheter and a 1- or 2-oz Asepto syringe barrel (minus bulb). Contrast material is poured by pitcher into the Asepto syringe. When approximately 1 to 1½ oz of contrast material is in the bladder, a low-pressure cystogram is obtained. The bladder is then further gravity-filled until it reaches the point where it no longer will accept fluid.

Following this one attaches the Asepto syringe rubber bulb filled with contrast material to the syringe and injects 5 to 15 ml more of fluid into the bladder, overdistending it. This added amount of fluid is aspirated and then again injected, the maneuver being repeated three to four times. The patient will usually develop bladder contractions.

The catheter is quickly removed and a voiding cinecystourethrogram is obtained. Patients will empty their bladders spontaneously at least 19 out of 20 times with this technique.

Method 2. Under minimal anesthesia the bladder is filled. For safety reasons loose restraints are applied, since the awakening child may be hyperactive. The patient is encouraged to void, and one waits until he voids to take the film.

Method 3. A suprapubic cystocath is introduced into the bladder of the anesthetized patient. The patient's bladder is filled through the plastic tubing, and one then waits until the patient begins to void. Fluid may be continually dripped into the bladder as the patient voids and the film is taken, or one may discontinue the addition of more fluid into the bladder.

These same techniques may be used with the regular X-ray process instead of the cineradiographic process. In using regular X-ray film the employment of a rapid cassette-changing apparatus will enable the taking of fast serial films which may demostrate reflux that would otherwise be missed.

Additional Helps in Cystourethrography

Knowing the patient's full bladder capacity before cystourethrography is of value. Before the day of the study one may instruct the patient to defer voiding until he feels quite full. The patient then voids into a container suit-

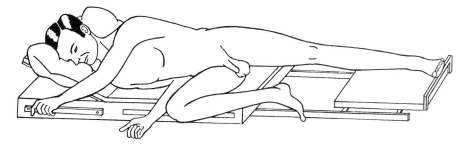

15. Positioning the patient for cystourethrography

able for measuring the urine. This test may be done on three to four occasions, recording the volume each time.

The patient then reports for his study. At that time one may have the patient void and then pass a catheter to note the residual urine. The residual urine volume may be added to the volume the patient has recorded as his bladder capacity. One may then ensure that this volume of contrast material, or air if this is the medium used, is placed into the bladder.

In filming the overdistended bladder it is helpful to place the patient in a lateral position, hyperextending the uppermost leg so that it is pointed somewhat backward, and bending the lowermost extremity as much as possible, so that the femur is not in the way of the urethra. One may take the urethrogram in the left or right oblique position (See Fig. 15).

Catheter for Use with Children in Cystourethrography

Use of a No. 8 French, 15-inch feeding tube (K-31) or a No. 5 French infant feeding tube for catheterization is helpful in doing cystography on children.

Chain Cystourethrograms

Some urologists still prefer the chain cystourethrographic technique in the female patient with stress incontinence. When properly placed in the bladder, the chain in a lateral view affords excellent visualization for both anterior and posterior urethrovesical angles on filling of the bladder. This procedure specifically indicates whether or not one should subject the patient to an anterior vaginal repair or an anterior urethropexy.

The chain itself is readily available since it is the same type as that utilized as a pull chain for electric lights. It may prove difficult to insert properly. The use of a cystoscopic rongeur type of forceps (with or without the use of the cystoscope) or of a resectoscopic utility forceps, by way of the resectoscope, facilitates its insertion.

Some urologists utilize a mosquito clamp to pass the chain into the bladder, grasping the distal end of the chain and placing it into the urethra and directly on into the bladder for a good depth. The flare of the clamp, however, is a hindrance. A uterine forceps may also be used.

An effective method of inserting the chain is to make a 10-cm slit down the axis of a 14 to 16 French Robinson catheter and insert the chain in the slit, with the last bead gently tapped into place at the end of the catheter. Using a generous amount of lubricating jelly, the catheter is then inserted into the urethra and on into the bladder with the chain held in place while advancing the catheter. Once it is in the bladder, the catheter is pushed while the chain is held, thus releasing it from the catheter. While still in the bladder the catheter may also be employed to instill the contrast medium.

The catheter is removed before the film is taken. A finger holds the chain at the bladder neck via vaginal pressure to keep the chain from slipping out of the bladder. It is secured to the vulva and thigh with adhesive tape. If the patient is not prepared on the X-ray table, she must be transported to the X-ray location by wheelchair.

Cystography and Contrast Cystography for Evaluation of Prostatic Hyperplasia and Diverticula

Cystography is often an important aid in the preoperative evaluation of the size of the prostate gland. The cystogram obtained as a part of intravenous urography is usually adequate for diagnostic needs. When not satisfactory, retrograde cystography can be performed. This involves the risk associated with the passage of a balloon-type catheter. The risk can be minimized by employing a small 12 French catheter and passing it gently and aseptically. If the balloon of the catheter is then distended with undiluted contrast medium, it is easily visualized on subsequent films.

The bladder may then be filled with air or diluted contrast medium and the patient placed in a semi-upright position, clamping with a hemostat the distal end of the catheter to pull the balloon down as far as possible. The position of the balloon as seen on X-ray thus becomes an important guide as to the degree of intravesical protrusion of the prostate. Confusing rectal gas shadows can usually be eliminated by passage of a rectal tube.

When bladder diverticula are encountered, combined air and opaque-medium cystography can be helpful. After the usual cystography has been done, about half of the opaque medium is evacuated through the catheter and replaced by an equivalent amount of air. Since most bladder diverticula appear off the posterior aspect of the bladder, the contrast medium is retained in a diverticulum when the patient is in the supine position. The size of the diverticulum and its relation to the air-filled bladder usually lying anteriorly to the diverticulum are easily discernible on X-ray. (See also *Identification of Urethral Diverticula*, Female, in Chapter Seven.)

Simplified Technique for Urethrography

Numerous methods are utilized for the filling of the urethra so as to obtain adequate films for urethrography. One may use any of the usual intravenous contrast media available in most departments of radiology. The contrast material may be diluted half and half with lubricating jelly. Prepared media in thick oils are also available for intraurethral use.

The contrast medium, in a quantity of about one-half ounce, may be injected into the urethra using a blunt-tip Asepto urethral syringe. While the injection is proceeding, the X-ray exposure may take place. Anterior-posterior and lateral films may be taken in this manner. A 20-cc piston syringe (without Luer lock) may also be employed for this injection.

Some urologists depend on the use of the Brodny clamp and a catheter in the urethra. Others use a No. 16 French balloon catheter or one even smaller. The balloon of the catheter is blown up with approximately 2 ml of sterile water after being passed just through the fossa navicularis. By thus filling the balloon with a small quantity of fluid there is no escape of fluid through the urethral meatus.

Voiding Urethrograms in Female Patients

Satisfactory investigation of the lower female urinary drainage system should include adequate visualization of the urethra. It is difficult for a female patient to void in a normal fashion on the cystoscopy or X-ray table. In this connection, please refer to the paragraph on *Collection of Urine Specimens on a Cystoscopy Table*, in Chapter Two.

A plexiglass saddle urinal is made for the specific purpose of obtaining female urethrograms. This was developed by the Picker X-Ray Corporation of San Diego, California, with the cooperation of local urologists and nurses.

Infusion Pyelography

For infusion pyelography a combination of approximately 150 ml of 30 percent meglumine diatrizoate (such as Reno-M-Dip, formerly called Renografin) with approximately 120 ml of 5 percent glucose in water is administered as rapidly as possible intravenously through an 18-gauge needle. It ordinarily takes from five to fifteen minutes for this volume of liquid to be infused intravenously. Films of good quality almost always result, without any special preparation whatsoever of the patient. Visualization of the pelvis, calyces, and ureter often appears even in patients in azotemia. Diagnostic films have been obtained in patients with blood urea nitrogen levels up to 85 mg percent.

While the contrast material is being administered intravenously, films may be taken at intervals of one, two, and three minutes to obtain a nephrogram for the purpose of assessing renal vascularity and parenchymal circulation. This technique of infusion pyelography often produces films of such diagnostic quality that the need for retrograde urography is lessened.

The increased use of infusion pyelography to more adequately visualize the ureters and decrease the incidence of suspected but undiagnosed ureteral calculi would also be valuable. It is estimated that from 5 to 15 percent of all renal or ureteral calculi are not seen on ordinary intravenous urography.

Infusion Pyelography and Nephrotomography

Infusion pyelography in conjunction with nephrotomography has been extremely valuable in differentiating cysts from neoplasia of the urinary tract. These two procedures in combination have also helped to eliminate the need of perirenal air insufflation in cases of suspected adrenal tumor. Infusion pyelography so well delineates the ureters that it is of special value in patients who have had testicular tumors with possible metastasis, or patients who need study for intra-abdominal masses in the region of the renal pedicle which stem from still other sources. Inward bowing of the ureters at the level of the promontory or midsacrum is very often found in carcinoma of the rectosigmoid with ileopelvic node involvement, and after abdominoperineal resection secondary to pelvic retroperitonealization.

Nephrotomography may be indicated under specific circumstances for better localization of certain pathologic lesions in the kidney.
(See also *Detection of Small Renal Tumors: a Method of Possible Value*, and *Localization of Kidney for Needle Biopsy Purposes*, in Chapter Four.)

Tomography or Planography for Renal or Ureteral Calculi

Tomography or planography may be useful in delineating soft tissue masses. However, the technique will also be of value in visualizing ureteral or renal calculi which may overlie a bony area. Under such circumstances one may be able to visualize a calculus which would otherwise not be demonstrated because of the underlying bony structures. One should therefore bear in mind the possibility of utilizing tomography or planography in instances of the presence of calculi.

Operating Table Pyelographic Visualization of Elusive Calculus

A small or semi-opaque stone, during the performance of a pelviolithotomy or a ureterolithotomy, may be elusive. One may be able to better visualize such a stone if air contrast is used in obtaining the X-ray. Therefore, if in the middle of a surgical procedure a calculus cannot be localized, injection by needle of approximately 10 ml of air, either into a ureter or into the pelvis, depending on the location of the calculus, may bring the stone into view.

(See also *X-Ray Localization of Renal Calculi in Surgery*, in Chapter Four, and *Aid to Visualization of Calculus in Lower Ureter*, in Chapter Five.)

THE KIDNEYS

DIAGNOSTIC CONSIDERATIONS

STANDARD DIAGNOSTIC TECHNIQUES are described in urologic textbooks. We make no attempt to discuss these universally accepted modalities. At the present time selective renal artery angiography, inferior venacavography and tomography are the favorite diagnostic approaches for renal tumor. The radioisotope renal scan done at progressive intervals is an important diagnostic aid. The recent use of ultrasound (echograms) may be effective in study of the functioning renal mass. Renal cystography as well as ultrasound techniques are being used to differentiate renal tumors from cysts. The latter technique may also be used to differentiate solid tumors from fluid. Future progress in this field appears promising.

The combined diagnostic studies of infusion excretory urography with the image intensifier and cineradiography demostrate well the dynamics of the ureteropelvic juncture.

This chapter mentions only a few of the considerations in diagnosis of renal pathology. Many other diagnostic concepts pertaining to other parts of the urological system will be found in the corresponding sections of the book. It is again emphasized that commonly accepted diagnostic methods are purposefully omitted in this volume.

Aids in Diagnosis

Pain in the Costovertebral Angle Area

When a patient has pain in the costovertebral angle area which on careful palpation seems to be elicited from the sacrospinalis muscle, about 10 ml of one percent Xylocaine may be injected into the sacrospinalis muscle at the area of maximum pain. When there is immediate relief one may rule out renal pain as the origin of the difficulty.

Split-Function Studies

When doing a differential kidney function test one may place a catheter in the bladder and aspirate with a two-ounce Asepto urethral syringe. This has a tendency to collapse the ureteral orifices around No. 5 French ureteral catheters. Two bottles, sealed and with a vacuum, then are used to collect the left and right urine specimens.

Contralateral Back Pain Possibly Relieved by Surgical Repair

Not infrequently patients with right renal pathology will present with left-sided back pain as their most prominent symptom, or vice versa. Surgical correction of the pathology may result in relief of symptoms on the contra-lateral side.

Reflux in Ileal Conduit Patients Lying on Abdomen

A possible overlooked cause for acute recurrent pyelonephritis in patients with ileal conduits could be reflux when the patient lies on the abdomen. This may be demonstrated on intravenous pyelography taken when the patient is turned on his stomach. Patients who wear ileal conduit devices should not sleep on their abdomen due to the possibility of increased pressure within the bag causing reflux pyelonephritis. This tends to defeat the purpose of dependent drainage without residual urine, for which ileal conduits have been so successful.

Incidence of Polycystic Kidney Disease

In instances of family history of polycystic disease the chances of a child having this disease would be approximately in the ratio of 1:4. The incidence would be higher with a history of the disease in both parents.

Renal Trauma—Aortography and Successive Renal Scans for Assessment

In the event of renal trauma, intravenous infusion pyelography often fails to reveal function in the involved kidney, especially in a patient in shock. When the vital signs are not of serious consequence one may determine early if there is any perirenal extravasation by aortography and by renal scan. The renal scans must be successive from a comparative standpoint. The aortography *per se* very often will reveal the presence of a ruptured vessel with bleeding outside of the kidney.

These diagnostic methods must be considered, therefore, in instances of renal trauma. If it is possible to delay several days before surgery, the chance of renal conservation often improves. An otherwise lost kidney could possibly be salvaged by vascular repair.

Detection of Small Renal Tumors: a Method of Possible Value

Small renal tumors are notoriously difficult to demonstrate by renal angiography. One diagnostic method which may warrant further trial is to purposely overfill the renal pelvis with contrast medium to produce pyelotubular backflow to outline the renal pyramids. Distortion of the usual pattern suggests the presence of a space-consuming lesion. If good pyelotubular backflow to demonstrate this is not obtained, then it may be necessary to resort to other diagnostic measures. (See additional aids in tumor diagnosis in *Infusion Pyelography and Nephrotomography*, etc., in Chapter Three.)

Presence of Varicocele in Carcinoma of the Kidney

Varicocele is often present, secondary to carcinoma of the kidney, due to vein invasion. Most physicians, under usual circumstances, examine their patients in the supine position. Were more of these patients to be examined in the standing position, it is felt that varicoceles might be found in a higher number of cases.

Value of Aortography and Venography in Space-Occupying Renal Lesions

Analysis of aortographic and venographic experience in the diagnosis of space-occupying lesions of the kidney parenchyma, in relation to the clinical and operative findings, demonstrates that one can often predict whether the tumor can be removed in very large lesions, whether otherwise unrecognized metastases are present, whether renal vein involvement is evident, and what the prognosis for survival may be. Some urologists feel that tumors over 10 cm in diameter are almost inevitably associated with a fatal outcome. Arteriographic-venographic-lymphangiographic examination can delineate and mirror renal vein invasion found at subsequent operation.

A number of unsuspected metastases and continuous tumor extensions cannot be discovered without arteriovenographic examination, as well as appropriate scans.

The many values of aortography and venography in the management of renal tumors, together with the relative benignity of the retrograde femoral procedure when properly performed, warrant inclusion of these procedures as a more routine part of the diagnostic approach to space-occupying lesions of the kidney.

Tomography in conjunction with infusion pyelography is also of vital importance.

Hilum Renalis Defect Suggesting Space-Occupying Lesion

A wedge-shaped filling defect occurring in the superior medial aspect of the renal pelvis and attributed to the overhanging lip of the renal parenchyma at the hilum compressing the renal pelvis at this point has been mistakenly interpreted as a tumor of the renal pelvis. The edges of the defect are smooth and are constant under minimal pressures of pelvic filling. However, when the *renal pelvis is overdistended,* this defect often will disappear. This is a point worth putting to the test.

Transureteral Biopsy of Upper Urinary Tract Neoplasm

In a suspected case of papillary tumors of the upper urinary tract the pathologist is always anxious to obtain sufficient cellular material to make a diagnosis of a renal pelvic or ureteral lesion. Cytological study results reported as suspicious create a quandary often resolved only by exploration. The nephroscope may be of value in establishing a diagnosis. Exploration frequently demands the removal of the kidney involved. Actual minute exploration must be done in the pathological laboratory.

Therefore, whenever urinary sediment cytology is inconclusive in instances of filling defects of the renal pelvis, one may pass a No. 6 or 7 French whistle-tip ureteral catheter and maneuver the tip until it lies adjacent to the filling defect as seen with the aid of the image amplifier. Normal saline, 5 or 6 ml, may be injected slowly into the renal pelvis or ureter. The solution may then be vigorously aspirated, creating suction at the catheter tip adjacent to the radiolucent area. If no large pieces are obtained in the aspirate, suction is maintained as the catheter is withdrawn. The catheter is then lavaged. Often papillary tumor fronds are trapped by this method.

In some instances one may insert a stone basket and run it up and down a ureter. On removal of the basket, tissue is often entrapped within the wires of the basket.

The above-described methods seem equally as valuable as the *Brush Biopsy Technique* described in Chapter Five. Use of the image amplifier for precise placement of probing instruments also affords greater accuracy.

Localization of Kidney for Needle Biopsy Purposes

Lead markers using numbers or letters may be placed on adhesive tape which in turn may be placed one inch apart along the vertebral column. At right angles lead markers may be placed one inch apart along the crest of the ilium. A posterior-anterior film and lateral nephrogram when then taken will serve as an accurate guide for the needle puncture site. One may scratch the film to desired intersecting line areas. Image amplification of these films is a further aid to needle orientation.

Percutaneous Needle Biopsy vs Open Renal Biopsy

Percutaneous and open renal biopsies have become commonplace procedures. Though most biopsies are done by the percutaneous route, usually under radiographic control by internists (nephrologists) and urologists, the open method is preferred by most urologists.

One of the authors (H.B.) experienced an instance of complete transection of the pedicle in percutaneous renal biopsy. Fortunately the biopsy was done in the operating room and the pedicle was clamped exactly three minutes following the incident. All renal biopsy patients are now subjected by us to the open technique. Patients with solitary kidney, advanced renal failure, history of bleeding tendency, severe hypertension, or small bilateral atrophic kidneys are definite contraindications for percutaneous biopsy.

Light microscopy, electron microscopy, and immunofluorescent studies are increasingly being done on biopsied specimens.

Open Renal Biopsy: Technique

The increased safety factor in open renal biopsy makes it preferable to percutaneous needle biopsy. The open biopsy may be simply performed by using the Simon vertical muscle retraction incision or the short subcostal incision. The exposure is simple and rapid. The biopsy may be expeditiously secured and bleeding adequately controlled under vision.

A subcostal paravertebral incision (10 cm long) is made down to the kidney. The lower pole is visualized after Gerota's capsule is opened. Chromic sutures (3-0 or 4-0) are placed about ½ to 1 cm apart through kidney substance and capsule. A ¾-cm incision is made in the capsule. While one flap of the capsule is elevated to expose renal parenchyma, the small cup biopsy forceps (V. Mueller) is used to remove three or four 1-mm fragments of surface tissue.

The outer surface of this tissue is densely populated with glomeruli. These small fragments invariably are excellent for evaluating glomerular structures. Tubules and small vessels are present as well. A small piece of Gelfoam ® is pressed upon this small surface area for five minutes, by the clock, and bleeding is easily controlled. There is more preservation of kidney tissue when biopsy is done in this manner, since suture over fat tabs into the kidney is obviated.

The wound is closed in three layers. One layer of interrupted No. 0 chromic suture is placed through all muscle layers. The second layer of closure consists of continuous No. 0 chromic suture through the external fascia. The skin is closed with mattress silk.

This procedure is preferably done under general anesthesia. Inasmuch as no major veins or arteries are encountered in this approach, there is no problem with arterial bleeding, extensive hemorrhage, or formation of arteriovenous fistula.

Hydronephrosis with Ureteropelvic Obstruction—Plastic Repair, Nephrectomy?

When ureteropelvic obstruction is present with hydronephrosis, numerous diagnostic criteria exist to determine the treatment of choice—pyeloplasty, nephrectomy, or continued observation. Should there be less than one centimeter of functioning cortex, nephrectomy may be the therapy of choice. Also, in patients in the older age group or poor-risk category, nephrectomy may be the best choice. Below this age group one is more prone to recommend plastic repair. Should the repair be unsuccessful, the patient is young enough to tolerate a secondary procedure (nephrectomy).

Individual urologists may make this determination on the basis of the patient's physical status rather than chronological age. The choice of type of definitive therapy is a decision for the surgeon.

Functional Aspect of Renal Mass

Of primary concern is consideration of the functional aspect of the renal mass. This is determined often by whether the pelvis of the obstructed kidney is intrarenal or extrarenal. Obviously, intrarenal types of pelves will have more destruction of renal mass. In the extrarenal type of pelvis, the hydronephrosis, largely extrarenal, will involve relatively less destruction of renal mass.

Renal function studies by numerous elective methods may be utilized to determine the function of the remaining renal mass. Selective renal angiography to outline the renal vessels is most useful to determine the extent of remaining renal mass and to outline the course of a vessel which may be producing the hydronephrosis. Functional renal mass may also be evaluated by renogram and scanning techniques. Very often the final decision is made at surgery.

RENAL SURGERY

Positioning the Patient for Renal Surgery

Orientation on the Operating Table for Most-Used Lateral Approach

The position most commonly used by urologists for renal surgery is placement of the patient in the lateral decubitus position with the kidney to be

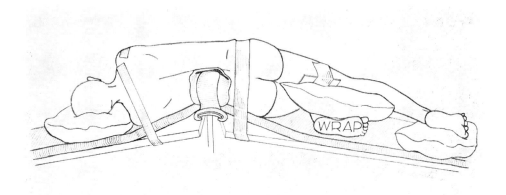

16. Surgical position for nephrectomy by lateral approach

operated upon in the upward position. The space between the twelfth rib and the crest of the ilium is positioned over the kidney lift. If the operating table has no kidney lift one may use a small rounded sandbag placed transversely between the twelfth rib and the crest of the ilium. A turkish towel rolled to resemble a sandbag may be used for the same purpose (see Fig. 16).

The Lower Extremities

The underneath leg is flexed, with the foot lying at the posterior edge of the table (from the standpoint of relationship to the body) and the knee to the anterior side. The foot is always completely wrapped in turkish toweling to prevent possible burn by grounding to the table with the use of the electrosurgical unit. The "top" leg is fully extended. A pillow is usually placed underneath the foot to prevent extension out into space when the table is flexed. A pillow is placed lengthwise between both thighs.

The electrosurgical unit grounding plate is placed under the thigh of the uppermost extemity. Adhesive is placed over the thigh and around the bottom side of the plate, holding it securely against the thigh and ensuring good contact. The adhesive should not run completely around the extremity and thus impair circulation.

The Torso

The short kidney brace is placed under the table pad on the kidney lift to brace the patient's back. This kidney brace must be covered with turkish toweling or plastic material to prevent grounding. A sandbag may also be placed under the patient's buttocks to immobilize him and keep him from rolling. Wide adhesive is placed over and below the crest of the ilium and attached to the table, preferably returning the tape around the rod arm of the operating table to further fix this adhesive.

Two lengths of adhesive are used loosely from the shoulder down to the operating table, one going forward loosely from its shoulder attachment and the other posteriorly from its shoulder attachment (see Fig. 16). The loose attachment prevents compression which would impair breathing.

The Upper Extremities

The underneath arm is extended outward. This arm is the one most frequently used by the anesthesiologist for administration of intravenous fluid and medication. Care must be taken that there is no pressure at the elbow and over the ulnar nerve. This is a common complication. One must be certain that there is no undue pressure on the patient's brachial plexus. The uppermost arm may be allowed to lie alongside the lowermost arm or preferably on a Mayo stand over a sheet, so that there is no contact with metal.

Variations for Improved Renal Exposure

One may vary the patient's position somewhat for better exposure. It is preferable that the kidney lift not be raised to its maximum, so that the patient's lung capacity is not impaired. The table break should be at maximum to obtain the widest possible amount of space between the twelfth rib and the iliac crest.

Better renal exposure may be obtained by tilting the patient slightly backward. Instead of having the patient's back and abdomen at an angle of 90 degrees with the flat surface of the operating room table, the patient's back may vary from 100 to 120 degrees. This tilt will expose more of the abdominal area. The 100-degree position seems to be the most satisfactory angle for placement of the patient's back.

Extension of the incision anteriorly allows easier access to the kidney pedicle area.

Incisions Used for Surgical Approach to the Kidney

Figure 17 presents incisions used in renal surgery throughout the years. In this volume no attempt is made to include or discuss all of the known renal incisions and their modifications.

Surgical Approaches—Lateral

Subcostal Incision for Rapid Renal Exposure

The incision of choice of most urologists under most circumstances is the subcostal incision. One obtains better exposure of the kidney, however, by extending the incision medially from the lower border of the twelfth rib more anteriorly than the usual incision and not as far back as the costovertebral angle.

This high transverse abdominal incision, with the patient tilted slightly backward on the table at the 100 to 120 degrees previously mentioned, allows better mobilization of the kidney under direct vision and avoids the neurovascular bundles posteriorly.

The anterior aspect of the kidney is thus more readily exposed. Individual ligation of renal vessels may be done more easily in nephrectomy cases. Patients seem to have a less painful postoperative course when this incision is employed.

Technique: The skin and subcutaneous tissues are cut and then in the region of the juncture of the external and internal oblique muscles with the latissimus dorsi muscle the incision is extended down through all layers of muscle through the transversalis muscle. One may insert a finger at this point and by blunt dissection reflect the peritoneum anteriorly. With one or two fingers holding the peritoneum anteriorly, scissors are used to cut through

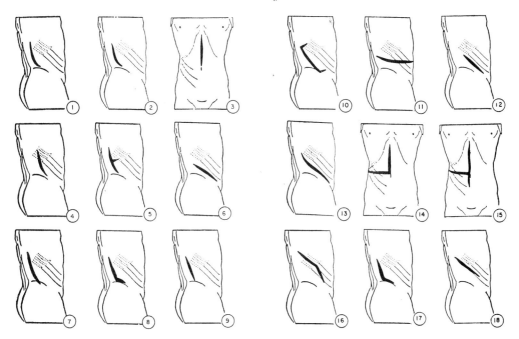

1. Simon, 1869
2. Bruns, 1871
3. Kocher, 1876
4. Czerny, 1879
5. Bergmann, 1874
6. Küster, 1883
7. Ceccherelli, 1884
8. Poncet & Guyon, 1887
9. Duret, 1887

10. Bardenheuer & Schmidt, 1890
11. Pean, 1894
12. Abbe & Mayo-Robson, 1898
13. W. J. Mayo, 1912
14. Cabot, 1925
15. Hugh Young, 1926
16. Fey, 1926
17. H. M. Young, 1937 & Furcolo, 1946
18. Hess, 1939

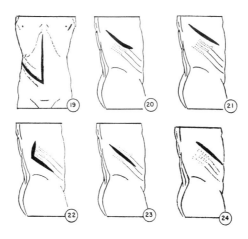

19. Sweetser, 1941
20. Marshall, 1946
21. Harper, 1947
22. Nagamatsu, 1949
23. Bodner & Briskin, 1950
24. Chute, et al., 1946. Marshall,
    1946. Harper, 1947.

17. Incisions for approach to the kidney

all three layers of abdominal muscles without fear of injuring any structures.

A rapid opening of the kidney incision is obtained in this manner. There is also less chance of injury to the ileo-inguinal and ileohypogastric nerves since one does not extend the incision backwards as far as the costovertebral angle. After the anterior aspect of the incision is opened, more deliberate care is used to open the posterior aspect of the incision under direct vision. In the manner described, the usual incision may be made in two to four minutes as contrasted with the longer period of time required to open the incision layer by layer. Some surgeons after incising the skin and subcutaneous tissue prefer to open the wound with the cutting blade of the electrosurgical unit. Others prefer use of the Turner-Warwick scissors activated by the electrosurgical unit.

For control of bleeding, one may find that by merely touching or "slapping" the hemostat with the electrode at the cutting current, hemostasis is obtained. Many surgeons use the coagulation current of the electrosurgical unit for hemostasis.

These are all acceptable modifications of standard techniques used by urologists.

Supracostal Approach, or the Eleventh Intercostal Space Incision

In most cases of renal exploration the orthodox lumbar subcostal incision is adequate. Where the kidney lies high or where it is necessary to approach the upper pole and renal pedicle, the supracostal approach of Pressman and Turner-Warwick has proven to be of great help (see Fig. 18).

An incision is made between the eleventh and twelfth ribs in the interspace. The intercostal tissue is divided along the length of the rib, avoiding the lower edge of the eleventh rib with its intercostal vessels and nerve. The incision is extended forward into the anterior abdominal muscles, including the external oblique, internal oblique, and transversalis. The diaphragmatic attachments to the rib are divided. The twelfth rib then swings downward out of the way. Anterior extension of the incision into the anterior abdominal muscles opens up this space widely and the pleura is gently pushed up out of the way.

Care must be exercised that one does not enter the pleura, which is adherent in the posterior aspects of the incision. To avoid this ask the anesthesiologist to make the patient breathe deeply while the pleura is identified and reflected. If accidentally opened the pleura may be closed immediately while the anesthesiologist keeps the lungs expanded. Complications when the pleura is accidentally opened and repaired are rare.

The renal pedicle is rapidly reached in this exposure. The operator is able in most instances to rapidly free the kidney and pedicle under direct

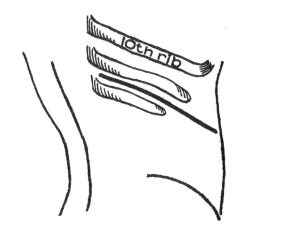

A

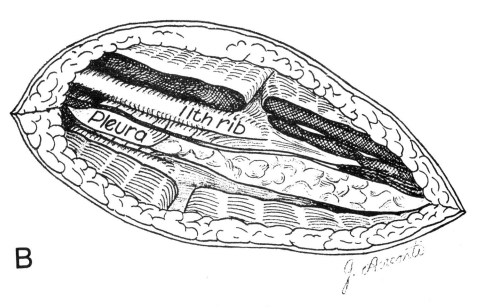

B

18. Supracostal approach
    A. Eleventh intercostal space incision
    B. Exposure completed. Edge of twelfth
       rib shown at lower margin of incision

vision. Another advantage of this approach is that, if unexpected pathology is encountered, the incision can be converted into a more radical one by extending it forward toward the midline and either removing the eleventh rib or extending the posterior aspect of the incision upward into a Nagamatsu approach.

This incision is particularly helpful in instances of large tumor, upper pole masses, secondary kidney operations, and radical node dissection. It is also of value in exposure of the spleen when splenorenal injury has occurred.

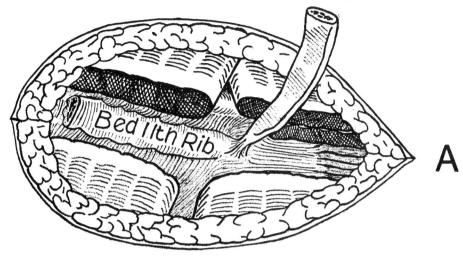

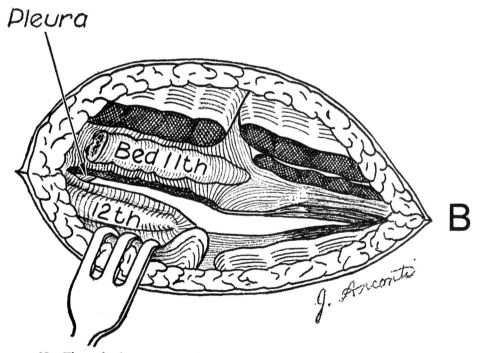

19. Eleventh rib resection with preservation of vessels (Bodner modification)
     A. Eleventh rib ready for resection
     B. Eleventh rib removed

An additional advantage is that this incision will usually not involve the nerves and blood vessels which run under the ribs.

Resection of the eleventh rib may also be done with preservation of the intercostal vessels, as described by one of us (H.B.) in 1950. See Figures 19A and B. Exposure of the aorta and vena cava are also afforded by the eleventh rib and eleventh interspace incision.

Thoraco-Abdominal Incision

The thoraco-abdominal approach is especially helpful for surgery in cases of very large renal tumors and lymphadenectomy. The exposure allows early visualization and clamping of the renal pedicle. Adrenalectomy and radical lymph node dissection may also be done by way of this exposure.

Technique: Following the skin opening the incision is extended along the course of the ninth or tenth interspace (cutting the costal cartilage) and across the abdomen to either above or below the umbilicus, depending on the location of the tumor. The pleural cavity is opened, the lungs packed away, and the diaphragm cut down to its posterior aspect, avoiding the phrenic nerve. The peritoneum is opened. On the right side the colon and duodenum may be reflected medially and the blood vessels of the kidney exposed. The splenic colon is mobilized on the left side (see Fig. 20)

Surgical Approaches—Anterior
(Supine Position)

Transperitoneal Renal Exposure, Anterior Abdominal

Some urologists prefer to place the patient flat on his back on the operating table and to utilize an anterior transabdominal kidney exposure. Others prefer to approach the kidney retroperitoneally with the patient also flat on his back on the operating table. With decreased fear of bacterial contamination of the peritoneum due to available antibiotics, the anterior approach has gained in popularity, especially in instances of tumor.

The vessels of the renal pedicle can be more adequately isolated and secured in this approach; bleeding can be more adequately controlled by individual ligations of the large vessels so frequently encountered in renal tumor surgery. The renal mass with its surrounding fascia, fat, and nodes may be completely and rapidly removed. Lymph gland dissection is also more accessible in the region of the aorta and vena cava.

The postoperative course of patients with large renal tumors operated upon with this approach is often smoother than that of patients on whom the lumbar approach is utilized. Infected kidneys, however, are still best not approached transabdominally.

Technique: The patient should preferably lie with the kidney lift between the iliac crest and the twelfth rib. The side to be operated upon in a uni-

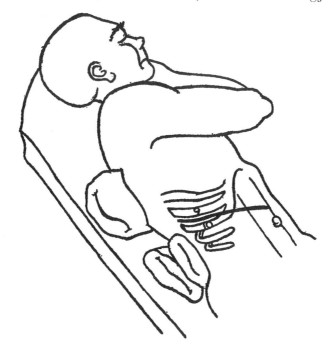

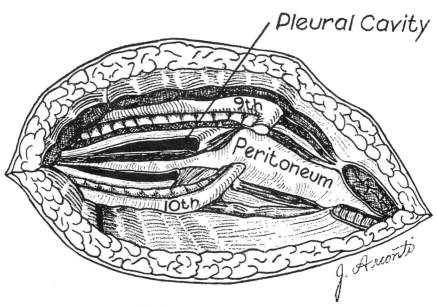

20. Thoraco-abdominal incision

lateral procedure should be elevated by sand bags or rolled-up toweling to facilitate rolling away of the bowel. The posterior peritoneum may be incised longitudinally between the aorta and inferior mesenteric vein along the route of the mesentery, or opened directly over the kidney; the blood supply to the colon, however, may thus be injured, and extreme caution is therefore mandatory. The lateral peritoneum may be opened along the paracolic gutter with mobilization of the colon medially and also mobilization of the duodenum on the right side.

There are definite advantages and disadvantages to the transabdominal approach. Improved accessibility to the vascular supply is especially useful in tumor cases and in previously operated-upon kidneys. However, the risk of bowel obstruction, contamination in renal stone cases, and intra-abdominal organ injury are factors to be considered also in the anterior abdominal approach. The decreased accessibility of the upper pole of the kidney in the transabdominal approach is evident.

Anterior Extraperitoneal Incision (convertible to transperitoneal incision)

The patient may be placed on his back and then elevated to an angle of about 30 to 40 degrees, with sandbags under the hip and shoulder on the side in which the incision is to be made. The incision is begun one centimeter below the subcostal margin, at the lateral border of the rectus muscle, and is extended straight laterally below the twelfth rib. Where limited exposure is necessary the internal oblique and transversalis may be separated rather than cut. The peritoneum is then reflected medially.

If desired, one may open the peritoneum, mobilize the splenic or hepatic flexure of the colon, and then proceed with the renal surgery after this exposure. If more exposure is needed, the internal oblique and transversalis may be divided and the incision extended more posteriorly.

With this approach all renal blood supply is easily identified and mobilized. Another benefit to be obtained from this incision is decreased postoperative pain. There is no compromise to the respiratory and cardiovascular function.

Combining Renal Surgery with Gallbladder Surgery

There are occasions when it may be necessary to do intraperitoneal exploration or even possible gallbladder surgery as a combined operation with renal exposure.

Under these circumstances the patient may be placed flat on the table as for any intra-abdominal operative procedure. An incision may be made along the right costal margin, but extended forward more than usual. The peritoneum is closed and reflected medially after the gallbladder surgery is completed. One then proceeds with the kidney surgery.

Anterior Abdominal Retroperitoneal Exposure

It may be necessary, in some situations, to place the patient in the flat position on the table and make the above-described incision without intra-abdominal exploration. Under these circumstances, one merely retracts the peritoneum medially and proceeds with the kidney surgery.

This incision may be used bilaterally in the event both kidneys need exploration. The incision need not be continuous for each side, and it is not necessary to change the position of the patient on the table. The kidney brace may be used on the lift so that, if necessary, one may slightly tip the table and roll away the intra-abdominal contents in order to obviate the presence of the peritoneum and the intra-abdominal contents while doing the kidney surgery.

The usual transabdominal approach may also be utilized for bilateral renal surgery.

Approach for Bilateral Simultaneous Subcostal Renal Surgery

The posterior approach for bilateral two-team simultaneous renal exposure is aided by the use of the Wilson frame, ordinarily used in orthopedic surgery. This jackknifes the patient in the prone position, thus facilitating flank exposure. Two operating teams may then work simultaneously.

Specialized Helpful Techniques in Renal Surgery
Skin Scratches at Incision for Proper Alignment in Closure

Whatever incision is used, proper alignment for closure is aided if one will make cross scratches over the line of the proposed incision, using the back edge of a knife blade. With the use of plastic drape, two opposing dots in the middle area of the incision may be made by pinpoint cautery or skin sutures. Following completion of surgery, Allis clamps in the subcutaneous fat at the cross marks help to obtain proper alignment for wound closure. A marking pencil or dye such as gentian violet or methylene blue, applied with an applicator stick, may be used in the same manner.

Methods of Mapping Plastic Flaps

Plastic surgeons outline skin flaps often with the aid of a marking pencil. Stay sutures are also utilized to outline a flap. This is done commonly for the flap in a pelvioplasty and also in the Y-V plasty of the bladder neck. Gentian violet applied with an applicator stick is very helpful. Another means may be that of using the tip of the electrode of an electrosurgical unit. By lightly burning the outline required, one may also mark the area well. Where the tissue is not dry a silver nitrate stick may also be utilized for the same purpose.

Electrosurgical Unit Precautions

One must be certain in usuing the electrosurgical unit that there are no portions of the body which have direct contact with the metal of the operating room table. This may serve as a ground and result in serious burns. The lower extremities are usually wrapped with turkish toweling or encased in leg and foot covers. The uppermost arm is also covered to prevent the possibility of grounding. Other exposed areas must also be covered. The patient's thighs are most often covered by sheets.

(See also *Safeguards in Use of Electrosurgical Units*, in Chapter One.)

Rib Retraction and Renal Exposure

The Burford-Finochietto rib spreader, which is usually employed in thoracic surgery, may be used for exposure of the renal fossa. This retractor serves to free the assistant's hands for other duties. It is supplied with two sets of detachable blades, the large blades being 3 inches deep and 2½ inches wide and the small ones being 1¾ inches deep and 2½ inches wide. The blades have protruding edges to prevent the spreader from moving during the operative procedure. The arms are curved to fit the contour of the body.

With high flank incisions involving the pleura, the pleura should first be well mobilized before insertion of the retractor. Otherwise, the pleura will tear when put on stretch by the retractor.

Gerota's Capsule (Perirenal Fascia)

Gerota's capsule may be opened in a number of different ways. Many surgeons open the capsule with a hemostat. One may pick up the fascia with two hemostats and cut the fascia with scissors between the clamps. One may very lightly cut Gerota's capsule with a scalpel and then with two fingers enlarge the opening. Scissors may also be used to cut open fascia without elevation of the capsule. The surgeon must be sure that Gerota's capsule is opened sufficiently far posteriorly so as not to open the peritoneum inadvertently.

Improving Exposure Without Extension of Skin Incision

A skin incision may be stretched somewhat larger than the actual incision made by the scalpel by utilizing a pair of towel clips and stretching the terminal ends of the incision when clipped to skin at a lower or higher level. This same method may be utilized for retraction to open up a wound. Using towel clips and attaching the incisional edge skin to the skin lateral to the wound frees the assistant from retraction. Some surgeons prefer to take a few sutures rather than using the towel clips.

Retraction of Kidney

It is often essential to be able to retract and hold the kidney in place when doing surgery either on the renal pelvis or the renal pedicle.

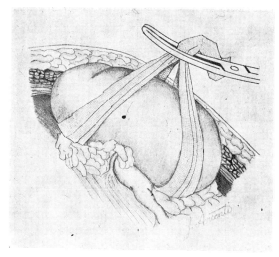

21. Kidney retraction by gauze sling technique

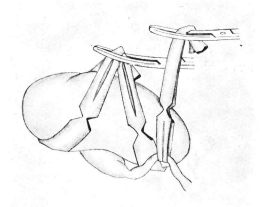

22. Kidney and ureter retraction by means of notched Penrose drains

One may accomplish this by opening up a wet 4- by 4-inch gauze square and placing this around the lower pole of the kidney. Another such square is placed around the upper pole of the kidney. A clamp * holding both these pieces of gauze is positioned so as to hold the kidney in a sling. In this way no slipping is encountered. See Figure 21.

An improvised fishnet sack with a drawstring has proved useful to some surgeons for kidney retraction. Plastic tape may also be used. Strips of

---

* Rubber-shod gastrointestinal clamps will occasionally slip. This may be avoided by covering the clamp with white "shoestring" material instead of rubber. Plastic material may also be used to cover the clamps. These coverings give enough friction to prevent slippage, and the clamps will still not crush tissue.

plastic material, which slide about more easily, may be preferred by some urologists for kidney retraction due to their ease of positioning.

Pinching or injury of the kidney by manual retraction is eliminated by the above techniques as well as by the method which follows.

Notched Penrose Drain for Safety in Traction

One may also use a Penrose drain wrapped around each of the poles of the kidney in the same fashion as just described, acting as a "cradle" for the kidney. A notch may be taken in the Penrose drain for one-half to two-thirds of its width as one does in a butterfly adhesive, so that in the event of excessive pull on the Penrose drain, the drain will tear rather than the kidney pedicle. This may also be done when retracting a ureter. See Figure 22.

Determination of Renal Tissue Supplied by Aberrant Artery

The amount of renal tissue supplied by an aberrant artery may be determined by clamping the aberrant vessel. This shows the area of potential infarction. However, by injection of indigo carmine through a fine hypodermic needle into the artery, that portion of the kidney supplied by the respective vessel is much more clearly demarcated by the blue dye, and the danger of infarction to the involved segment is diminished.

Irrigation of Open Wounds in Cancer Surgery

For wounds in which cancer surgery is done, the area should be irrigated because of possible loose malignant cells. Sterile water is preferable. Sterile saline may be used for its washing effect only. Sodium oxychlorosene (Clorpactin) and n,n',n'',-triethylenethiophosphoramide (Thiotepa), 60 mg in 60 ml water, are used by some surgeons for their tumoricidal effect. A 1 to 10 dilution of ordinary sodium hypochlorite solution such as Clorox ® may replace Clorpactin.

The danger of absorption of the chemotherapeutic agent must be considered. Repeated mechanical washing with sterile water would appear to be the most desirable method. Sterile water will more readily "rupture" carcinoma cells than will saline.

Control of Odor in Carcinomatous Wounds

Sugar placed on an open carcinoma wound will decrease odor. This should be borne in mind in instances where there is carcinoma involving the skin surface or an area suitable for the application of sugar. Granulated sugar may be "blown into" some wounds by utilizing an Asepto syringe and bulb.

One must also consider using topical antibiotic creams in such cases, due to surface slough and infection.

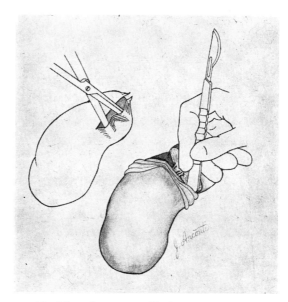

23. Blunt dissection of kidney parenchyma

Cutting Kidney Parenchyma in Partial Nephrectomy or Heminephrectomy

In performing heminephrectomy or partial nephrectomy, vascular clamps or bulldog clamps may first be placed around the renal artery or in some instances across the entire pedicle. *This clamping, en masse, however, is undesirable and should be avoided if at all possible.* The capsule over the pole of the kidney to be resected is cut and peeled away from the kidney. The kidney is then cut, wedge shaped (see Fig. 23). A strand of No. 0 chromic suture, a strand of sterile rubber band on stretch, or the back end of a scalpel may be used to cut the renal substance, shearing the renal tissue away from vessels and avoiding the cutting of the vessels themselves.

The vessels may be individually clamped, cut and tied, effecting a relatively bloodless procedure. The clamps controlling bleeding may then be released to see if there are any bleeding vessels. If so, these are individually tied.

Guillotine Partial Nephrectomy

A simple and effective guillotine partial nephrectomy can be performed safely without first isolating and compressing the renal artery. The renal capsule over the portion of the kidney to be removed is incised and peeled back. Instead of peeling back the capsule, a circumferential incision can be made through the capsule at the desired point of amputation (Fig. 24) but this does not permit covering the stump when closure is made. Covering the stump probably adds to hemostasis.

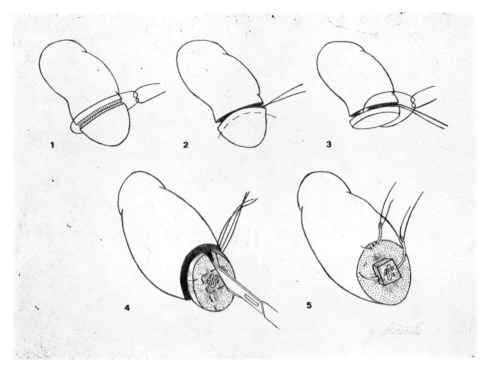

24. Arconti guillotine method for partial nephrectomy

A No. 1 chromic catgut suture is then placed in the groove made by the capsular incision, or at the desired point of amputation if the capsule was peeled back (the suture must not compress the capsule). The suture is then tied firmly. The suture will cut through the renal parenchyma and engage the major calyx or infundibulum with the adjacent blood vessels. The diseased portion of the kidney is then excised with a scalpel about one centimeter distal to this tie by a second parallel guillotine incision. This is necessary to later develop a ligature stump that will not allow the ties to slip off, with resultant bleeding.

After excising the parenchyma there will be some heavy oozing of blood from the area of the calyx. This occurs because the original tie cannot be pulled tightly enough to compress the pericalyceal vessels while the kidney tissue to be removed is still attached. This oozing is quickly controlled by placing another No. 1 suture over the original tie. The collar of parenchymal tissue distal to these two ties is then excised, taking care to leave a generous central stump, thus preventing the ties from slipping.

At this point there will be noted some oozing of blood from two or three small vessels on the cut surface of the parenchyma. A warm pack to the cut surface usually controls this, or a fine catgut figure-of-eight suture can be placed for hemostasis. A No. 0 or 1 chromic catgut "sticktie" is then placed through the calyceal stump to further assure hemostasis. If the renal capsule was preserved this is brought over the stump of parenchyma and closed with 4-0 chromic catgut continuous suture. The area is drained.

Should the ties slip off during the procedure, bleeding can be controlled by sandwiching and compressing the renal parenchyma between the thumb and index finger just proximal to the guillotine incision. A suture ligature can be placed while compressing the parenchyma.

Positioning the Kidney After Conservative Renal Surgery: Nephropexy

To hold the kidney in position after surgery, a suture is placed through the lower-pole capsule of the kidney in criss-cross fashion or figure-of-eight fashion and tied over a pad of fat. This same suture is then sewed to the psoas or quadratus lumborum fascia and tied. Two such lower-pole ties should be used to keep the kidney from rotating. The sutures are placed preferably less than 4 to 7 mm apart in and out of the renal capsule. Sutures placed more widely will tear through the capsule.

Immobilization of the kidney is further ensured by suturing of the perirenal fat with 2-0 chromic suture to the fascia of the muscles under the lower pole of the kidney. It is helpful if the assistant holds the kidney in place with a sponge holder while sutures are tied.

Pyeloureteroplasty

The urologic surgeon should be acquainted with all types of pyeloureteroplasty: (1) the dismembered type of repair, (2) the Foley-Y-Plasty, (3) the Culp-Scardino technique, (4) the Davis intubated ureterostomy, (5) the side-to-side anastomosis, etc. A recent innovative method employs parallel incisions, beginning at the superior part of a dilated pelvis, leaving the dependent portion attached. Out of this, one may fashion a tube. The distal ureter is then telescoped into the distal end of this flap tube and sutured with 4-0 or 5-0 chromic suture. See Figure 25.

In performing pyeloureteroplasty the authors invariably anchor the kidney as previously described. Straight takeoff of the ureter to prevent buckling is of paramount importance.

Pyeloureteroplasty Drainage—Nephrostomy

The drainage of a kidney pelvis may be accomplished by one of several methods. Whether one should or should not use splinting catheters in renal plastic surgical procedures is arguable. Some urologists use no splints—some do not use nephrostomy or pyelostomy tubes.

The most desirable method for drainage in pyeloureteroplasty in our hands has been nephrostomy. Pyelostomy drainage is also done, but much

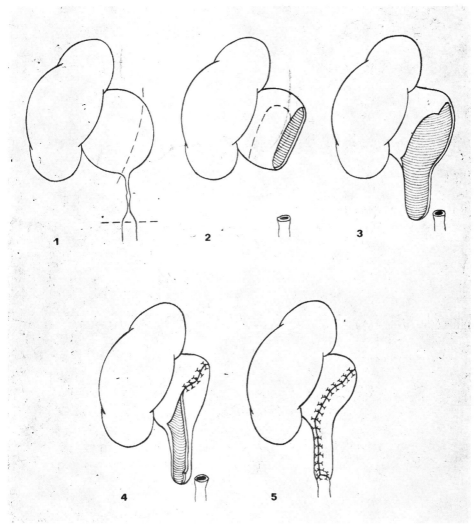

25. Production of tubular flap by parallel incision method for pyeloureteroplasty

less frequently. The use of Hemovac ® drainage is invaluable in keeping the wound dry.

T-Tube Splinting in Pyeloureteroplasty

Whenever urinary diversion and ureteral splinting are necessary, the T-tube has been useful for both applications. The T-tube should have extra holes cut in the upper arm of the tube so that there may be more adequate drainage of the renal pelvis. The tube may be clamped off so that there may be passage of urine down the ureter. A wedge is cut out of the tube at the junction of the horizontal and vertical arms to facilitate removal of the T-tube.

The T-tube may be easily removed as an outpatient office procedure during the postoperative period.

T-tubes made of Silastic® tubing with multiple openings and added length of the arms of the tube within the ureter would allow for tailoring the tube to the needs of the operator.

Additional Uses for T-Tubes in Urology

A T-tube may be used for ureteroureteroanastomosis, ureteroneocystostomy, and emergency ureterostomies as well as for the previously mentioned applications. The T-tube is usually placed in the ureter proximal to the site of repair (i.e., closer to the kidney to divert urine).

Catheter Splinting in Pyeloureteroplasty

Through the same nephrostomy site and at the same time as the balloon catheter is positioned, one may lead down into the pelvis and down the ureter beyond the site of repair a No. 8 or 10 French rubber ureteral catheter which serves well both as a splint and as a nephrostomy tube. A Robinson catheter (No. 6, 8, or 10 French) may be used in like manner. One must cut multiple holes in the splint in the region of the pelvis and use this for drainage, in addition to using the remainder of the catheter down the ureter as a splint. Plastic infant feeding tubes of varied size are the choice of some urologists.

The rubber splint, serving also as a nephrostomy drainage tube, may exit the kidney through a second site so that one then has a "double-barreled" nephrostomy. The No. 16 French, 5-ml balloon catheter, distended with 2 to 3 ml of water in the balloon, may serve as the second nephrostomy tube.

Silastic tubing with multiple holes is favored by some. The Silastic tubing or the rubber splint may be utilized without the balloon catheter as a nephrostomy tube. However, should this tube slip, the drainage site relationship is then lost, so that the entire operative procedure may be jeopardized.

Many other variations are used for drainage. A four-wing Malecot (with two wings cut) or Pezzer catheter may be preferred. Robinson catheters with extra draining holes are the choice of others. Many varied types are available.

Fixation of Drainage Tube, Splint; Dye in the Balloon Catheter

If a balloon type of catheter is used, the balloon is distended with approximately 1 to 3 ml of water depending on the size of the renal pelvis. The splinting catheter is placed alongside the nephrostomy tube and down the ureter to its lower one-third or even into the bladder. The splint and nephrostomy tube are tied to each other in several places with 3-0 chromic suture and sutured to the adjacent fascial layers to ensure that neither catheter comes out. The nephrostomy tube and splint are both brought out together through a stab wound.

A skin stitch is placed and tied to the tubes to further ensure their staying in place should the balloon of the catheter deflate. Several drops of indigo carmine or methylene blue are put into the balloon to indicate any deflation of the balloon due to a perforation.

All of these precautionary measures are necessary to assure good drainage from a kidney which has been subjected to repair.

Alternate Source of Drainage

When Silastic tubing or any other type of tubing is used as a splint, additional holes made in the splint in the region of the pelvis serve as "safety valves" and an alternate source of drainage in the event the pyelostomy or nephrostomy tube fails to drain the kidney pelvis properly.

Fitting a Proper Draining Apparatus to a Rubber Catheter

Occasionally one has difficulty in fitting a proper drainage apparatus to a rubber catheter or other type of small-lumen catheter. A mosquito clamp may be placed inside of the rubber catheter and the blades of the clamp opened from a lateral-to-lateral position. Another mosquito clamp in the vertical or opposite direction may be used to open the end of the splint catheter in the top-to-bottom direction.

With the end of the catheter thus opened, one may place the plastic connector end of the intravenous drainage tubing into the catheter. The hemostats are then withdrawn. In this manner a good snug fit is obtained. The opposite end of the plastic drainage tubing, which with the "Murphy drip" plugs normally into the intravenous bottle, is then cut off. The cut end is placed into any type of sterilized glass bottle or plastic bag for drainage collection, taking care that the end of the drainage tube is never immersed in the urinary drainage.

A large-gauge needle, such as a No. 13 or 15, may be used also as a connector. One must bear in mind that any step down in connector size may serve as a trap. Too small a lumen must be avoided.

Replacement of Ureteral Catheter by Silastic Catheter

If one wishes to place a splinting catheter in a ureter instead of an already emplaced ureteral catheter, Silastic tubing (or a Silastic catheter) or another type of plastic tubing which is just large enough to fit over the ureteral catheter may be used. The Silastic tubing or catheter is well lubricated, led over the guiding ureteral catheter and pushed up to the kidney

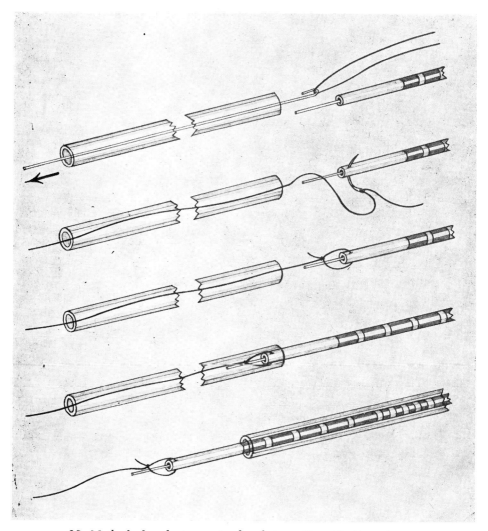

26. Method of replacing ureteral catheter with a Silastic catheter

pelvis. The ureteral catheter may then be removed, assuming the Silastic catheter is shorter than, and pushed beyond the ureteral catheter.

If a metal ureteral catheter stylet is put in place to stiffen the ureteral catheter, the outer Silastic catheter will more readily be passed. Care must be exercised that the stylet is not pushed far enough to pass out the end of the ureteral catheter.

To prevent the splinting catheter from being pushed further up into the ureter, one may place a black silk suture through the distal end of the splint (using a fine needle and tying it in), and then with a wire stylet or straight needle lead the silk suture through the distal end of the Silastic tubing. See Figure 26.

Nephrostomy Placement

It is most desirable to place the proximal end of a nephrostomy tube into the lowermost calyx. However, in a patient confined to bed, the superior calyx is the most dependent one. Needle aspiration of a quantity of urine in the pelvis, and then palpation of the softened area are first performed to indicate the site of the lower calyx. A 1- to 2-cm incision is made in the renal pelvis, following which a small hemostat, tonsil clamp, right-angle clamp, Randall stone forceps, nephrostomy hook, probe, or trocar is passed through the opening in the pelvis and guided to the lowermost calyx.

The pointed end of the instrument used is directed just posterior to the midline of the kidney, ideally, and then pushed through the parenchyma so that there may be the least amount of bleeding. When the clamp is in the lower calyx, it is pushed out to the capsule and an incision is made in the capsule over the clamp.

Nephrostomy catheters or drainage tubes include silicone catheters, ordinary rubber catheters, Malecot or Pezzer catheters, and infant feeding tubes (American Hospital Supply Company No. K-31). An old-time favorite of some urologists is a combination single-unit balloon-type catheter and ureteral splinting catheter called the "Thackston Tube."

Use of a Probe for Leading the Catgut and Catheter

One may use the small, narrow, blunt end of a probe, passed through the opening in the pelvis and guided to the lowermost calyx, rather than the clamps previously mentioned, to lead a nephrostomy catheter into the renal pelvis.

The probe, prior to its insertion, is bent at what appears to be the proper angle. The pointed end of the instrument is directed just posterior to the midline of the kidney and pushed through the parenchyma. One end of a piece of catgut may be securely tied to the end of the probe and the other end fixed through the tip of the nephrostomy catheter with a cutting-edge

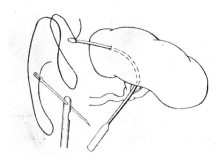

27.   Positioning of nephrostomy tube by means of probe and catgut leader

needle. The probe is then withdrawn from the renal pelvis, pulling the catgut along with it. This in turn guides the catheter into the lower calyx (see
Fig. 27).

Extraction of Blood Clots in Nephrostomy Tube

After a nephrostomy tube has been put in place, bleeding from within a
kidney may plug the tube so that vital urinary drainage is blocked. One
cannot safely remove a recently installed tube with the expectation of re-
anchoring another tube without resorting to open surgery. The following
measures may be taken in attempting to maintain drainage via the nephrostomy tube:

1) Irrigate and aspirate frequently with a 10-ml syringe and normal saline.
Aspiration must at first be carried out with extreme delicacy; later more vigorous
aspiration may be done.

2) Pass a stone extractor into the nephrostomy tube and attempt to "basket
out" the clots.

3) Insert a Fogarty catheter (preferably under fluoroscopic control), blow up
the balloon 1 to 2 ml, and while holding the nephrostomy tube in place, pull out
the Fogarty tube with clots therein. The Fogarty catheter must be easily maneu-
verable within the nephrostomy tube. It is a simple matter to irrigate the nephrostomy tube following this maneuver.

4) Pass a small ureteral catheter into the nephrostomy tube and irrigate and
aspirate, 2 to 3 ml at a time.

5) Pass a ureteral catheter alongside the nephrostomy tube and irrigate and
agitate.

6) If using a balloon catheter as the nephrostomy tube, deflate the balloon
and further irrigate and agitate.

7) If the tube must be removed, maintain suction as it is withdrawn and frequently the clots will come out with the nephrostomy tube. Then immediately
try to anchor a smaller nephrostomy tube.

8) Inject contrast material into the nephrostomy tube or ureteral catheter
passed alongside the nephrostomy tube to determine if the tube is in proper position.

Excessive Urine Drainage from a Splinting Catheter

At times, in placing a splint down the ureter into the bladder, there may
be drainage, by way of the splint, of urine from the opposite kidney. When
there is this profuse urine drainage through a splint, one must always consider the possibility that the splint is either in the bladder and also draining
the opposite kidney content of the bladder, or that there is reflux up the
ureter. For this reason, when also using a nephrostomy tube, one may wish
to clamp off or tie off the splint.

(See also *Post-Nephrostomy Clot Dissolution*, in Bleeding section of this
chapter.)

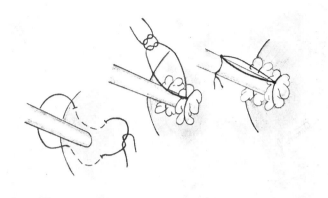

28. Method of anchoring splint and/or drainage catheter

Multiple-Knot Procedure for Anchoring Splint and/or Drainage Catheter

The splinting catheter and the balloon catheter should be tied at the nephrostomy exit site from the kidney by mattress suture, over fat pads, through the kidney parenchyma, and then tied to the catheter. The technique is as follows (see Fig. 28). Place one side of each mattress suture (using 2-0 suture) around the catheter. Place a piece of fat about 2 cm long and 1 cm wide under the looped end of the suture and under the knotted end of the suture. Cinch up the suture snugly and tie.

A loop is then made and the suture tied again. At the distal end of this loop, the suture is wrapped tightly around the nephrostomy or splinting tube and then tied.

If both nephrostomy tube and splint emerge from the same opening, the suture is wrapped tightly again around the second tube and tied. Instead of a wraparound tie, one may *spiral* the suture around the tube tightly and then tie (as described in *Anchoring Cystostomy Tubing*, in Chapter Six. See Fig. 43A).

Splinting Catheter from Renal Pelvis to Bladder

A splinting catheter placed in the renal pelvis and led down into the bladder is the technique used by some surgeons. At a future date the catheter is removed by use of a cystoscopic rongeur or forceps. This may be satisfactory in many instances. One must be certain, however, to anchor the catheter because of the possibility of its moving down the ureter by reason of ureteral peristalsis. On the other hand, when there is a catheter in the bladder, the patient frequently will have a good deal of bladder spasm and bladder discomfort which can be relieved only after removal of the splint.

Decreasing the Capacity of the Renal Pelvis

Usually only 2 to 3 ml of fluid are utilized to inflate the balloon of the renal pelvis catheter. Five milliliters is often too large a volume to be utilized. If the renal pelvis is of such size that a volume of 5 ml or more may be placed into the balloon of the catheter, a good rule of thumb is that there is too much pelvis.

Should the excess pelvis be extrarenal, much of the enlarged pelvis must be trimmed away, if at all possible, and the pelvis then closed with interrupted 3-0 or 4-0 chromic suture. The extrarenal pelvis should be of such size as to barely accommodate a 5-ml balloon catheter.

If the excess pelvis is intrarenal, a large volume of residual urine may result in infection with subsequent failure of the plastic procedure. Nephrectomy may have to be resorted to at a future date if infection cannot be controlled.

Relief of obstruction also allows a distended pelvis to decrease in size, usually within a period of about nine to twelve months.

Pyeloureteroplasty Drainage—Pyelostomy

Most urologists prefer nephrostomy over pyelostomy. Some, however, claim to obtain equally good drainage results with pyelostomy, without destruction of any renal parenchyma.

For pyelostomy the balloon catheter, preferably the Silastic-coated or nylon-coated type, is recommended. The balloon of this type of catheter will usually remain in one good position and drain well.

Some surgeons prefer a straight catheter such as the Robinson, which has been tied in. The straight catheter may, however, change its position and fail to provide good pyelostomy drainage.

Other urologists use a four-wing Malecot, with two wings cut off, or a Pezzer catheter for pyelostomy. One of us (H.B.) has an aversion to the use of the Malecot or Pezzer catheter in the kidney as tubes for *either* nephrostomy or pyelostomy because of the occurrence of secondary hemorrhage on two occasions when the tubes were removed.

Balloon Catheter as a Pyelostomy Tube

When a balloon catheter is used as a pyelostomy tube instead of a nephrostomy tube, it is preferably placed in the renal pelvis through a separate stab wound of the pelvis rather than being part of the repair of this pelvis. A splinting catheter may be tied to the balloon catheter and led down the ureter and out through the same opening in the pelvis.

Some question has been raised by authors in the past as to whether one should or should not lead the splinting catheter all the way into the bladder or leave it someplace in the ureter. Some urologists claim that stricture occurs at the end site of the splinting catheter. The authors have never seen secondary stricture at the end of a splinting catheter in their many years of urological surgery. The splint, therefore, is led down the ureter to somewhere in the region of its lower third and left at this site.

Continuous Suction Drainage for Post-Renal Surgery

Continuous suction by way of the Hemovac or Stedman pump has been advocated to help keep the renal surgical patient and wound dry. However, negative pressure produced by such a pump can conceivably evert the edges of the incision in the ureter or pelvis, holding them open long enough to establish a fistulous tract, and often prolonging drainage. Therefore, the use of negative pressure equipment for drainage in instances in which an incision is made into a secreting organ or its tributaries must be carefully evaluated in each individual case. Many surgeons do use Hemovac and are pleased with its function.

Post-Pyeloplasty Manometry

Management of the post-pyeloplasty patient should include nephrostograms to determine if there is any drainage of contrast material down the repair site around the ureteral splint (this should be done with the patient in the semi-upright position).

The physiologic function of the healing pyeloplasty can be determined by water manometry. After placing the patient in a supine position, the splinting catheter may be removed. The nephrostomy catheter is then connected to a Y-tube attached to short pieces of connecting rubber tubing.

An Asepto syringe is connected to one arm of the Y-connector, and a 30- or 50-ml syringe barrel (only) attached to the second arm of the Y-connector. A metric ruler is then taped to the side of the glass syringe with the 0-cm mark at approximately the level of the renal pelvis. Sterile water poured into the Asepto syringe is measured several minutes later at the resting level.

The normal physiological level at the pelvis is from 0 to 8 cm. If the level is 15 cm of water pressure or less, the nephrostomy tube may be removed and there will be little or no drainage from the nephrostomy wound. Should the pressure be between 15 and 20 cm, there may be prolonged drainage.

When the pressure is above 20 cm, the nephrostomy catheter must not be removed. The passage of days, or even weeks, may be necessary before healing progresses and edema decreases to the point where the resting water level is below 15 cm.

Further definitive surgery may be necessary if the pressure remains above 20 cm.

Bleeding

Clamping the Renal Pedicle in Nephrectomy

A number of different types of pedicle clamps are suggested for handling the renal pedicle in nephrectomy. The 8-inch Carmalt clamp has been for us the most preferable. The Mayo and Guyon clamps are favored by many—others are the Herrick, Walther, Young and Ockerblad, Wertheim-Cullen and Wertheim-Reverdin, Jeppesen, Kutzmann, etc.

Some urologists use no clamps and remove the kidney after the pedicle has been tied with heavy silk, chromic, cotton, or synthetic suture. Most urologists will separately clamp the pedicle artery and vein. The artery is by preference clamped first. However, we have not seen the kidney expand to unusual size by first clamping the renal vein.

In tumors of the kidney the artery must be clamped first to prevent possible increased intrarenal pressures and dissemination of tumor cells. *A renal vein with tumor thrombus presents a precarious situation which requires minimal handling—sudden fatal tumor emboli have been reported.*

Ties placed about the entire pedicle have been known to result in arteriovenous fistulae. Whenever possible, therefore, the pedicle vessels in all patients subjected to nephrectomy should be individually tied.

Three pedicle clamps are generally used by most urologists in clamping the entire pedicle. The following variations are used: some surgeons merely place a double tie around both the first and second of two clamps which remain on the pedicle after the third clamp has been removed with the kidney; other surgeons place a tie around the pedicle before applying the clamps.

A safe procedure has been to apply three clamps in the following manner, if at all possible. The clamp designated as #1 is closest to the kidney and clamp #3 is closest to the aorta and vena cava. The kidney is removed by cutting between clamps #1 and #2. Care is taken that the pedicle is cut closer to clamp #1 so that if there is slippage of the pedicle this occurs on the specimen side. A chromic 2-0 suture is then stitched between the two remaining clamps in mattress fashion, around the artery if possible. The suture is placed in a loop as though to tie the knot, but not tied. The loose ends of the tie are held with a Mayo clamp.

In this manner, should there be any slippage whatsoever, the suture is around the artery and loosely looped once, and may easily be grasped and held. A chromic 2-0 tie is placed underneath clamp #3. The tie is looped and pulled tightly as the clamp is loosened and removed, so that the tie falls within the groove of the clamp closest to the cava and aorta. The suture ligature previously placed loosely around the artery is then tied. The pedicle vessels are therefore tied with two sutures each, one being a free tie and the other a suture tie. See Figure 29.

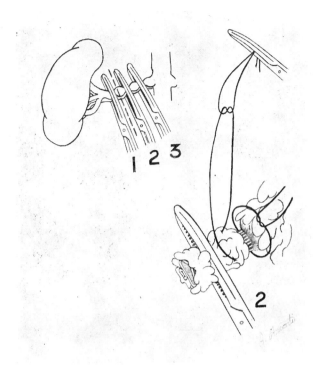

29. Method of tying off renal pedicle

Some surgeons will tie between clamps #2 and #3 and then remove clamp #2; others prefer to tie between clamps #2 and #3, but first remove clamp #3.

Hemorrhage from the Renal Pedicle

On rare occasions one may be exposed to the shocking occurrence of profuse bleeding of the renal pedicle. Two choices of remedial action are here described.

One may quickly grab large abdominal laparotomy sponges, place these hurriedly into the wound, and exert with the sponges a good deal of pressure on the presumed source of the bleeding. One must be sure that pressure is placed on the vena cava below the renal vein, and also that pressure is placed in the region of the aorta above the renal artery. The pack is left in for a period of at least ten to twelve minutes. In the meantime, attempts are made to stabilize the patient's blood pressure and to rapidly replace blood loss.

One then very carefully packs away all bowel and places carefully all retractors. Clamps are in readiness to quickly grasp the bleeding site as the packing or large laparotomy sponges are removed. From the time all packs are removed to the time bleeding will begin again from a renal artery, renal vein, or vena cava, there is often a lapse of approximately 10 seconds. In this period of time, the bleeding site must be grasped with a clamp. The bleeding vessel or vessels are then tied off, or the vena cava or aorta repaired, etc., depending on the cause of the bleeding.

A second approach may be used. The hand is placed in the depths of the wound. A fluttering type of sensation is felt when the bleeding is arterial. This area is grasped and finger-squeezed as the blood is aspirated and wiped by laparotomy sponges, and then a clamp is placed around the renal artery. This direct approach is obviously much more rapid than the previously described action. The bleeding areas are then handled as described above.

One may feel the site of vena cava or renal vein bleeding and compression with one or two fingers may successfully control this. The site of the bleeding is then searched for and clamped. Umbilical tapes or Penrose drains may be placed above and below the bleeding site if vena caval or aortal.

When one is attempting to control bleeding from a renal pedicle, a Rumel flexible cardiovascular tourniquet with one-eyed obturator stylet may be very helpful. One should always note the time at which the artery is clamped, so that avascularization is minimized. The occlusion is best limited to periods not longer than 10 to 15 minutes. *Vital signs must be carefully noted when laparotomy sponges are tightly placed and packed; one may completely occlude the vena cava and cardiac blood flow return.* (See also section on *Control of Renal Bleeding in Partial Nephrectomy and Related Procedures*, this chapter.)

Tumor Thrombus in Renal Vein

The following method of freeing the renal vein from possible tumor thrombus may be helpful where renal vein involvement with tumor complicates nephrectomy. After first tying the renal arteries individually, the renal vein and/or veins and vena cava are widely exposed and isolated. Vascular clamps or tapes are applied beyond the palpable tumor thrombus. Previously made inferior venacavograms are of great value and mandatory in such cases. A longitudinal venotomy is made in the renal vein. The tumor thrombus or clot is removed or aspirated, followed by irrigation with heparinized saline. Aspiration is continued until there is a free flow of venous blood.

If the tumor thrombus is located in the vena cava, the cava is clamped with vascular clamps at least 1 cm caudal to the takeoff of the renal vein. Again the venotomy is done, thrombus removed, and the cava irrigated with weak heparin solution and then closed with 5-0 continuous silk or 6-0 polyester fiber material such as Tevdek ®.

At times it may be necessary to tie off the caudal vena cava. The cephalad cava may be closed open-end with the same 5-0 silk or 6-0 polyester material. The clamp on the cephadad cava above the renal veins must not be left on for any period of time, but removed quickly.

Some surgeons have grasped the renal vein with small Kocher clamps after wide exposure of the vena cava and renal veins. Venotomy is done and the tumor thrombus removed. *This is a dangerous approach* due to the frailty of the renal vein and its tendency to tear. The vena cava with tumor thrombus must be handled most cautiously. A tumor thrombus may float loose and result in instant fatal embolization. Tumor thrombi have reportedly been removed from the cava, extending into the atrium of the heart.

Control of Renal Bleeding in Partial Nephrectomy and Related Procedures

To control bleeding from the kidney in partial nephrectomy or related procedures requiring equal control, one of several techniques may be utilized:

1) The assistant may place his fingers around the entire renal pedicle, squeezing the vessels between his fingers. This generally is not too satisfactory.

2) One may isolate separately the vessels, and then place a rubber-shod clamp or bulldog clamp on the renal artery or arteries depending on the renal arterial supply, as determined by dissection of the pedicle area or as shown by preoperative aortography.

3) One may place a Penrose drain around the pedicle, gently pulling downward.

4) Wide plastic tape may be used in lieu of a Penrose drain (above), in the same manner.

5) One may place a hemostat on the drain at the inferior aspect of the pedicle, occluding the blood supply to and from the kidney (it is preferable to occlude only the renal arterial supply).

The definitive surgical procedure is then accomplished.

Again, one should always be certain that a notation is made of the time at which the artery is clamped, so that avascularization is kept to a minimum. The occlusion is preferably limited to periods not longer than 10 minutes. This period could be longer with perfusion of iced solution. Oliguria during the first 24 to 72 hours has occurred with longer length of time of renal ischemia. However, 250 ml of 10 percent or 500 ml of 5 percent mannitol solution prior to clamping the artery helps to prevent oliguria. High-molecular dextran also would serve the same purpose.

Simplified Method for Renal Hypothermia

Effective renal hypothermia can be accomplished with equipment readily available in any hospital. Bottled sterile saline is preferably cooled in advance. A Y-type intravenous tubing set is connected to two bottles of sterile saline to allow for continuous lavage of the kidney. The intravenous tubing is then coiled, making several loops that are immersed in a basin of ice

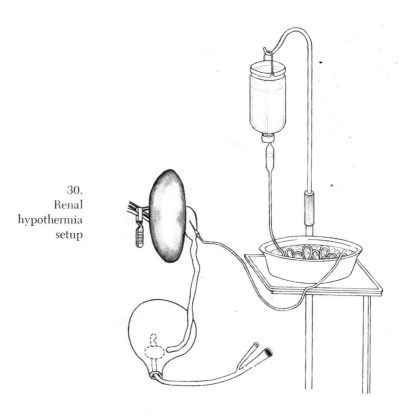

30.
Renal
hypothermia
setup

water. It is usually necessary to use the tubing from two intravenous sets
to obtain sufficient length to permit coiling of the tubing. See Figure 30.

From the ice bath the intravenous tubing runs directly to the kidney
pelvis. An 18-gauge needle is connected to the needle adapter, and the
needle is inserted into the kidney pelvis, directing it toward the center of
the kidney but only into the pelvis. A balloon retention catheter is inserted
into the bladder preoperatively to collect the saline that will drain into the
bladder during the lavage (see Fig. 30).

The saline lavage may be started as one is nearing the actual corrective
procedure to be performed. The renal artery is then temporarily occluded
and generally within 5 minutes the kidney has cooled satisfactorily. The
actual kidney temperature can be determined by placing a temperature
meter on the upper or lower pole of the kidney.

While the authors prefer clamping the renal artery for very short periods,
there are times when the period must extend far beyond 10 minutes. Some
urologists feel that the renal artery may be occluded up to 2 hours without
hypothermia if the patient is well hydrated the evening before surgery and
receives mannitol the morning of surgery, as well as heparin (0.5 mg/kg).

Control of Bleeding in Instances of Short Renal Pedicle or Injury to Vena Cava

When there is a large renal or adrenal tumor on the right side one frequently is faced with the problem of a short renal pedicle, with possible injury to the vena cava. In addition, occasionally there is need to open the vena cava for removal of tumor thrombi. For these reasons, urologists must be prepared to repair a vena cava. Pressure below the bleeding site will control much of the hemorrhage.

Vascular clamps, such as a Satinsky clamp or Johns Hopkins bulldog clamp, should be available as well as 5-0 arterial silk, 6-0 Tevdek or Polydek ®, or other synthetic suture. Back bleeding from the renal mass may be controlled by placing a figure-of-eight heavy transfixion suture before the vein is incised.

Slight oozing, if present, may be controlled with pressure on Gelfoam or gauze, or a laparotomy sponge. Vascular clips may be helpful in multiple bleeding sites in tumor cases. These clips are also timesavers in doing deep pelvic node dissections and node dissections around the great vessels.

Repair of Vena Cava

Care must be taken not to blindly clamp tissue in the region of the vena cava. A rent in the cava, for example, may be made longer, compounding the situation, if clamps are injudiciously utilized. One may loosely grab a rent in the cava with Babcock or sponge forceps. *Extreme caution* must be used so that the forceps themselves do not cause further tear in the cava. If the clamp is closed loosely, it may be sufficient to control the bleeding in the cava and at the same time steady the structure to facilitate its repair. It is safer to use umbilical tape above and below areas of tear. The use of special vascular or bulldog clamps, of course, is preferable.

It must be emphasized again that the described methods are presented as practical aids for the urologist and not as authoritative techniques utilized by the vascular surgeon.

Suturing the Vena Cava

Arterial 5-0 atraumatic silk suture or synthetic suture placed as a continuous suture, is utilized to repair a rent in the vena cava. Closure is preferable to ligation of the inferior vena cava.

Suture of Aorta or Other Large Artery

In the event of tear of large arteries or aorta, control of bleeding may be done by repair. Closure of the thick-walled aorta is usually easier than repairing the thin-walled vena cava. Continuous everting suture interrupted in one-third sections, and overlapping of the ties, will usually suffice. Satinsky clamps must first be placed on the aorta at the site of the tear before attempts are made at repair.

Heparinization

Intravenous heparin in dosage of 50 to 75 mg is often administered to prevent clotting when performing vascular surgery. For irrigation locally, a weak irrigating solution may be prepared by dissolving 10 mg of heparin in 100 ml of normal saline.

Repair of Injury to Diaphragm During Renal Surgery

Injury to the diaphragm or pleura during rib resection in renal surgery is of little significance if the incident is noted and appropriately treated. Repair is done while the anesthetist keeps the lungs expanded.

If pulmonary leak persists, then a chest tube with water seal drainage must be used. Chest X-ray, in either event, must be done immediately after surgery to be certain that there is lung expansion. Pleural air, if still present, may be aspirated through an upper anterior interspace with syringe and needle. Injuries to other organs of the abdomen must be recognized and appropriately treated.

Repair of Carcinomatous Pedicle

In renal carcinoma, with severe invasion of the pedicle and surrounding aorta and vena cava, severe bleeding may dictate the need to remove the kidney. One may apply clamps to the pedicle and remove the kidney. The clamps may then be slowly and carefully opened, one by one. Frequently the pedicle may be so severely involved by tumor that one may cut across the pedicle with no ensuing bleeding. If bleeding occurs and is uncontrollable by suture due to the massive tumor involvement, etc., the clamps may be left on and treated as described in a succeeding section.

Again, *one must be aware that clamping across the renal vein may invite embolization.* However, circumstances may dictate the necessity of across-the-pedicle clamping.

Secondary Nephrectomy for Control of Bleeding with Difficult Pedicle

When faced with a severely fibrotic wide pedicle, usually in repeat renal surgical approach and when the pedicle can be approached en masse only, the vessels often may be closed individually with the use of large metal vessel clips. Thus, the following procedure of leaving hemostatic clamps on the pedicle is obviated.

Hemostatic Clamps Left in Wound for Interim Period

On extremely rare occasions, one is faced with a severely fibrotic or tumor-invaded pedicle in secondary nephrectomy (usually) in which the wide mass makes it impractical to tie off the pedicle or place vascular clips across the vessels. A clamp, or clamps may be applied to the pedicle and the kidney removed. The wound is then closed, allowing the handles of the pedicle clamps to remain outside of the wound.

On the fourth postoperative day, *in the operating room*, the clamps are loosened notch by notch every fifteen to thirty minutes until they are completely loose, watching the wound for bleeding. Should bleeding occur, the clamps are quickly closed again, and the process repeated again in about 48 hours.

If no bleeding occurs, the clamps are then removed.

Intracapsular Nephrectomy

When one is dealing with a kidney previously operated upon, it may be extremely difficult to mobilize the kidney for nephrectomy. The capsule of the kidney may be opened along the external border and the kidney mobilized by stripping the capsule down to the region of renal sinus. This decapsulation of the kidney results in bleeding from the parenchyma. An incision at right angles should then be made through the capsule, and with blunt dissection the individual vessels may be clamped and ligated. The capsule is then cut away and the pedicle approached as in any other secondary nephrectomy.

Control of Bleeding from Inoperable Carcinoma of the Kidney

In bleeding from an inoperable carcinoma of the kidney, one may ligate the ureter in the region of the brim of the pelvis, or any other readily accessible portion of the ureter. There is increased formation of erythropoietin, and subsequent increased red blood cell count and rise in hemoglobin. A hydronephrotic atrophy may subsequently occur with loss of blood supply to the kidney. This kidney, in a subsequent operation, then is easily removed with less bleeding.

Use of G-Suit ® in Severe Pelvic and Abdominal Bleeding

Though clinical data in abundance is lacking, the G-Suit apparently works well in hemorrhage control. Whenever all methods for control of hemorrhage have failed, one must consider use of this device.

The suit, a heavy plastic envelope which extends from lower chest to mid-thigh, is obtained through the Kendall Company, of Chicago, Illinois. The usual recommended pressure within the suit should be in the range of 20 to 30 mm of mercury.

This equipment could prove to be a very valuable adjunct in control of urinary tract bleeding.

Post-Nephrostomy Clot Dissolution

Streptokinase and streptodornase have been utilized in the dissolution of bladder clots and the liquefaction of heavy infectious material in the bladder. The same regime may be useful in instances of intrarenal bleeding, with clotting, in cases of nephrostomy. The usual dosage schedule consists of one ampule of the streptokinase or streptodornase in 5 to 10 cc of saline, injected through the catheter two to three times daily. The application of pancreatic dornase, increased to instillations of every hour, has resulted in prompt resolution of renal pelvis bleeding.

Wound Closure

Suture of Kidney: Suture Buffer

The kidney may be sutured by employing a continuous stitch through the capsule and through the renal parenchyma, utilizing pads of fat or Oxycel ® underneath the sutures to prevent them from pulling through the capsule. One may in this manner obtain a tight hemostatic closure.

When fat is not readily available for buffering renal sutures, one may use Oxycel. One-inch strips of catgut arranged into sheaths of six or eight pieces, or one piece folded over six or eight times, in addition to muscle, make excellent suture buffer material.

Triple-0 chromic suture is utilized for the continuous stitch through the capsule and parenchyma; either 4-0 or 5-0 chromic on a swaged-on needle is best used for the capsular closing.

Closure of Kidney in Heminephrectomy or Nephrotomy

Closure of a kidney may be facilitated by utilizing a number of sets of spinal needles instead of the usual circular needles with the swaged-on suture. Prior to the renal incision, a number of 18-gauge spinal needles may be threaded with 3-0 or 4-0 chromic catgut sutures. Half-length suture material doubled back on itself is used. When the two halves of the kidney are approximated, the threaded needles are placed all the way through the cut end of the kidney substance (Fig. 31). If desired, a piece of fat placed in the bisected kidney for hemostasis may be penetrated by this needle.

The doubled suture is grasped, not clamped, by an assistant and a piece of fat or a roll of Oxycel is included in the looped end. The needle is removed and the suture is tied over fat or Oxycel. Two rows of suture are used, one

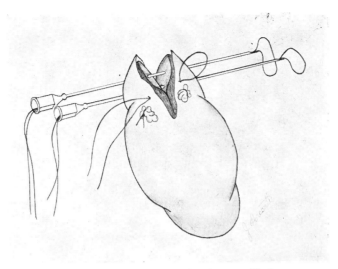

31. Use of spinal needles for closure of kidney

on either side of the incised kidney. By utilizing several sets of needles, sutures may be placed into the renal parenchyma rapidly, thus decreasing operating time. Fewer holes are made in the kidney substance, thus also minimizing necrosis of renal tissue.

Renal Surgery Wound Closure

Meticulous care in wound closure is as necessary as the technical repair in pyeloureteroplasty or other carefully executed renal procedures. Special care is required in flank incisions because the peculiar contour of the flank and the great amount of motion in the flank subject the closure to unusual stress. Moisture from drains and tubes may further contribute to unsightly and uncomfortable scars.

In children and in women, one can make a special attempt at cosmetic results by use of subcuticular monofilament nylon suture which can be left *in situ* for much longer than can the standard sutures. This prevents also the slow separation of the skin edges commonly seen in the flank which results in a broad bridging of fibroblasts, producing a wide scar.

By following the well-established skin incision lines, by using good supportive subcutaneous sutures and subcuticular closure, and by bringing drains and tubes out through separate stab wounds, the incision can be nearly invisible, as well as much more comfortable. For the girl who wishes to wear a bikini, the separate stab wound scars can be excised later.

Monofilament nylon is difficult to tie securely and must be held with a lead bead. The bead will make a pressure mark on the skin. To avoid this, one may place five or six Steri-Strips ®, one on top of the other, under the bead; the suture may pass right through the Steri-Strips.

Alternative Rapid Incision Closure Techniques

Renal surgery wounds are most commonly closed layer by layer, utilizing various techniques and types of sutures. One may use interrupted sutures or continuous sutures on each one of the layers.

A rapid alternative technique consists of placing interrupted suture through all layers. Chromic suture may be used, or nonabsorbable sutures such as Polydek, Tevdek, wire, nylon, or silk. After these sutures are placed, fairly close together, with the patient still in the operative position (i.e., with the table flexed and the kidney rest up), one may drop the kidney rest, unflex the table, and then "cinch up" and tie these sutures.

On completion of the tying of the sutures the external fascia may be closed with a continuous suture of one's preference, of absorbable or nonabsorbable material. The skin is then also closed with the suture and method of one's choice.

This type of closure is timesaving and the incidence of herniation is no higher than with the layer-by-layer closure. A Penrose drain is brought out through a stab wound.

Another alternative in critical situations (e.g., with poor-risk patients who must be subjected to minimal operating room time) is to place polyester stay sutures or other nonabsorbable heavy sutures through all layers and then unbreak the table, cinch up the sutures, and tie them over a 2- to 3-inch-wide polyfoam pad or over rubber tubing. These sutures are left in for twelve to fourteen days before removal.

Skin Closure in Children

In closing the skin of children, interrupted nonabsorbable suture may be used. The sutures are cut off long (i.e., 7 or 8 cm). All of the sutures are twisted together and a tie is placed around the site of the twist. When the time comes for skin suture removal, all sutures are cut at the skin and then,

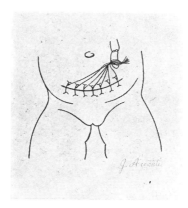

32. Simultaneous removal of skin sutures in children

because they are tied together, with one pull all are removed at one time. In this manner the patient is subjected to only one period of pull on suture instead of having each one of the sutures removed individually.

One may use skin clips, Steri-Strips, or a subcuticular stitch. Fine wire or plasticized material may also be used as a continuous suture and removed as one unit. See Figure 32.

Collection Device for Excessive Postoperative Drainage

The pediatric urine collecting bag is ordinarily used to collect urine from infants. In certain patients with excessive postoperative urinary drainage due to, for example, a ureterolithotomy wound, the pediatric bag has been used to collect the drainage. The patient is much more comfortable because the dressings are kept relatively dry.

Some Postoperative Complications

Wound infections nonresponsive to appropriate antibiotic therapy should make the urologist suspicious of: (1) possible foreign body (such as unabsorbed suture); (2) possible fistula; (3) diabetes or other systemic disease; or (4) carcinoma. Postoperative gastrointestinal complications require the usual appropriate therapy, as do cardiovascular complications.
Important Note: See also *Surgical Removal of Calculi in the Renal Pelvis or Ureteropelvic Junction Area*; this section includes many additional aids in Renal Surgery, specifically with reference to calculi.

RENAL CALCULI

Conservative Therapy

Etiology of Calculi in the Urinary Tract

Many factors relate to the formation of calculi. Much experimental and clinical work has been done to study this problem; the literature is extensive with reference to calculi and its matrix. The role of calcium, phosphorus, magnesium, colloids, hydrogen ion concentration, dietary factors, stasis, infection, parathyroid disease, Fanconi syndrome, renal tubular acidosis, sarcoidosis, multiple myeloma, milk alkali syndrome, cystinuria, uric acid diathesis, oxalosis, nephrocalcinosis, etc., are all extensively recorded.

Dilution of Urine

The first morning voided urine (the night urine) is obviously the most concentrated of any during the 24-hour period. It is felt that a large number of patients develop their recurrent calculi during the night hours. Accordingly, the authors feel that more emphasis than one normally sees in the literature should be placed on attempting to dilute the night urine and renal excretion.

Our practice, therefore, is to advise patients who have had recurrent calculi to drink at least two glasses of water immediately before retiring. Should these patients be forced to empty their bladders during the night hours (by virtue of one-time nocturia), then they are urged to again drink approximately two glasses, or sixteen ounces, of water. This usually will carry the patient to morning. On this type of regimen, the night urine concentration frequently will approach that of the day urine concentration. Emphasis should be placed on comparative specific gravity determination.

The incidence of calculi in recurrent stone formers should be decreased if the reason for the repetition of stone formation is relative to colloid-crystalloid imbalance or the concentration of electrolytes in the urine.

Stone Formation Due to Recumbency

Patients with stones which form due to recumbency should have a trial of therapy consisting of: (1) increased activity, (2) correction of urinary infection, (3) forcing fluids orally, and (4) lowering of the pH of the urine. Patients should have an output of at least 3,000 ml of fluids per day (with intake adjusted to insensible water loss through perspiration, diarrhea, and vomiting). They should be maintained on a low-calcium diet; acidifying agents may be necessary to obtain a urinary pH of 5 to 5.5.

Methylene Blue Dye as a Kidney Stone Solvent

In a recent study it was found that methylene blue, in oral doses of 65 mg two to three times a day, may dissolve calcium oxalate stones. The continued use of the methylene blue orally has also been shown to prevent formation of new stones in some patients. The methylene blue does not cause anemia, and it has not caused hepatomegaly or splenomegaly. Patients must be warned, of course, of the fact that their urine will be blue in color.

In the series followed, one patient with a great number of calculi had all of these stones disappear after two years of methylene blue treatment.

Surgical Removal of Calculi in the Renal Pelvis or the Ureteropelvic Junction Area

Exploring Inside the Kidney

In a patient with a large extrarenal pelvis, one may explore the kidney by placing one's finger on the inside of the pelvis, calyces, and infundibula. Caution is necessary to avoid tearing the infundibulum of a calyx. Bleeding may be profuse. The renal pelvis is best opened on its posterior side because there is less danger of injury to the pedicle vessels.

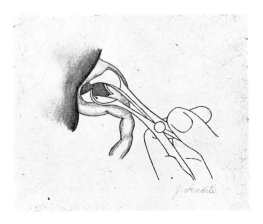

33. Visualization of renal pelvis and calyces by use of nasal speculum

Methods for Effective Visualization of the Renal Pelvis and Calyces

The new fiber optic renoscopes or nephroscopes are probably the most satisfactory instruments for visualization of the innermost recesses of the pelviocalyceal system at the time of surgery. However, with an extrarenal pelvis, a small nasal speculum may also be very helpful (see Fig. 33). The speculum may be introduced through the pyelotomy or nephrotomy opening and cautiously manipulated to afford maximum visibility. A spotlight, flashlight, or preferably the cystoscopic fiber optic cord with light at the terminal end serves well to shine through the open blades of the nasal speculum. A long-bladed speculum permits good visualization quite deeply within the kidney.

One may also make good use of a panendoscope with foroblique lens for visualization of a stone in the pelvis. Should a stone be viewed, one may pass a Randall stone forceps alongside the endoscope to grasp it. The renal pelvis may be irrigated while sucking up the irrigating fluid with an aspirator, when the endoscopes are used.

The infant vaginal speculum with fiber optic light may also be used in an extrarenal pelvis. The otoscope and battery handle have been utilized also for this purpose.

Intrapelvic Insertion of Stone Forceps

Stone forceps should always be inserted through the pyelotomy incision into the renal pelvis *with the jaws already opened* as widely as possible. Only too often the stone forceps is introduced into the pelvis with the jaws closed, and then when the forceps is opened the stone is pushed away from the forceps into another portion of the pelvis or into a calyx. This then makes search for the stone all the more difficult.

Conversion of an Intrarenal into an Extrarenal Pelvis to Facilitate Surgery

A pelviolithotomy must occasionally be done in a patient with an intra-renal type of pelvis. One may possibly convert this type of pelvis into an extrarenal type by placing a Dourmashkin bag catheter below the uretero-pelvic juncture area about one hour before surgery. The renal pelvis is filled to capacity with saline and is allowed to enlarge further by the secretion of urine. This procedure may be considered too time-consuming by many urologists.

Another method of dilating the pelvis is to use the Fogarty balloon cath-eter. This catheter is a single-lumen type; thus, the balloon may be filled and there is no other drainage through the catheter. (Note: the Fogarty catheter is made in sizes 3, 4, and 5 French.)

Surgical Approach to Intrarenal Pelvis

Whenever the renal pelvis is intrarenal and more exposure is necessary, one may mobilize the pelvis from the renal parenchyma at the sinus area. By gentle finger pressure, or with a "peanut" sponge, the pelvis is separated from the renal parenchyma on the posterior aspect of the kidney. Two or three small perforating vessels may be clamped, cut and tied, or fulgurated. The pelvis now may be completely free on one side. The renal parenchyma may be lifted away from the pelvis by the use of vein retractors or lid retrac-tors. It is possible, by this technique, to extend the pelvic incision as far as the infundibulum of a calyx.

This area may also be sutured by raising the parenchyma with retractors. One should be very careful not to injure a relatively large vein crossing the renal sinus along the hilar-pelvic juncture.

In some instances, it may be necessary to cut the parenchyma. The bleed-ing vessels may be clamped and tied, and this flap lifted up so that the intra-renal pelvis may be easily inspected. Visualization of the infundibuli and calyces is enabled by this maneuver.

Location of Calculi in Intrarenal Pelvis

If at all possible, it is better to avoid intrarenal manipulation with the surgeon's finger. However, when calculi are not readily found in the renal pelvis, one may insert a finger through the pyelotomy opening and into the calyces to palpate for stone, after unsuccessful probing with stone forceps.

Pelvionephrotomy

There may be times when one cannot readily separate the renal pelvis from the parenchyma. The deliberate insertion of the surgeon's finger into a small pyelotomy incision will enlarge the opening by blunt dissection;

however, this maneuver will frequently tear the parenchyma, though there is less bleeding than when parenchyma is cut by scissors or scalpel. Often the parenchyma will tear, leaving the vessels intact. If small, the vessels may be clamped, cut, and tied.

The capsule may be opened extending from the renal sinus towards the outer renal border and downward in the direction of the lower calyx. The renal parenchyma may then be opened down to the pelvis by using the blunt end of the scalpel, or by "sawing through" with 2-0 chromic catgut. By this means, vessels are usually not cut, and may be grasped with hemostats, cut, and tied. Bleeding is minimized. This elevated flap will allow intrarenal visualization and easier access to the calculus. After removal of the stone, the parenchyma may be closed with chromic suture over fat pads.

Aid in Removal of Stones from the Kidney

By making an incision in the renal pelvis in the renal sinus area higher toward the cortex of the kidney after the renal parenchyma has been gently stripped away from the renal pelvis, as previously described, one may obtain an opening into the renal pelvis large enough and high enough to be able to see directly into the minor calyces. One may also be able to palpate readily into the calyceal cups to feel a stone.

Spot Nephrotomy for Intrarenal Stone

When a stone is palpated, gentle pressure may be maintained over the calculus to keep it from moving, and the surgeon may then make a small incision in the capsule of the kidney, preferably in the lateral border, directly over the stone. With a forceps, the renal parenchyma is separated to the calyx where the stone is lodged; a small incision is then made into the calyx. A stone forceps may be introduced through the nephrotomy incision to grasp the stone as it is held in place with the finger.

A large dilated calyx with calculus (i) may require segmental renal resection for prevention of future difficulties.

Management of Small Stones Entrapped in a Calyx with a Narrow Infundibulum

A calculus frequently may not be removed through the pyelotomy incision because the stone cannot be grasped with a stone forceps or hemostat, even though the stone may be small enough to come through the infundibulum. The operator may insert his little finger through the pyelotomy incision and into the infundibulum of the calyx. The stone in the calyx is often readily palpated. While maintaining gentle pressure of the finger within the renal pelvis, the blunt end of a straight needle or of a large spinal needle may be inserted through the convex surface of the kidney directly opposite the finger inside the kidney. The tip of the needle is directed to contact the stone.

By advancing the needle and gently releasing the pressure of the finger inside the kidney simultaneously, the stone may be brought into the renal pelvis and then easily removed. The pyelotomy incision may be closed in the usual fashion. The needle site bleeding will frequently be controlled by a few minutes of compression with a sponge.

Calculi in Renal Pelvis and Lower Ureter

One may occasionally have a calculus in the renal pelvis associated with a calculus in the lower ureter. If a high subcostal incision has been made, and it is difficult to approach the lower ureter, one may pass a Johnson, Dormia, or other type of stone basket down through the opening in the pelvis to an area estimated to be beyond the ureteral calculus or preferably into the bladder. The basket may then be expanded and pulled upward toward the renal pelvis. Frequently the lower stone is engaged and pulled up out of the ureter.

Of course, one may always extend the incision and expose more area of ureter, and thus do a direct approach to the stone. If one cannot reach the lower calculus and "milk" it upwards, one may then make an incision extending from the tip of the twelfth rib downward and anteriorly to end, if necessary, in the area near the midline of the symphysis. This incision is utilized for retroperitoneal exposure. (Please refer to the section on *Incisions* in this chapter for further suggestions relative to this approach.)

Exposure of Stone Area with Minimal Manipulation

A calculus is frequently impacted at the ureteropelvic junction. The most gentle manipulation may dislodge the stone. It should be a standing rule that the surgeon alone (not his assistant) must palpate the ureter and the ureteropelvic junction to immobilize the stone. (*See Fixation of Stones During Open Surgery,* in Chapter Five.)

Too vigorous and anxious manipulation by assistants, or carelessness with placement of retractors, may change the position of a readily accessible stone.

X-Ray Localization of Renal Calculi in Surgery

X-ray of a patient in the operating room can pinpoint exactly the needed operative site. The sterile-sheet-covered cassette is placed in front of the patient on the abdominal side, and the X-ray tube is placed so as to expose the patient in a posterior-anterior view. Localization of the calculus may be facilitated by placing a long skin needle (e.g., a Keith needle) into the kidney in a specific region, and then taking the X-ray. The stone may be localized in relation to the needle.

X-rays (K.U.B.) taken immediately prior to surgery must be routine procedure for all stone cases—these films must be on the view box in the operating room.

Aspiration Technique for Elusive Stones

In spite of all attempts, a calculus within the pelvis may not be readily located. The following approach may then be tried. The pelvis may be irrigated with excess pressure using an Asepto syringe. About one ounce of sterile saline may be injected as rapidly as possible. The tip of the Asepto syringe is placed within the pelvis and the bulb squeezed as firmly as possible. Pressure is slowly released on the bulb so that fluid is aspirated. As one aspirates, the stone frequently is sucked to the opening of the Asepto syringe, which may be gently withdrawn from the pelvis when one suspects the stone is at the syringe opening.

Suction Through Laparotomy Pad to Facilitate Aspiration

Excess fluid may be removed by suction through the laparotomy pad. With this method, fat particles do not plug up the openings in the suction tip. Careful search must be performed after such irrigation to be certain that no calcific debris is left behind in the kidney wound.

Routine Irrigation of Renal Pelvis in Stone Cases

Following removal of stones from a renal pelvis, copious irrigation is indicated, preferably with an Asepto syringe or with a Toomey syringe. The irrigation may be somewhat vigorous. Little stones or debris will wash off of the mucosa of the pelvis or infundibulum or calyx. Under such circumstances it is well to place a laparotomy pad outside the pelvis so that any stones washed out may be recovered.

Alternatively, one may place a No. 10 or 12 French Robinson catheter in the renal pelvis and into each individual calyx. Irrigation may then be done through the catheter. Malleable metal catheters are also available for this manipulation.

The "Water-Pik®" Spray in Renal Pelvis Irrigation

The innovative high-pressure spray system widely used in dental care may be adapted to irrigation of the renal pelvis to loosen up an adherent stone trapped in a calyx. This should be used with minimum pressure and extreme caution, since serious bleeding and tissue damage may result from improper use of the spray. Cautious experimentation should precede its use—the fine swirling spray may be either helpful or dangerous, depending on its application.

Purposeful Failure to Close Pyelostomy to Allow Passage of Calculi

If all attempts to locate a calculus are unsuccessful, the following method may prove helpful in rare instances. A lower-pole nephrostomy and a pyelostomy may be done, placing No. 28 French catheters through each site. The renal pelvis may be irrigated copiously with saline or one-fourth percent acetic acid solution for the next 10 days.

The nephrostomy tube is then removed, maintaining negative pressure on the tube by suction with an Asepto syringe. The calculus, if small enough, will often present itself at the opening of the sinus tract. If the stone if larger, irrigation through the pyelostomy tube may wedge the stone in the sinus tract. It may on occasion be forcibly removed with a hemostat, or even crushed and irrigated out.

Additional Maneuvers for Removal of Calculi

Should the lower-pole nephrostomy and irrigation technique prove unsuccessful, one is still in a position to insert a panendoscope or nephroscope through the nephrostomy site to visualize the stone and remove it with the aid of a cystoscopic rongeur. A stone forceps may be passed blindly through the panendoscope sheath into the nephrostomy site. If one feels the grating of a stone, it may be grasped and removed.

Bleeding is often initiated by stone forceps manipulation so that endoscopic vision is disturbed. Therefore, this should be done only if all other methods fail.

Renal Papilla May Simulate Grating Sensation of Stone

Blind palpation into each separate, distinct calyx with a Randall forceps will often reward one with the grating sensation of the stone. One must remember, however, that contact with the renal papilla (calyceal cup) very often will simulate a grating sensation. One may in error grasp the papilla and attempt to remove the "calculus." The mucosa is often torn in this unfortunate accident and severe bleeding occurs. Bleeding under such circumstances may be controlled by pressure with a peanut sponge against the involved area. Most often this bleeding will stop spontaneously.

It may be necessary, on occasion, to do a nephrotomy through the involved calyx so that the pressure of the balloon catheter may control the bleeding. Excessive uncontrolled hemorrhage may necessitate nephrectomy on a rare occasion.

Spontaneous Rupture of the Kidney with Ureteral Stones

Spontaneous rupture of the kidney secondary to ureteral stones occurs more frequently than suspected. There is wide divergence of opinion regarding the need for surgical intervention in these patients. Conservative measures, with the prime object the removal or passage of the obstruction, are advocated by some. Other urologists report extensive damage from the extravasation following the rupture and claim that the drainage of this is paramount in importance, with removal of the obstruction secondary.

It should be noted that removal of the obstruction often results in prompt resolution of the parenchymal rupture. If rapid resolution of the rupture, as shown by diagnostic studies, does not occur, nephrectomy may become necessary.

The importance of close follow-up should be stressed. The decision to observe or treat the patient surgically will depend on the clinical course. An afebrile patient whose pain has subsided can be observed.

Ileal Ureter for Repeat Stone Formers

The anastomosis of an isolated loop of ileum to the renal pelvis or to the dilated lower calyx should be considered in instances of markedly hypotonic and dilated ureters. This loop of ileum (in the isoperistaltic direction) may serve as an ileal ureter or as an ileostomy to allow passage of repeated large stones in patients who are chronic stone formers.

Completion of Pelviolithotomy or Nephrolithotomy

Pelvio- or nephrolithotomy is not complete until all fragments of calculi are removed. The calyces are then repaired with fine catgut suture. Bleeding from a small nephrotomy wound is controlled by fat tabs fixed in place with mattress sutures through the capsule. X-rays of the kidney should be taken before the patient leaves the operating room.

Small sterilizable films, placed under the kidney, are of tremendous help in this type of X-ray. One can, of course, wrap the X-ray cassette in sterile sheets or pillowcases as previously noted.

Calculus in the Solitary Kidney

A more conservative viewpoint must be maintained in the treatment of calculi in solitary kidneys. Repeated bouts of pyelonephritis or hematuria may prompt one to intervene surgically. The patient often accommodates well, however, to the decreased renal function. It is recommended that these patients be treated by long-term courses of antibiotic or chemotherapeutic agents.

In the event this solitary kidney has been previously operated, the indications for conservative management are all the more accentuated. Surgery on this solitary kidney is fraught with the danger of its loss as a result of secondary surgery. Under circumstances like this, one is faced with the need for possible reimplantation of this kidney to a lower site in the patient, or if this is not practicable, placement of the patient on a dialysis program.

Pregnancy and Renal Calculi

Obstetrician-gynecologists should be encouraged to obtain postpartum flat plate films and intravenous pyelograms on those patients who were treated for "pyelitis of pregnancy." Staghorn calculi are treated much more frequently in the multiparous female than in the nulliparous one. The multiparous patient also has stones ten times more frequently than the nulliparous patient. It is best that these pyelograms be done about eight weeks postpartum.

Chapter Five

THE URETERS

THE TRICKS OF the trade applicable to diagnosis and treatment of renal pathology are closely allied to those dealing with the ureters. There are, however, specific aids applicable to the ureter which warrant detailed description.

Again, as in previous and future chapters of this book, procedures of common acceptance and use will not be emphasized. Some generalities in the management of ureteral calculi are, nevertheless, reviewed.

CONSERVATIVE MANAGEMENT OF URETERAL PATHOLOGY
Ureterolithiasis
Introduction

Detailed etiology and symptomatology with reference to ureteral calculi are not discussed in this book. It is well recognized that most ureteral stones 6 mm or less in diameter will pass spontaneously, assuming that the calculi are smooth and free of spicules. Pure uric acid calculi are non-opaque and small. Therefore, a patient who gives a history of having passed such calculi rarely requires cystoscopic instrumentation or open surgery.

Approximately 50 to 60 percent of ureteral calculi 8 mm or less in diameter will pass spontaneously within three weeks. The stones are usually about 1 mm smaller in actual size than those one can see and measure on the X-ray film.

While awaiting the passage of a small stone one may medicate for relief of pain and ureteral spasm. Opiates for pain and tripelennamine (Pyribenzamine) or large doses of intramuscular propantheline bromide (Pro-Banthine) are all occasionally effective in decreasing ureteral spasm. Intravenous mannitol to promote increased urinary output volume in hospitalized patients has also been utilized. Intravenous valethamate bromide (Murel), in 20-mg doses, may be administered prior to transurethral manipulation of calculi.

Spinal anesthesia will allow more ureteral relaxation with occasional passage of a calculus. Intraluminal ureteral topical medications have been advocated, with controversial acclaimed success.

Generalities in Small Stone Management

A "watch-and-wait" position is usually taken in most instances of small stones. Estimates are that 75 to 80 percent of all stones pass spontaneously. In occasional cases, stones greater than 1 cm in diameter do pass.

On rare occasions, stones as small as 3 or 4 mm in diameter may become impacted and will not pass. Such an obstruction (due to calculus plus edema) may cause rapid progressive hydronephrosis. Cystoscopic manipulation is then indicated.

A stone impacted in one location for six to eight weeks may result in stricture at the site of obstruction. Therefore, instrumental intervention or eventual surgery is indicated in a calculus which is not progressing downward. Calculi impacted in the ureter may produce various other pathological changes, dependent on the size of the calculus in the specific area of the ureter, the absence or presence of infection, etc.

Indications for surgery, when cystoscopic methods fail, include stones approaching 1 cm in diameter, or smaller stones of irregular contour which seem to be impacted. Additional indications for surgery are sepsis, rapidly progressive ureterectasis or pyelectasis, continuous and intractable pain, and long-term immobility of calculi.

Atypical Symptoms with Stones

About 20 percent of patients with urinary calculi have symptoms not referable to the urinary tract. These situations may be very confusing. In complete ureteral obstruction with no drainage down the involved ureter, the urinalysis also may be entirely normal.

Calculus, Appendicitis, or Other Diagnostic Pathologic Entity

On occasion, the differential diagnosis of a possible right ureteral calculus versus possible ruptured appendix is presented. The plain X-ray may not be informative if the calculus is nonopaque, or is not visualized over bone. An intravenous pyelogram may be helpful—intravenous pyelography with tomography is more useful. A rectal examination should always be performed. Sometimes a high rectal mass will lead to the correct diagnosis. Pelvic inflammatory disease by virtue of its proximity to the ureter frequently simulates urinary tract disease.

One will occasionally encounter a dissecting aneurysm which will simulate completely a ureteral obstruction. When nonfunction of a kidney is thought to be due to a nonopaque stone not visualized on pyelography, the actual diagnosis may be dissecting aneurysm or massive renal infarction. The diagnosis of a dissecting aneurysm is only too frequently made at autopsy.

Seminal vesiculitis must also be considered as a possible differential diagnosis. Other less common differential diagnostic possibilities must be recognized depending on the site of pain and the side involved. Such remote conditions, on rare occasion, as black widow spider bites and herpes zoster may present diagnostic problems.

Undiagnosed Microhematuria May Herald Nonopaque or Early Calculus

An occasional patient with microhematuria and minimal symptoms of costovertebral angle pain may exhibit a normal pyelogram. After a period of one or two years, these patients have been known to spontaneously pass calculi, or a previously nonopaque stone may become radiopaque by virtue of being coated by calcium salts. These possibilities must be considered and discussed when one first sees a patient with undiagnosed microhematuria. The referring physician is impressed by the wisdom of his urological consultant when the patient with undiagnosed hematuria passes the discussed possible calculus of a year previous.

Diagnostic studies such as air pyeloureterograms may demonstrate a nonopaque calculus in the renal pelvis.

Calculi Causing Sepsis

It has been axiomatic throughout the years that infected urine must be drained. Basically this axiom remains unchanged, but with the availability of broad-spectrum antibiotics, it is often rewarding to start the patient on an antibiotic, waiting 48 hours before considering manipulation or open surgery when dealing with a stone that one would otherwise expect to pass. In the majority of cases, the infection will be controlled and the patient will subsequently pass the stone.

If the patient does not quickly respond to antibiotic therapy, open surgery or manipulation can then be performed. Chemotherapy for 24 to 48 hours before ureteral manipulation will reduce the possibility of bacteremic shock secondary to the manipulation.

Where the calculus has been lodged in one position for a long time, suggesting impaction, or in situations where the stone's size suggests undue time in passing, the urologist must follow the time-honored maxim that infected urine must drain and immediately institute drainage.

Cystoscopy, with passage of a ureteral catheter or a ureteral stone extraction instrument beyond the stone, is indicated for calculi in the lower one-third of the ureter. For stones in the upper or midureter under the same circumstances, ureteral catheter drainage or, if unsuccessful, immediate open surgery, is indicated. Once manipulative methods are begun, the watch-and-wait position must be abandoned for definitive therapy.

Air Disimpaction of Ureteral Calculi

Air disimpaction of ureteral calculi is utilized by some urologists to dislodge stones in any location in the ureter. Since air is compressible, it will readily rise above a calculus if enough is injected (10-15 ml). Air is less apt to rupture a ureter than is water under hydrostatic pressure. Even large stones in the ureteropelvic junction may be successfully dislodged by the introduction of approximately 5 ml of air through the ureteral catheter to the region of the stone.

This method is less successful in the intramural ureter because of difficulty in passing the catheter far enough to obtain a satisfactory seal. As the injected air goes by the stone, a gush of urine through and around the catheter follows. If the air does not pass around the stone, a larger catheter or a Braasch bulb is utilized and 5 ml of air is again injected. Even though the stone may not pass, dislodging it by this method affords relief until other conservative measures may be tried, or until the patient can be prepared for surgery.

Should the above methods fail, and if the stone is not removed on the second passage of a Dormia or Johnson basket or a bulb or looped catheter, depending on the patient's age, general physical status, size of the calculus, etc., one has the options of either attempting to pass and anchor ureteral catheters again or, if unsuccessful, performing open surgery.

Aid to Visualization of Calculus in Lower Ureter

An opaque stone in the lower ureter may be better visualized by injecting air by means of a catheter into the bladder. This has the effect of pushing the bowel out of the field and makes for stronger contrast of the stone. Another method is to fill the bladder to capacity with sterile water—the water-filled bladder displaces the intestines upward. Therefore, the lower 4-5 cm of ureter is no longer obscured by bowel. (See *Operating Table Pyelographic Visualization of Elusive Calculus*, in Chapter Three.)

Indications for Manipulation of Calculi in Lower Ureter

If with conservative treatment there is no progress in the downward passage of a ureteral calculus, and there is increasing ureteral dilatation, the stone located in the lower one third of the ureter may be manipulated. The ideal calculus for manipulation is round, smooth, and less than 5 mm in diameter. However, some urologists will manipulate calculi up to 1 cm in diameter as seen on X-ray.

Some urologists consider stone extraction in female patients easier and more successful than in the male patient. It is felt also that complications are greater in the male patient.

Major Surgery Preparation Necessary Before Instrumentation of Stones

Whenever a calculus is scheduled to be manipulated cystoscopically, one should also schedule the patient for major surgery and so inform the patient. The possibility of being unable to pass the stone basket or like instrument beyond the calculus, or of perforation or avulsion of the ureter, must always be considered. The patient, therefore, may by necessity or preference be subjected to open surgery immediately after stone manipulation.

Post-instrumentation infection should always be guarded against and anticipated. With the current state of the art in antibiotic therapy, some margin of safety is afforded the patient who has an unsuccessful stone manipulation. As noted, antibiotic therapy, started several days before cystoscopic manipulation, protects against acute bacteremic shock.

Frequently, after unsuccessful stone manipulation, the ureter is dilated to such an extent that the stone will pass spontaneously.

Initial Instrumentation with Stone Basket

The Dormia stone basket has proved most helpful in the authors' armamentarium. The Johnson basket, due to the stiffness of the basket wire seems to be more traumatic.

Should the stone fail to be removed on first or second passage of a stone basket, ureteral catheters may be passed beyond the stone and left in place from 48 to 72 hours. Preferably a No. 5 or 6 French * ureteral catheter is first passed beyond the calculus. Attempts at passing a second catheter of the same size should then be made if the first catheter has passed the stone.

With one catheter inserted beyond the stone, one has the option, after 48 to 72 hours, of removing the catheter and hoping the stone will pass spontaneously through the dilated ureter, or manipulating the stone secondarily. If two or more catheters were passed, one has the additional option of twisting, trapping, and extracting the stone.

After the first passage of a ureteral stone basket beyond a calculus and unsuccessful extraction, it is not always possible to pass any instrument or ureteral catheter beyond the stone for the second time. This is usually due to ureteral edema from trauma. Therefore, "the first pass may be the only pass."

Second Attempt at Calculus Extraction with Stone Basket

Having failed to insert any instrument beyond the stone with the primary manipulative attempt, a second manipulative procedure is scheduled. If able to pass and anchor one or preferably two ureteral catheters, these

---

* The No. 4 French ureteral catheter *per se* drains inadequately; however, there is some drainage *around* the catheter. Therefore, *two* No. 4 French catheters may well permit sufficient drainage. The No. 5 French ureteral catheter drains at the minimal adequate flow; the No. 6 French (or larger) ureteral catheter is most satisfactory.

catheters may be left in place from 48 to 72 hours. At the end of that time, one of the catheters may be removed and a stone basket passed be- yound the stone, after which the second ureteral catheter may be removed.

Some urologists prefer the passage of ureteral catheters as the primary maneuver in stone manipulation, following this with passage of the Dormia basket and attempted extraction—catheter passage tends to dilate the ure- teral orifice and ureter and is less traumatic than extraction of the stone without preliminary dilatation.

Traction on Stone Extraction Instrument

A spiculated or flat stone may turn sideways in the basket and be im- pacted in the ureteral mucosa. If the calculus is engaged in the basket but does not come down readily, the instrument may be left indwelling with *light* rubber band traction applied for 24 to 48 hours. The rubber bands are attached to the distal end of the basket instrument and the distal ends of the rubber bands may be placed on stretch, pulling on the stone extractor. The rubber bands at their distal end are taped securely to the patient's lower extremity. One or two ounces of traction is preferable. Up to one pound of traction has, however, been used.

Some urologists, after sedation of the patient, exert traction once or twice per day for a stone enmeshed in a basket. This may be continued until the stone is removed or the empty basket is extracted.

Many urologists are strongly opposed to any traction for removal of a ureteral stone because of possible ischemic changes occasioned by the continuous pulling and pressure of an impacted stone. Avulsed ureters, ureters denuded of mucosa, etc., have been reported secondary to ag- gressive traction. Other urologists oppose any type of basket manipulation— these questions continue to be debated.

Impaction at the Ureteral Meatus

Should calculus impaction occur at the ureteral meatus, a ureteral mea- totomy can be done with the basket in place, avoiding contact with the basket if performed by electroresection. An arcuate artery which runs across the top of the meatus may bleed readily. Fulguration of this vessel may be necessary.

Ureteral Stone Basket Modification to
Accommodate the Urethral Filiform Tip

When attempting to remove a ureteral calculus with a stone basket, it is a distinct advantage to use a long filiform attached to the stone basket. If one does not engage the stone, as noted when the basket is withdrawn into the bladder and viewed through the cystoscope, the long filiform is still in the ureter beyond the stone. It is then much easier to again manipulate the stone basket beyond the calculus. For this reason, long filiforms should be utilized. There are, however, no long filiform attachments for the Dormia or Johnson baskets.

A local instrument man can change the screw tip on these instruments to that of the thread of American-made instruments. Thus one may have available the filiforms ordinarily used for passage beyond urethral strictures in male patients which readily fit the screw thread of the Phillips catheters or Le Fort sounds. This makes repeat manipulation for the stone much easier.

One disadvantage to the filiform technique is that less direct traction may be applied while viewing endoscopically the basket as it is withdrawn. The manipulative procedure as originally described by Dormia called for removing the endoscope and applying traction, which permits movement of the ureter downward toward the bladder neck. Using this technique, the calculus usually falls into the surgeon's hand as the basket is withdrawn from the urethral meatus. The filiform may be a safeguard for those who have a tendency toward impatience and are tempted to "lean on the basket" using the original technique. An avulsed segment of ureter on the stem of the basket is a frightful sight.

Use of Ellik Loop Catheter for Ureteral Calculi and Stricture

For a patient with recurrent ureteral calculi and consequent ureteral stricture, one may pass an Ellik loop catheter up the ureter into the renal pelvis where a loop is carefully formed. The looped catheter is then brought down very cautiously and slowly. This is most successfully performed as a staged procedure, first merely engaging the stone in the loop and on subsequent days intermittently applying traction after the stone is "glued" to the loop. The bulk of the loop precedes the calculus down the ureter acting as a dilator. Extracting the calculus intermittently affords a better dilating effect.

A 2-oz fishing weight may be attached to the distal end of the looped catheter and left for one to three days, exerting minimal traction, in order to further dilate the stricture.

Use of Fogarty Catheter in Ureteral Manipulation

A No. 4 or 5 French Fogarty catheter may in certain instances be passed beyond a stone and the balloon inflated above it so as to permit manipulation with a stone basket without the risk of pushing the stone back into the dilated ureter.

Fixation of Ureteral Stone with Multiple Ureteral Catheters

When one has several ureteral catheters around a ureteral calculus, twisting the catheters about each other may entrap the calculus. In most instances the catheters will not entwine about the calculus due to the limited space available for catheters to move around a calculus in the ureter. The emplaced catheters, however, serve to dilate the ureter about the stone. The calculus therefore more readily passes spontaneously on removal of the catheters.

Medication to Facilitate Passage of Calculi and Prevent Infection

The emergent situation present with an impacted ureteral calculus is relieved after passage and anchoring of a ureteral catheter(s) and the establishment of good renal pelvis drainage. One may leave such catheters in position for three to four days.

Appropriate effective gram-negative chemotherapeutic and antibiotic medications may be used, such as the ampicillins, nalidixic acid, the nitrofurantoins, cephalosporins, etc. Some urologists prefer the instillation of neomycin sulfate in 0.5 percent solution into the renal pelvis several times per day via the ureteral catheters.

There are clinicians who feel that instillation of a 1 to 2 percent procaine solution will diminish ureteral spasm, facilitating passage of a calculus. Sterile olive oil, 2 to 3 ml, has also been employed. The use of these medications is of questionable value. Following spinal anesthesia, however, a number of instances of passage of ureteral calculi are documented.

Parenzymes for Inflammatory or Reactive Ureteral Edema

Edema due to trauma caused by a calculus may in itself create complete obstruction where previously the calculus was only partially obstructing. The use of sterile chymotrypsin (Alpha Chymar), an enzyme capable of selectively reducing inflammatory or reactive edema, is therefore recommended. The drug, in reducing the edema, may also permit the spontaneous extrusion of the stone. The recommended dose is 0.5 ml intramuscularly twice a day. These enzymes are also beneficial in reducing edema following ureteral surgery or retrograde pyelography.

Additional Ureteral Pathology
and Therapeutic Aids

Tests for Ureteral Fistulae in Females

When intravenous pyelography and cystoscopy do not clearly indicate the presence of a suspected ureteral fistula, one may pass a bulb catheter into the ureteral orifice and through the catheter inject indigo carmine or methylene blue in the dilution of 5 ml per 100 ml of water or saline. At the same time, one may inject boiled milk into the bladder. If blue dye is found in the vagina, this is proof that the fistula is a ureterovaginal one.

If one is certain he is not dealing with a vesicovaginal fistula, but not certain as to which ureter communicates with the vagina, then one may inject phenolsulfonphthalein (diluted 1 ml to 100 ml sterile 5 percent sodium bicarbonate solution) into one ureter and methylene blue into the opposite ureter, using a bulb ureteral catheter first in one ureter and then the other. By the color of the dye in the vagina one determines which ureter has the ureterovaginal fistula. Usually, the routine intravenous pyelogram will demonstrate changes in the ureter on the involved side.

Differential diagnostic studies must often be done when the fistula is in the intramural ureter.

Visualization of Upper Tract and Ureter in Ureterocele Patients

In patients with ureterocele, the ureteral opening at times may not be visualized, or impossible to catheterize, so that evaluation of the upper tract is prevented. One or the other of the following steps may be tried:

1) One may watch the ureterocele until there is bulging outward during a peristaltic wave and then with a Bugbee electrode cut over the maximum point of the bulge to open up the ureterocele (ureteral reflux may occur with this maneuver).

2) One may pass a needle on a flexible shaft through the panendoscope and inject the bulge of the ureterocele at the time of the peristaltic wave, in order to instill the contrast material. The orifice, if seen, may be enlarged with cystoscopic scissors.

Ureteral Biopsy

If prior to excision surgery one suspects polyp or tumor of the lower ureter, pathological diagnosis can often be made by cystoscopic biopsy of the lower ureter. Under adequate anesthesia, a ureteral stone basket may be passed above the area that is under suspicion. Following the passage of the basket, the bladder is emptied. The basket is then rotated (always clockwise to prevent filiform from coming loose on its thread) and withdrawn into the bladder. Tissue of sectionable size is frequently obtained.

After a few minutes, allowing the renal urine to flush out the curetted ureter, the bladder contents are again removed. The material obtained is promptly sent for tumor cell stains, or sections can be made of the material. Bleeding is usually minimal.

Brush Biopsy Technique

An innovative method for trapping ureteral biopsy tissue employs the passage of a large open-ended catheter up to the lesion with a smaller catheter temporarily within it to provide a smooth tip. Retrograde pye-lography, aided by image-intensified fluoroscopy, may be used to check the positioning. The small inner catheter is then replaced by a disposable wire with a tiny nylon or steel bristle brush at the tip. The lesion is brushed back and forth from three to five times to trap biopsy material in the bristles.

This maneuver may succeed in trapping fragments which would other-wise never be available for biopsy. It has proved of significant value in certain cases.

High-Pressure Irrigation and Aspiration Biopsy

One may instill vigorously and aspirate vigorously, via whistle-tip ure-teral catheter and 10-ml syringe and needle, sterile saline into the ureter (or as mentioned previously, into the renal pelvis). Tiny pieces of tumor and tumor cells are obtained from the aspirated fluid. These are then sub-jected to tumor cell stain and microsection study.

Length of Infant Ureter for Catheterization

A simple rule of thumb to determine how far to insert a ureteral catheter in an infant is to measure the distance from the suprasternal notch to the symphysis. One half of this length will represent the length of the ure-ter in the infant and the distance to insert the catheter. A tape measure, or preferably a ureteral catheter, may be used to determine this measurement.

Fixation of Length of Ureteral Catheter Stylet

When using ureteral catheter stylets to facilitate passage of a ureteral catheter, one must use caution not to pass the stylet beyond the eye of the catheter. When the stylet is passed to the distal tip of the ureteral catheter,

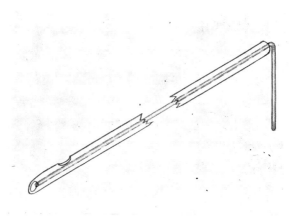

34. Bend in proximal end of ureteral catheter stylet

one may bend the stylet back on itself at the proximal end of the catheter, as shown in Figure 34. This will prevent excessive length of the stylet in the ureter and fix the site of the stylet in the catheter.

Connecting Ureteral Catheters for Drainage

There are many methods for connecting a ureteral catheter for drainage. In one procedure, a needle of adequate caliber is inserted into the lumen of the ureteral catheter for tight-fitting, leakproof drainage. The filter end of intravenous tubing is cut off and the needle end of the tubing is connected to the needle which is in the catheter. A finger cot is then placed over an empty intravenous bottle and a hole is made in the finger cot of such size that the plastic tubing fits snugly into it. This makes a tight, satisfactory collection device, and prevents the end of the tubing from pulling out of the bottle. However, the needle in the ureteral catheter serves as a trap and prevents free and adequate drainage. A needle also may be placed into the collection bottle to provide an airway.

Another method of connecting a ureteral catheter for drainage is the following: Depending on the size of the ureteral catheter, a 1¼- to 1½-inch needle is placed from within the balloon catheter at its distal end outward and threaded into the ureteral catheter. The needle then serves as a stylet to help guide the ureteral catheter end into the lumen of the balloon catheter. The ureteral catheter is then pushed through the needle lumen pathway of the balloon catheter.

With the above method, one must be sure that the entire length of the needle remains within the lumen of the ureteral catheter for adequate reinforcement in pushing the ureteral catheter through the wall of the urethral catheter.* The ureteral catheter then drains into the urethral catheter. The standard urethral catheter drainage tubing and bottle (plastic closed type) is then connected to the urethral catheter; a leakproof connection results. See Figure 35.

Other methods include the use of perforated cystoscopic rubber tips which can be easily attached to both the catheter and the plastic intravenous tubing. A rubber cap on a medicine dropper may be perforated at its end and the catheter threaded into the medicine dropper. This can then be inserted into latex tubing which is in turn connected to a Gomco suction pump. The tip of the medicine dropper, if such is used, must be filed off with an "ampule file" to make it impossible for the dropper lumen to also serve as a trap.

For better fixation of the ureteral catheter and bladder drainage, a bal-

---

* Note: A small safety pin tip heated to "red hot" may be used to burn a tiny hole in the wall of the balloon catheter to facilitate passing the ureteral catheter through the latex of the urethral catheter. This union is not as leakproof as when no hole is burned through the catheter.

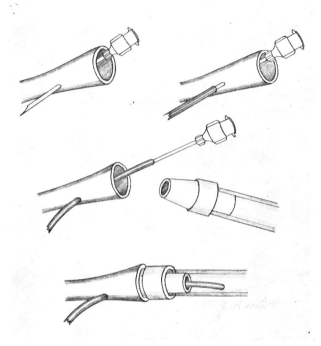

35. Method of connecting ureteral catheters for drainage

loon catheter is passed into the bladder and the ureteral catheter is
tied to the balloon catheter in several places with silk or cotton suture material. The urethral catheter is then connected to gravity drainage.

Anchoring Ureteral Catheters for Drainage

When it is vital to drain a kidney with a ureteral catheter, reliance on a
balloon-type catheter alone to maintain the position of the ureteral catheter
is unsatisfactory. One can tie the ureteral catheter to the balloon-type
catheter, leaving the tie long, and then tie the string ends to a suspensory. Should the balloon bag rupture, both the balloon-type catheter and
the ureteral catheter remain anchored in position to the suspensory. The
balloon catheter may then be replaced without removal of the ureteral
catheter.

Long-Term Catheter Drainage for Ureteral Obstruction

The long-term use of indwelling catheters of Silastic tubing or other
inert plastic material, introduced at cystoscopy, has not been adopted generally by urologists. Nephrostomy, cutaneous or loop ureterostomy, ileal
conduits, etc., for ureteral obstruction due to cancer, particularly carcinoma
of the cervix, continue to be diversionary methods of choice. In se-

lected cases, however, Silastic catheters may be well tolerated, and since they are worn internally there is no need for a collecting device.

A catheter of the largest size feasible, usually 0.125 inch (9.6 French) outer diameter and 28 to 29 cm long, should be used. A catheter of smaller size may be required. The tubing is beveled at its proximal (kidney pelvis) end, sealed with silicone rubber cement, and allowed to set for 24 hours. Three to four drainage openings are made, and it is then gas-sterilized.

The catheter is passed, with a smaller ureteral catheter inside acting as a marker and providing rigidity, all the way up to the 26- to 28-cm level, for good drainage, and the cystoscope is then removed. In the female (where this procedure is especially valuable) a hemostat is then placed blindly * transurethrally, grasping the Silastic tube and holding it in place while the ureteral stylet catheter is withdrawn. The Silastic tube is then appropriately cut and coiled back into the bladder. The tubing length of 28 or 29 cm should allow 1 or 2 cm to protrude into the bladder distal to the ureteral orifice.

This is a simple, practical means of drainage in some instances. The catheter may remain in place for a number of months, with minimal incrustation.

Drainage Holes Made in Silastic Tubing

Small drainage holes made in Silastic tubing near the sealed end may be made using a very small scissors or by use of a No. 12 or 14 needle heated to a red heat. Holes burned into the Silastic by this latter method are smoother than those cut by scissors.

Removal of Silastic Tubing Inserted Beyond the Orifice

Occasionally Silastic tubing is inserted beyond the ureteral orifice. In one such instance, suspected incrustation warranted removal of the catheter. A No. 6 French Dormia basket was passed about 8 to 10 cm and the basket opened. The snug gripping of the tubing by the basket (or vice versa) allowed the tubing to be withdrawn from the ureter.

Small (No. 6 French) cystoscopic alligator forceps or cup biopsy forceps may also be used; the intraluminal tightening resulting from the insertion and attempted opening of jaws of such an instrument may aid in the gripping and extraction of the tubing. Use of the last-mentioned instruments should be done with the utmost caution—such maneuvering is extremely limited in its application.

---

* The cystoscope and flex grasping forceps may be used in place of the blind procedure to grasp the Silastic tube.

Passing Ureteral Catheter Beyond Obstructed Area

When true obstruction does not exist, one may still find it impossible on occasion to pass a ureteral catheter cystoscopically due to angulation or to a mucosal fold just within the orifice. Passage of two small olive-tip catheters into the ureteral orifice, alternately probing each catheter, will sometimes allow one of them to pass.

This is analogous to the bypassing of an area in the urethra when one experiences difficulty in passing a filiform—at times the passing of a second or third, or even a fourth filiform, may enable the passage of one instrument. The same technique will work very much the same way in the ureter, but limited to two catheters.

Reinsertion of Anchored Ureteral Catheter to Higher Level: Determination of Proximal End Site of the Catheter

It is necessary at times to maintain a patient on indwelling ureteral catheter drainage. After 24 to 48 hours the drainage openings of the catheter may slip down out of the renal pelvis. Pushing the catheter, *per se,* does not move the catheter up the ureter. It is quite easy to pass the catheter back up to the kidney by inserting a wire ureteral catheter stylet which will stiffen the catheter sufficiently to allow the catheter to be reanchored in its original position. Caution must be exercised to avoid passing the stylet beyond the eye of the ureteral catheter.

One encounters considerable resistance to the passage of the stylet at the ureteral orifice site of the ureteral catheter. If the stylet cannot be advanced it may be held in place while the ureteral catheter is fed up over the stylet. The support afforded the ureteral catheter in its course through the urethra and trigone by the stylet prevents the catheter from coiling up in the bladder.

The proper repositioning of a ureteral catheter is best determined by X-ray. When positioned correctly, the catheter is then reanchored at the meatus to a balloon catheter by tying one to the other with heavy black silk or cotton suture.

Care of Indwelling Ureteral Catheter

When the ureteral catheter is left indwelling, irrigation of the catheter by nursing personnel, though undesirable, sometimes becomes necessary, especially where there is a considerable amount of mucus and pus present. The irrigation by staff nursing service has always presented the danger of cross-infection, contamination, etc. The following orders should therefore be given for the care of indwelling catheters.

> Irrigate ureteral catheter q ——— hours with strict aseptic
> precautions, using:

1) sterile water for injection, USP;
2) a *new* disposable 2-ml or 5-ml syringe each time;
3) sterile 22-gauge needle for 4 French,
          20-gauge needle for 5 French,
          18-gauge needle for 6 French,
          16-gauge needle for 7 French.*

There may be substituted for the sterile water for injection a solution of any antibiotic used for intravenous or intramuscular injection which comes in a rubber-capped vial or bottle, or a powder that can be dissolved in water or saline and kept in a rubber-capped vial until used.

This method assures the least possible chance of contamination, as the nursing staff will treat it just as they would an intramuscular or intravenous injection. Neomycin, 3 to 5 ml of a 0.5% solution, serves as an excellent irrigant or as an antibiotic instillation measure. Furacin ® solution as a 1:6 dilution in distilled water or saline also is a very useful irrigant.

Ureteral Catheter Perforation of Ureter

The lower one third of the ureter damaged or perforated by ureteral catheterization will almost invariably quickly seal. The patient should be maintained on antibiotics for prevention of possible periureteral abscess. If a catheter can easily be redirected and passed up into the renal pelvis, it should be left indwelling for 48 hours or longer. Where damage to the ureter is in midureter or the upper one third of the ureter, drainage of a subsequent periureteral abscess often becomes necessary. A trial of conservative observation and antibiotics is warranted. Should sepsis and pain persist, T-tube splinting and repair of the ureter over the lower limb of the tube are advisable.

Good rules to follow are that: (1) perforation of the lower one third of the ureter may be treated by broad-spectrum antibiotics; (2) middle or upper one-third ureteral perforation may be treated like (1) for 24 to 48 hours. If sepsis and pain continue, surgical drainage and antibiotics are necessary.

OPEN SURGERY

Ureterolithiasis

Fixation of Stones During Open Surgery

When seeking a ureteral calculus by palpation, the operator, on palpating the stone, grasps it with his index finger and thumb so that it does not slip up or down. It is important that assistants do not attempt to palpate the stone before it is immobilized. Many operations for ureteral calculi

---

* These figures may vary slightly depending on manufacturer and type of catheter.

have been complicated, or the stone lost, because of needless or inopportune palpations.

After the stone has been located and immobilized, Babcock clamps may be placed above and below the calculus. When the surgical approach to the ureter is simple and the ureter is easily visualized, with the calculus "bulging," the operator should immediately place the Babcock clamps, avoiding the possibility of the calculus slipping up out of the operative area on palpation. The upper clamp should be placed first. The ureter is then incised over or above the stone as it is removed. Special instruments such as the Lewis ureteral stone isolation forceps have been devised to hold the calculus in place.

When a calculus has been impacted for a long period of time, it is desirable to move the stone upward and to do the ureterotomy in an undamaged section of the ureter.

Extraperitoneal Surgical Approach

The surgical approach to the ureter may easily be done extraperitoneally. Though the normal ureter is rather elastic and resistant to injury, the presence of long-standing infection or a stone in the ureter for any length of time causes the ureter to become thickened and friable so that traction on it may cause it to tear. To minimize the danger of a ureteral tear, one may use a small Penrose drain above the calculus, after first incising the two outer edges of the drain to almost two thirds of the way across its diameter. When cut thus, the exerting of traction will cause the Penrose drain to give way before the ureter (as mentioned in Chapter Four with reference to the kidney; see Fig. 22).

Location of Ureter in Pelvis

The lower one third of the ureter should be exposed always in the region of the promontory of the sacrum. In the usual extraperitoneal approach, one looks for the ureter as it crosses the iliac vessels. The ureter is frequently pulled out of the field with peritoneum. If one will expose the iliac vessels at the promontory and allow peritoneum to fall back on to the vessels, the site of peritoneum meeting the vessels may be grasped with Allis forceps. The ureter is almost invariably found within the grip of the forceps.

Transperitoneal Approach for Ureteral Calculi

Although the ideal method of exposing the ureter for a stone is extraperitoneal, there are certain occasions in which transperitoneal approach is necessary. In patients who have had two or three or more stones removed from the same site, it sometimes is impossible to mobilize a ureter.

Therefore, a transperitoneal approach may be made, extracting the stone and closing the peritoneum over the incised area with drainage retro-peritoneally.

This approach has been utilized on occasion in patients who had been subjected to previous ureterolithotomies. The surgical approach was further complicated in several instances in patients suffering from severe Marie Strümpell arthritis, with marked fixation of the spine. The transperitoneal approach allowed the removal of stones with ease under these circumstances.

The ureter is best located at the pelvic brim crossing the iliac vessels. One looks to the left of the sigmoid colon on the left side, to avoid damage to the blood supply to the colon entering medially.

Calculus Location in Ureter: Measurement Relative to Self-Anatomy

A calculus is often lower in the ureter than one suspects from X-ray visualization. To accurately pinpoint the location of a stone, the graduates on the ureteral catheter may be utilized as a ruler, with measurements taken on the X-ray film from specific other reference points, e.g., the lower edge of a vertebral body or sacral promontory, etc., to stone site.

As previously mentioned, use of known measurements from a surgeon's own anatomy—distal phalanx width, thumbnail diameter, index finger length—as measuring guides can be very helpful.

Muscle-Splitting Incision for Stone in Upper Ureter

A large stone fixed in the upper ureter may be readily removed through the flank, muscle-splitting incision described by Dr. F. Foley many years ago. For details, the reader is referred to a standard textbook. We mention here five points of particular importance:

  1) Positioning—patient not flexed to the usual degree used in renal surgery, in order to more easily retract the muscles;

  2) Location of ureter—usually attached to the peritoneum, and not found posteriorly;

  3) Placement of clamps—accomplished early in operation because of limited operative area;

  4) Incision convertibility—if inadequate, can be easily converted to subcostal incision;

  5) Approach—more suitable for stones near L3 and L4 than for calculi in the uppermost ureter (L2).

The usual procedure, after splitting the muscles and incising the lumbodorsal fascia, is to push the peritoneum forward with a sponge stick until the ureter is found on the peritoneal side. If the vena cava or aorta are visualized, "back up." This is more a visual procedure than a "finger" procedure. Palpation of the stone, though frequently possible, is usually unnecessary. Without mobilizing the ureter, a Babcock clamp can be placed above the ureter or the Lewis ureteral stone forceps can be placed directly over and under the stone. The ureter is incised and the calculus removed. Closing of the ureter is optional. A drain is placed down to the site of the incision in the ureter.

Transvesical Removal of Impacted Lower Ureteral Calculi

Impacted stones in the lower ureter, 1 to 2 cm above the ureteral orifice, may present a difficult surgical approach. This is especially true in obese patients. There usually is a considerable amount of inflammatory process around the thickened adherent ureter, and the calculus may be partially embedded in ureteral mucosa. This type of ureteral stone, impacted in or just above the intramural ureter, may be approached transvesically with less difficulty than when one attempts to do a ureterolithotomy from behind the bladder.

A cystotomy is done. One may palpate the stone through the bladder, or one may palpate intravesically and with the other hand palpate the intramural ureter in the extravesical position. If the stone is not palpable, the juxtavesical ureter may be exposed by incising the bladder mucosa and muscle in the line of the ureter. The ureter is grasped with a Babcock forceps. Plastic or umbilical tape or Penrose drain is placed around the ureter to prevent the stone from moving upward, the exposed ureter being pulled downward into the bladder.

The ureter may then be opened, the stone removed, and the ureter closed with fine absorbable catgut. After ureteral closure, adequate length of muscularis of bladder is closed behind the intramural ureter to prevent reflux if the original incision was made low enough to disturb the previously normal passage of the ureter through the bladder wall. The mucosa is then closed over the ureter.

A splinting catheter may then be passed up the ureter and brought out suprapubically or through the urethra. To bring the splinting catheter out via the urethra, one may first pass a catheter into the bladder transurethrally. The splinting catheter is tied temporarily to the transurethral catheter which, when removed, pulls the splint easily to the exterior transurethrally. The tie is then cut. A urethral balloon catheter may be reintroduced and tied to the splinting catheter to ensure its position (see *Anchoring Ureteral Catheters for Drainage* in earlier part of this chapter).

Modification of Transvesical Approach to Calculi in the Lower Ureter

Another approach to the lower ureter begins with opening the bladder in the usual manner. An incision is made in the *posterior* wall of the bladder about 2.5 to 5 cm above and lateral to the ureteral orifice, in an oblique fashion. The lower ureter is then exposed readily through this bladder

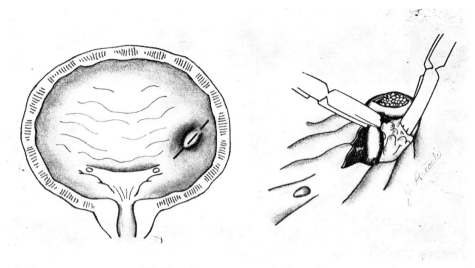

36. Posterior incision in bladder for access to calculi in the juxtavesical or intramural
    ureter

incision. The ureter can be further fixed by passing a catheter up to the
point of obstruction.

With this technique the stone is removed transureterally via the transvesical approach. The incision is also helpful if there is considerable inflammatory change in the lower ureter. Since the ureter has been mobilized,
it can be reimplanted into the bladder if necessary. See Figure 36.

Ureteral Stone Forceps

The Lewis ureteral stone isolation forceps is a very helpful instrument
in the performance of ureterolithotomy. When the calculus is located, it
may be immobilized by using the forceps. A small incision may be made
over the calculus, and the posterior blade of the stone forceps then used
to quickly and easily force the calculus out of the ureter. Keeping the instrument in place facilitates closure of the ureterotomy.

The Babcock forceps also may be used for this purpose. One may twist
them one-half turn and maintain them thus, one above and one below, to
prevent the calculus from moving upward or downward. Some surgeons
use umbilical tape, ¼-inch Penrose drains, or plastic tapes above and below the calculus to maintain its position.

X-Ray Localization of Ureteral Calculi in Surgery

Occasionally it is impossible to palpate the stone in the operative field.
One may not be certain whether the calculus is above or below the area
exposed. A small silver McKenzie brain clip or Samuels blood vessel clip

the anatomical relations in the pelvis. The infusion pyelogram usually visualizes the ureters vividly. *The passage and anchoring of ureteral catheters will facilitate the surgery.*

The surgeon performing pelvic surgery should be advised not to have a false sense of security on completing the removal of the diseased organ as all too often the ureteral injury occurs during closure of the pelvic peritoneum. On withdrawing the ureteral catheters, previously labeled right and left,* at the end of the operative procedure, the surgeon should realize that any resistance to their withdrawal could indicate ureteral damage by suture. If resistance is met, the catheter should be left indwelling and correction immediately instituted.

In cases of iatrogenic ureteral injury, the best results in repair are obtained when the injury is discovered in the immediate postoperative period, before extravasation of the urine produces a considerable amount of inflammatory reaction and scarring. A slight temperature elevation, pain or tenderness in either flank and persistent ileus should alert the consultant to order an immediate intravenous pyelogram (preferably infusion) and further diagnostic studies. If an obstruction is noted, immediate cystoscopy with attempts to pass a ureteral catheter will help localize the problem. Repair should be done without delay. Occasionally both ureters will be involved, with resultant anuria. This is an obviously emergent problem.

Forcible Breaking of Ureteral Catheter Tie

On occasion, a catgut tie around the ureter may be forcibly broken by passage of a No. 8 to 10 French wedge-shaped-tip ureteral catheter. This maneuver may spare the patient the need of open surgery. The procedure must be performed before ischemic necrosis of the ureter from a tie has occurred. It is imperative that identity of the suture material used in the vicinity of the ureter be known. Following passage, a ureteral catheter should be left indwelling. It is assumed, too, that there will be excellent urinary drainage through the catheter passed into the renal pelvis.

Pyelostomy or nephrostomy may be a lifesaving procedure if obstruction is not immediately relieved. Frequently corrective surgery, including deligation, is necessary. At times ureteral reimplantations are required, etc., depending on time factors and etiology and size of the obstruction.

Stylets to Facilitate Palpation of Ureteral Catheters in Pelvic Surgery

In certain cases, especially where there is a considerable amount of pelvic inflammatory disease, suspected tumor, or extremely large uterine fibroids, the gynecologist will request the presence of inlying ureteral

---

* See *Identification of Anchored Ureteral Catheters*, soon to follow.

catheters during pelvic surgery. The added use of a ureteral catheter stylet to stiffen the indwelling catheter is an aid both in passing the catheter up to the desired length, and also in palpating the ureteral catheters at the time of surgery.

Identification of Anchored Ureteral Catheters

If color-coded catheters are used, the *red*-tipped catheter is used for the right kidney (*R* for *Right*). If no color-coded catheters are employed, the beveled-end catheter is used for the left side, the *right* or *unchanged* catheter is used for the *right* side.

Ureteroneocystostomy

In pelvic surgery, ureteral damage is most frequently located close to the bladder. The problem may be rectified by any one of a number of techniques for ureteroneocystostomy.

Under general or spinal anesthesia, a midline suprapubic or transverse suprapubic (Pfannenstiel) incision is made to expose the bladder and perivesical spaces. The lower ureter may be identified and the involved portion examined. Occasionally it may be necessary, where part of the ureter has been destroyed, to use a rectangular flap of bladder as a ureteral tunnel (Boari flap) and anastomose this to the remaining ureter in an antireflux fashion. Portions of ileum have been used when long portions of ureter are necessary, or ureteroureterostomy.

T-tube splinting or transureteral splinting may be utilized. Some urologists use no splints. At times, one may suture the bladder on tension to the posterior pelvic wall musculature, so that less ureteral length is required for ureteroneocystostomy.

URINARY DIVERSION
Cutaneous Ureteroileostomy

Urinary diversion by means of cutaneous ureteroileostomy has proven to be a satisfactory means of diversion. The following considerations may be of interest in regard to this subject.

Preoperative Preparation for Ileostomy, Colostomy, and Incontinence Devices

Of extreme importance is the proper location for a proposed ileostomy or other 'ostomy device. The patient, whether adult or older child, should wear the chosen device for two weeks prior to surgery, finding the best eventual position for the 'ostomy.

This trial is especially important because of belt lines for panty tops and girdles in female patients, and the belt line in the male patient. The exact preferred position of the device can be marked for this two-week preoperative trial, so that the location of the stoma is determined before the patient undergoes surgery. One may be misled as to the 'ostomy site with the patient prone on the operating room table.

By following this regime, many problems of type and fit of the device, comfort, etc., that commonly occur in the postoperative period are eliminated.

Skin Site for an Ileal Loop Stoma: Skin Incision

One may mark off a skin site for an ileal loop stoma by cutting around the edge of the barrel of a large drinking glass or plastic syringe. Any other sterilized circular object of the surgeon's choice may be used, including a clamp opened and employed as a compass for marking purposes.

An abdominal wall punch is now manufactured in five standard sizes which produces a symmetrical tubular channel through all layers of the abdominal wall. Hopefully this will minimize the complication of stomal conduit stenosis.*

Changing the External Appliance

When a patient with an ileostomy is undergoing change of the external appliance, a sudden gush of urine may completely undo a meticulous skin preparation and application of cement. To prevent this, a Pyrex ® glass tube may be placed over the stoma, packing cotton loosely around the stoma. A tampon may be used in place of the Pyrex tube. The skin can thus be prepared in an unhurried fashion without danger of urine spillage.

Adhesive Discs for Ileostomy

One of the more difficult problems encountered with ureteroileostomy is the finding of the proper adapter for the cutaneous ileostomy. Many patients develop excoriation and dermatitis with the use of the skin cement that is necessary to hold the adapter over the ileostomy.

Double-faced adhesive tape discs which adhere to the rubber or plastic 'ostomy appliance as well as to the skin are made by specialty manufacturers such as Marlen Manufacturing and Development Company and the 3 M (Minnesota Mining and Manufacturing) Company. Should skin excoriation remain a problem, sterilized treated powder pads are available which give complete skin protection, eliminating irritation and promoting healing of sore skin areas.

---

* N. L. Bosworth and P. D. Stull, "Conduit Stenosis Prevented by an Abdominal Wall Punch," *Journal of Urology*, 108:413 (1972).

Additional Sources of Appliances for Urinary Diversions

Disposable and permanent types of appliances and accessories for urinary diversion may be obtained from the following manufacturers:

Atlantic Surgical Company
1834 Lansdowne Avenue
Merrick, New York 11566

Marlen Manufacturing and Development Company
5150 Richmond Road
Bedford, Ohio 44146

Nu Hope Laboratories
2900 Rowena Avenue
Los Angeles, California 90039

Torbot Company
1185 Jefferson Boulevard
Warwick, Rhode Island 02886

United Surgical
Division of Howmedica, Inc.
Largo, Florida 33540

Disposable appliances may be obtained also from:

Hollister, Inc.
211 East Chicago Avenue
Chicago, Illinois 60611

The above companies constantly upgrade their merchandise and keep abreast of new developments to make the life of the 'ostomy patient more comfortable and secure.

We are aware of the existence of similar firms. The above listing is not intended to be complete, nor does it constitute an endorsement. It simply indicates that we know and have experience with these firms and their products.

New Paramedical Discipline*

The International Association for Enterostomal Therapy, Inc. (IAET) was conceived at the United Ostomy Association annual convention in 1968 at Phoenix, Arizona, by enterostomal therapists under the guidance and inspiration of Rupert B. Turnbull, Jr., M.D., colon-rectal surgeon at the Cleveland Clinic. Dr. Turnbull trained the first enterostomal therapist in the late

---

* Information courtesy of Mrs. Patricia Klemens, Certified Enterostomal Therapist now in private practice in the Los Angeles, California area.

1950's, and a training program was begun at the Cleveland Clinic early in the following decade.

The International Association for Enterostomal Therapy now recognizes five institutions as accredited to train therapists. The association has approximately 150 members at the present time in all parts of the world.

Accredited institutions are as follows:

Ferguson-Droste-Ferguson Hospital
Grand Rapids, Michigan 49502

Harrisburg Hospital
Harrisburg, Pennsylvania 17101

The Cleveland Clinic
Cleveland, Ohio 44106

Emory University Hospital
Atlanta, Georgia 30322

Roswell Park Memorial Institute
Buffalo, New York 14203

The authors feel that it is most helpful to call upon an enterostomal therapist to guide and instruct patients who are to be subjected to 'ostomy surgery. This instruction should begin several weeks prior to the scheduled surgery.

Chapter Six

THE BLADDER

BLADDER SYMPTOMATOLOGY AND DIFFERENTIAL
DIAGNOSTIC PROBLEMS

MANY CONDITIONS ENTIRELY unrelated to obstructive genitourinary tract pathology may make themselves evident by primary urinary
tract symptomatology, for example, herniated disc, diabetes mellitus, multiple sclerosis, etc. Urinary tract symptoms may also be manifested as a result
of the use of anovulatory medications or other drugs. Drugs and drug
categories that have been implicated in urinary tract and bladder symptomatology were listed in Table III, Chapter II.

One should bear in mind such related situations as are known to cause
urological symptoms. For example, frequency, dysuria, and urgency of urination may be markedly improved by the administration of estrogens to the
patient with postmenopausal cicatricial atrophic vaginitis and urethritis.

Bladder symptomatology may be due to myriad causes; many diverse
problems requiring a multitude of orthodox and unorthodox approaches
are presented by the *vesica urinaria*. A urological outlet obstructive disease
in combination with a neurological process may be impossible to differentiate.

Again, it is stressed that no attempt is made herein to cover all of the related subjects under a specific heading. Only a limited number of aids considered applicable in light of the book's purposes and aims are presented.

Some Nonurological Nonobstructive Causes of Bladder Symptomatology

Bladder Dysfunction Due to Herniated Disc or Other Neurologic Disease

Any type of bladder dysfunction which cannot be explained by thorough
urologic evaluation must be considered as possibly secondary to central and
peripheral neurologic lesions. A herniated disc is a commonly missed neurological lesion which may involve the bladder, with neurological findings
from nil to minimal. One must consider, too, the fact that the first and only
presentation of neurovesical dysfunction often occurs many years before
the actual disease itself. This is especially the case in patients with multiple
sclerosis.

Unsuspected diabetes mellitus must also be included in this large elusive
group of neurological vesical dysfunction diseases, as well as the cerebrovascular accidents, combined sclerosis, etc.

Urinary Tract Infection Associated with Hematuria During Menses

Women subjected to pelvic surgery who thereafter have symptoms of recurrent urinary tract infection and hematuria associated with menses must be suspect for the possibility of uterovesical fistula. The patient may often confuse severe hematuria with her menstrual bleeding. One should, therefore, have an awareness of possible uterovesical fistula under these circumstances.

Eosinophilic Cystitis

A patient may present with marked hematuria several months after the performance of suprapubic prostatectomy, vesical diverticulectomy, or other bladder surgical procedure. Resection of the bleeding area may reveal eosinophilic cystitis—presumably a hypersensitivity reaction to the chromic catgut used in the procedure. This is another reason for postoperative bleeding which must be borne in mind.

Hematuria Due to Cyclophosphamide (Cytoxan)

Patients with treated or untreated carcinoma who are on long-term chemotherapy with cyclophosphamide (Cytoxan), a nitrogen mustard compound, will often have hematuria of very severe degree involving bladder mucosa. Though the serum half-life of the compound may be about 4 hours, the drug or metabolites are detected in serum for as long as 72 hours. Therefore, the hematuria may be prolonged in some instances.

It is imperative that the patient be informed of the need of ample fluid intake and frequent voiding.

(See also *Control of Bladder Hemorrhage Due to Cytoxan Therapy, etc.,* this chapter.)

Urinary Leakage vs Vaginal Discharge

An occasional female patient may complain of urinary leakage shortly after voiding. Examination may be entirely uninformative, revealing no evidence of a urethral diverticulum, vesicovaginal fistula, stress incontinence, or other urologic problems such as ectopic ureter. Patients with urethral diverticula may have slow leaks to account for the continued moisture.

One may try giving the patient phenazopyridine hydrochloride (Pyridium), making certain the patient wipes after voiding. If no orange stain is later found in the patient's panties, one may presume that the moisture complained of is probably due to a vaginal discharge. One may place a cotton pledget into the vagina and remove this before the patient voids. Lack of color usually eliminates any possible ureterovaginal or vesicovaginal fistula. Discharge from a diverticulum may not be stained, however, nor may drainage from an ectopic ureter where a double kidney segment is nonfunctioning.

The patient found to be voiding into the vagina may, to eliminate her leakage problem, be advised to do forceful evacuation of the vagina after voiding by increased intra-abdominal pushing.

Additional Causes for Bladder Symptomatology

Various medications or foods may account for urinary tract symptoms or signs, e.g., dysuria following medication, or red urine following the ingestion of beet soup. Other symptoms and causes are acute retention due to hematocolpos, rectal spasm, or local abscess; pressure sensations and urgency due to pelvic extravesical masses, etc.—the list may be endless. (See also *Urine and Symptomatology* section in Chapter Two.)

DIAGNOSIS AND THERAPY OF BLADDER PATHOLOGY AND DYSFUNCTION

Diagnostic Aids in Study of the Bladder

Air Cystometry

Since the development of automatic-recording cystometry the use of air as the filling medium in cystometry has proved advantageous. Air need not be sterilized, is more comfortable for the patient, and can be instilled much faster due to lack of viscous drag. A formerly time-consuming procedure is now done quickly and easily with the use of an air cystometer. Introduction of this instrument has made cystometry in infants and children practicable.

Universally Available and Disposable Cystometer

Cystometric studies are often not made despite indications for their performance and their obvious value diagnostically, because of the immediate unavailability of a cystometer. Disposable spinal manometer units may be used, or the apparatus may be constructed from readily available material (see Fig. 38).

The items necessary are a balloon-type catheter, a meter or yard stick, an intravenous unit (1000 ml of sterile water or saline and plastic tubing with 18-gauge needle), and clear plastic tubing of the kind in common use for bedside catheter drainage (to be used for manometer).

A 20 French balloon-type catheter is inserted transurethrally into the bladder and the bag distended with 5 ml of sterile water. The meter stick is fastened to an intravenous standard with the bottom of the meter stick at the estimated level of the bladder neck. One end of the clear plastic drainage tubing is taped along the meter stick and the other connected to the

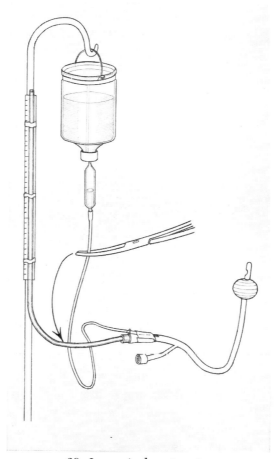

38. Improvised cystometer

catheter. The 18-gauge needle of the intravenous unit is inserted into the lumen of the urethral catheter, *directed toward the bladder*, proximal to and on the opposite side of the "Y" used to fill the balloon of the catheter. The needle is anchored to the catheter with a piece of adhesive tape.

The urethral catheter is clamped distal to the needle, and solution is allowed to flow into the bladder in increments of 25 to 50 ml. At the end of each 25- or 50-ml increment, the intravenous tubing is clamped and the urethral catheter unclamped. Readings are taken of the height of the liquid in the column. The results are plotted on a graph, pressure against volume, and the curve is interpreted.

If cystograms are desired during the same examination, radiopaque material should be used as a substitute for water or saline. When cystometry is completed, the cystogram may be taken. The urethral catheter is then removed and a voiding cystourethrogram is taken, followed by a postvoiding cystogram. Evidence of possible ureteral reflux is thus noted.

The described apparatus is also useful for closed bedside irrigations, with the drainage tube diverted to a dependent collection bag.

Instrument to Measure Bladder Neck: Kollmann Dilator

A simple device to measure accurately the dynamics of the vesical outlet is lacking. No instrument precisely measures bladder neck contracture or vesical outlet stenosis, hypertrophied internal sphincter, etc. One may examine a bladder neck with an endoscope and estimate the size of the bladder neck, but it is difficult to appraise the diameter within several millimeters.

If one will pass a well lubricated and normally working Kollmann dilator and then slowly open the blades, the slightest increase in resistance of the bladder neck can be felt; by then looking at the dial on the instrument, the diameter of the bladder neck may be determined. The Kollmann dilator, therefore, used in this manner may also serve as a diagnostic instrument. It is assumed that the determination is made with the patient under anesthesia.

Calibration in this fashion is unreliable in the presence of urethral strictures. In situations where the tapered portion of the dilator is not located within the urethral meatus where the caliber of the urethra is often normally smaller, the examiner may meet urethral meatal resistance before encountering bladder neck resistance.

Bladder Tone Determination

Determination of bladder tone may be accomplished simply by inserting a balloon-type catheter and then filling the bladder slowly by gravity through an Asepto glass syringe until the patient experiences the urge to void. The syringe, still attached to the catheter, is lowered or raised till the water level in the syringe is on a plane with the bladder level. If the bladder tone is adequate, the fluid rises in the Asepto syringe when the patient attempts to void, perhaps running over the top of the syringe. In patients with poor bladder tone, the water in the syringe will rise only a slight amount.

Alternatively, plastic drainage tubing can be attached to the balloon catheter and held up about 24 inches; water will rise up the tubing if bladder tone is adequate. This rather crude cystometric test is of practical value in determining when to remove indwelling balloon catheters in patients with urinary retention on a myogenic basis.

Flat Film of Abdomen for Bladder Size

Urinary retention may be suspected in a patient in whom catheterization may be contraindicated. A plain film of the abdomen may be taken over the bladder area. If the bladder shadow does not appear on the first film, a second film with different X-ray penetration may be done. Usually, in the event of a full bladder, the X-ray will demonstrate an appreciable bladder shadow suggesting residual.

More accurate estimate of residual urine is obtained by pyelography and the postvoid film over the bladder area.

Bladder Infections

Bladder Infections Associated with Adjacent Structures

One must assume that under usual and normal circumstances the urinary tract does not become infected. Recurrent cystitis, therefore, in addition to the many urinary tract factors *per se*, may be caused by conditions outside of the urinary tract. Some patients void large volumes of urine into the vagina during urination, only to have this urine wash back again into the bladder.

One may demonstrate this by placing about 100 ml of 20 percent sodium methiodal, NF (Skiodan Sodium), or other contrast material into the vagina and asking the patient to gently adduct her legs and then extend them. Fluoroscopically intensified observation may demonstrate reflux of this contrast material into the bladder.

Alternatively, one may place blue vegetable dye in a bathtub full of water. The patient may flex her legs upward toward the abdomen and then slowly extend the legs downward (assuming that the bladder has been previously emptied). After douching the vagina to be certain all of the coloring material has been eliminated from this area, the patient may then carefully empty her bladder into a bedpan. Blue dye in the bedpan is an indication that the colored material has entered the bladder from the tub water.

Frequent detergent douches and vaginal chemotherapeutic or antibiotic creams are required to prevent recurrent infections in these patients. Therapy thus directed towards the vagina decreases the vaginal bacterial flora concentration and the possibility of bladder implication.

Voiding while swimming or just before swimming may result in aspiration of water into the bladder through the urethra, since exercise may cause negative intra-abdominal pressures.

The increased trend of rectal coitus in the younger generation demands that the urologist be aware enough to direct his history to obtain this information. The increased incidence of rectal gonorrhea should alert the urologist to consider this possibility and to perform more rectal cultures.

Despite instruction to female patients concerning proper drying techniques after voiding and bowel movement, vaginal contamination by Escherichia coli remains exceedingly common. The proximity of the rectal and vaginal areas and the movement of bacteria by underclothing or iatrogenic causes demands more attention by the urologist to minimize bacterial contaminating flora by advocating the use of antiseptic vaginal creams, suppositories, and improved mechanical cleansing methods. Women will often report the onset of bladder symptomatology following coitus.

Our simple expedient advice consists of the following:

1) Douche two to three times per week regularly, at bedtime. The douche may consist of 2 to 3 drops of a surgical detergent soap to 2 quarts of water, or ⅓ cup vinegar to a douche bag of water.

2) Follow douche by antiseptic cream or tablet, such as triple sulfa vaginal cream, nitrofurantoin suppository, Vagisec ® Jelly (polyoxyethylene nonyl phenol, edetate sodium, dioctyl sodium sulfosuccinate, aminacrine hydrochloride), Gynben Vaginal Inserts (diiodohydroxyquinoline, sulfadiazine, diethylstilbestrol in a base containing sodium lauryl sulfate, tartaric acid, boric acid, dextrose and lactose, and koalin), or another vaginal antiseptic cream of equal efficacy.

The patient should be advised to wear loose clothing, to avoid panty hose (especially in hot weather), panties of synthetic fabrics, hygienic sprays to vaginal area, bubble bath, strong soaps, etc. (See *Etiology of Dysuria*, in Chapter Two.)

Infections in Neurogenic Bladder: Means of Decreasing Residual Urine and Clearing Infection

In patients with neurogenic bladder who have residual urine and infection resistant to therapy, one should predetermine the amount of residual urine. The patient should be asked to void, and a catheter then passed into the bladder and the residual urine removed. The latter is replaced with air of a larger volume. For example, if the residual urine is 90 ml, one may place into the bladder 120 to 150 ml of air (which will compress to a smaller volume of space). The air will gradually be replaced or absorbed over a period of two or three days.

In the meantime, the air replaces the residual urine in the bladder. The patient voids without carrying residual urine to serve as a bacterial culture medium. Air occupies the highest area of the bladder and is expelled *last* during the emptying phase of a normal bladder which carries no residual urine.

This procedure, done on one or two occasions, may result in spontaneous clearing of infection, even though on a temporary basis. Moderate success has been obtained with this method of treatment on selected patients. Some exceedingly resistant neurogenic bladder infections have been cleared by this means.

Bladder Calculi

Television Monitoring in Bladder by Image Amplification

Some urologists prefer crushing a large bladder stone with a blind lithotrite. Calculi must either be crushed in this manner or removed surgically when they are too large in size to be crushed by the observation lithotrite.

One may visualize the lithotrite and the stone by placing the patient under the image amplifier, especially when there is an associated television monitor. The grasping of the bladder stone and crushing may be monitored under vision. With the availability of the portable image amplifier and television monitoring operating room equipment, this method is now much simplified.

It is probable that standard operating cystoscopy tables will in the near future be equipped with image amplification equipment. This will greatly facilitate the placing of catheters in the *renal pelvis* and the visualization of *ureteral instrumentation.*

Transrectal Alignment of Lithotrite

Most urologists have a favorite instrument for crushing calculi in the bladder. The Hendrickson lithotrite affords good visibility. However, the metal catch holding the sleeve attached to the lower jaw may spring loose and cause the jaws of the instrument to turn at right angles, so that the lithotrite cannot be closed for its removal per urethra. The position of the jaws may be visualized by an X-ray film or by fluoroscopy. With a gloved finger in the rectum, the jaws of the instrument may be most adequately manipulated and properly aligned under image amplification, and then successfully removed, thus obviating cystotomy.

New Method of Lithotripsy

The innovative technique of stone crushing by ultrasound recently described by Russian urologists has been introduced into this country. This should encourage the development of advanced instruments for the employment of ultrasonic energy for stone disintegration.

The small, broken-up pieces are irrigated out of the bladder.

Interstitial Cystitis

Diagnostic Signs

When a patient gives a history of urinary frequency, and the urologist on distending the bladder to capacity with fluid finds the fluid volume to be smaller than normal, along with terminal bleeding upon emptying of the bladder, interstitial cystitis is suggested. Most normal bladders will not bleed on overdistention.

Patients with interstitial cystitis also find distention of the bladder very painful even before capacity is reached.

The typical stellate vessel findings of interstitial cystitis described in most standard textbooks are not always seen. Biopsy of these bladders is also frequently misleading as to the diagnosis of interstitial cystitis. However, biopsy is favored by many as a means of differentiating interstitial cystitis from the occasional case of carcinoma of the bladder that does not present itself as the usual mucosal lesion but, instead, is located beneath the mucosa.

Possibility of Perivesical Fluid Extravasation with Hydrostatic Bladder Dilation

One must be well aware that the mucosa is the water barrier and that with mucosal distention and tear following hydrostatic bladder dilation, perivesical fluid extravasation may occur. An occasional patient with severe suprapubic pain following such dilation must be suspected of having extravasation. These patients, fortunately, almost invariably improve on catheter drainage and complete bladder decompression over a two- to three-day period. A rare patient may become infected and require perivesical drainage.

Treatment Modalities

Bladder dilation at repeated intervals, under anesthesia, will often dramatically improve for a time the symptomatology of a patient with interstitial cystitis. Dilation followed by thorough and wide fulguration or transurethral resection of the lesion also will give dramatic and long-standing relief up to six months or longer. Some patients, however, have symptomatic relief from the above therapy for only short periods of time. For those patients requiring frequent bladder dilation—for example, once a month—subtotal cystectomy with either a small or large intestine patch must be considered.

Tumors of the Bladder, and Sequelae

Aid to Staging of Bladder Tumors

Visualization of the bladder wall in the presence of bladder tumors is sometimes aided by injection of air into the space of Retzius, followed by hypogastric angiography bilaterally by way of percutaneous femoral catheterization.

Injection into Bladder via Cystoscope

Cortisone, Thiotepa, or even radiotherapeutic solution may be injected into the bladder by means of the flexible shaft needle, which may be used through most cystoscopes. One must be on guard as to the depth of insertion of the needle. There is no way to prognosticate the thickness of the bladder wall. The needle must therefore be inserted very close to the bladder mucosal level.

This needle and shaft were developed years ago for the injection of adrenalin and other medication directly via cystoscope into the prostate.

Control of Bladder Hemorrhage Due to Cytoxan Therapy, Telangiectasia from Radiation, or Bladder Tumor: Use of Glucose, Olive Oil, Formalin, and Normal Saline Filling

Bleeding from any of the above causes may occasionally be difficult to control. Fulguration, if possible to perform, will be helpful but there are instances in which it is impossible to control the hemorrhage. The use of 50 percent glucose, sterile olive oil, or 4 to 5 percent formalin in the bladder may then be tried. One should use 25 to 50 ml of the 50 percent glucose, and clamp off the catheter for 20 minutes. About 2 to 4 ounces of sterile olive oil placed in the bladder, with the catheter clamped off for 15 to 20 minutes at a time, may also be useful if the glucose therapy is not successful.

Should both the above methods fail, one may use formalin. *When using this solution, anesthesia prior to the introduction of formalin into the bladder is necessary.* The bladder may be gravity-filled with a solution of 4 to 5 percent formalin (30 to 50 ml). Some urologists have used up to 10 percent formalin for short instillation periods. The general anesthesia must be carefully maintained to prevent the patient from spontaneously emptying the solution into the urethra. The bladder must be emptied of formalin *by the same* CATHETER since *there is danger of severe stricture of the urethra should the patient void out the solution.* Some men place mild traction on the balloon catheter to prevent urethral spillage.

The formalin is left in the bladder for 20 to 30 minutes. Depending on the bleeding site, the patient may need to be turned to one side or the other, or on his back or abdomen, for periods of 5 to 6 minutes. After the formalin is emptied out of the bladder, BY CATHETER, the bladder is irrigated with several hundred milliliters of 10 percent alcohol, followed by irrigation with large amounts of normal saline.

The disadvantage of the use of formalin is that the bladder volume is markedly decreased due to severe fibrosis.

As a last resort, before undertaking cystotomy, one may use intravesical pressure from saline. The bladder may be distended with normal saline until the pressure is great enough to keep blood from coming into the bladder. The catheter in the bladder may then be connected to an open-end Y-tube placed in the inverted position. This Y-tube is kept at the height necessary to maintain the intravesical pressure at a level to prevent bleeding (see *Y-Tube Gradual Decompression Apparatus,* near the end of this chapter). After the urine becomes clear, the Y is lowered an inch or so every day until it is completely at bladder floor level.

For refractory Cytoxan cystitis, methylene blue solution instilled into the bladder and retained for about one-half hour may markedly improve symptomatology. Orally administered methylene blue tablets are also helpful.

Patient Follow-Up for Bladder Carcinoma

It is the practice of the authors to repeat follow-up cystoscopy on patients who have had bladder carcinoma every three months for the first five years. If there has been no recurrence, cystoscopy is done every six months for the second five years, and once a year thereafter. When recurrences take place, the three-month follow-up regime is again instituted.

This policy or a similar one should be the rule of all urologists. Numerous instances are reported of recurrence after ten to twenty years in patients with no other interval recurrence.

The tumor file follow-up and sending of recall cards, with first-class letters if no response is obtained, should be rigidly adhered to by all urologists and medical facilities.

Use of Papanicolaou Smear in Bladder Carcinoma

The follow-up care of patients who have had no recurrence of treated carcinoma of the bladder should include a Papanicolaou smear of the bladder urine sediment. In those cases in which there has been a suspicious or positive "Pap" smear, despite negative cystoscopy, further observation eventually shows the presence of a recurrence. In many cases, Papanicolaou smears foretell the recurrence of disease prior to its appearance on cystoscopy. We therefore suggest that the frequency of cystoscopy should be determined not only by visual findings in the bladder, but by findings on Papanicolaou smear.

Ultraviolet Tetracycline Fluorescence for Localizing Abnormal Mucosa for Biopsy

Ultraviolet tetracycline fluorescence studies have been used as a technique for localizing areas of abnormal mucosa for biopsy. Their usefulness is limited since carcinoma *in situ* is rarely found without some visible mucosal abnormality detectible with ordinary incandescent light cystoscopy.

Neurogenic Bladder

Bethanechol Chloride (Urecholine) Test for Neurogenic Bladder

It has been shown that when an organ is chronically without its motor nerves there develops an increased sensitivity to normal stimuli, as well as to calcium, potassium, tyramine, acetylcholine, etc. This response is demonstrated by striated muscle, smooth muscle, glands, and ganglia.

Stretching bladder muscle with fluid results in muscle contraction, with a rise in intravesical pressure. This stretch response is markedly exaggerated by bethanechol chloride (Urecholine) in the sensory and motor neurogenic bladder.

For the Urecholine test a 16 French balloon-type catheter is placed in the bladder, and 100 ml of saline is instilled into the bladder at the rate of 20 ml/minute. Urecholine, 2.5 mg, is administered subcutaneously and a continuous pressure recording is taken for a period of 30 minutes.

If the greatest intravesical pressure rise over control is less than 15 cm of water, no neurogenic disease in the sacral spinal cord area or the lower reflex arc is indicated. If there is pressure response greater than 15 cm over that of control and *not associated* with uninhibited neurogenic bladder, then there is disease involving the lower motor neurons or the afferent part of the lower reflex arc.

If uninhibited contractions of the bladder are present, the test may be done using spinal anesthesia. Should the response then be over 15 cm over control, the diagnosis is motor or sensory paralytic bladder. Many lower motor neuron patients will show increases of 40 to 60 cm of water pressure.

Clearing Infection in the Neurogenic Bladder

(See *Bladder Infections* section presented earlier in this chapter.)

Incontinence

Incontinence in Children Following Surgery

Instances are seen of children becoming incontinent following Y-V plasties and internal urethrotomy. To remedy this unfortunate problem, a Marshall-Marchetti-Krantz procedure may be performed.

Plication just proximal to the bladder neck, by placing a suture in the bladder musculature, lengthens the urethra. The suture is placed just proximal (3-5 mm) to the urethrovesical angle at the 3, 12, and 9 o'clock positions. When tied, this suture will plicate the bladder and create an elongation of the urethra by making the bladder neck closer to the interureteric ridge by 3 to 5 mm. This new "bladder neck" is then sutured to the midline fibrocartilage of the underside of the symphysis.

This technique has proved helpful for amelioration of incontinence in a great many cases by elongating the urethra and angulating the urethra at the bladder neck.

Bowel Training of Fecal-Incontinent Children with Myelomeningocele

Urinary diversion patients with conus medullaris lesions of myelomeningocele often become continent (even when there is a lax rectal sphincter and fecal incontinence) following bowel training.

A patient with this problem may be trained to react to irrigation of soapsuds or tapwater enema just as do colostomy patients. A daily enema, with the buttocks held firmly together to hold the liquid content, will train this bowel to empty in response to such irritation as the enema. In some instances, a suppository such as bisacodyl (Dulcolax) may be used daily in lieu of the enema. The bowel, of course, must first be well cleaned out before starting the training program.

Adult Urgency Incontinence: Use of Imipramine Hydrochloride (Tofranil), Anticholinergics, and Chlorpheniramine Maleate-Phenylpropanolamine Hydrochloride-Isopropamide (Ornade Spansules)

An occasional adult patient may have sufficient urge incontinence to confuse both the patient and the physician as to the possibility of the presence of a vesicovaginal fistula. Many patients have severe urge incontinence due to urethritis or trigonitis. Prostatectomy patients often have poor urinary control for several weeks postoperatively due to severe urge incontinence. Many of these adult patients will respond favorably to imipramine hydrochloride (Tofranil) therapy. Contraindications should be carefully followed; in particular, it is contraindicated for women of child-bearing age.

Tofranil may be started as a 25-mg dose and increased up to 100 mg three times daily. Often there may be no response to the minimal dose schedule, with resultant need to increase the dosage as indicated.

Anticholinergic therapy is also helpful for the urge-incontinence patient. Most post-prostatectomy urge-incontinence patients show marked improvement in symptomatology by the time six to eight weeks' postoperative healing has taken place. An occasional post-prostatectomy patient may have stress incontinence up to one year postoperatively.

If Tofranil and anticholinergics have not been successful, chlorpheniramine maleate-phenylpropanolamine hydrochloride-isopropamide (Ornade Spansules) may be utilized. Some patients respond to one or another medication on this type of regimen. In some instances, combinations of the above medications may be helpful.

Male Incontinence, and Measures for Control

True incontinence in the adult male patient is often of iatrogenic origin. Medical means are employed to treat urge incontinence. The problems of neurologic incontinence have been adequately described in most textbooks and in the literature. Anterior cystourethroplasty (Marshall-Marchetti-Krantz) procedures and modifications are less successful in the male than in the female. The recent perineal pressure plastic devices such as polyurethane foam-covered silicone gel prostheses are going through extensive clinical evaluations. Immediate results appear successful ·in a very commendable percentage of cases; long-range results must still be evaluated.

Angulation or elongation of the urethra; bladder neck wedge resections; bladder flaps; modifications of sling operations for application in the male;

creation of new vesical outlets sewed to the prostatic urethra; support, compression, and plication of the external sphincter; symphysiotomies; the Kelly plication operation and perineal pressure by use of varied types of appliances (including the silicone gel types mentioned above)—all are valuable aids in our armamentarium of surgical approaches to this unfortunate problem.

Some patients are relegated to use of one of the many incontinence devices such as the McGuire urinal. Others tolerate well a penile clamp like the Cunningham clamp. A wide-banded athletic support maintaining pressure against the penile urethra lying against the abdominal wall may be helpful. Some patients must resort to use of highly absorbent diaper-like material (such as the commercially available EVER-SAFE® and similar products). Others depend on this material inside a condom or plastic bag held on the penis by adhesive tape or suspended by string around the waist. Male patients may use the Fuller shield, reversing it from the position used by women. This shield (or belt), obtainable from surgical supply houses, is often used for a postoperative dressing in patients who have undergone combined abdominoperineal resection.

Eventual urinary diversions such as uretero-ileal cutaneous diversion are necessary in some instances. Urinary incontinence remains a problem which exacts a highly devastating emotional toll of the patient and the physician.

Female Incontinence, and Measures for Control

The incontinence problem is especially difficult to handle in the elderly female patient. Several methods for urine control are suggested:

1) Tofranil, anticholinergics, and Ornade may be tried, as suggested previously.

2) A urethral catheter may be emplaced and hooked up to a leg bag or to bedside drainage. Leakage around the catheter, however, often remains a problem.

3) A device called the Pilcher bag (now difficult to obtain) may be placed in the vagina to exert pressure against the urethra. Rubber tubing placed through the loop of the bag and brought to a belt around the waist, front and back, holds the bag in place.

4) A donut type of pessary, inserted in the vagina, may exert enough pressure against the urethra to control urine in some patients.

5) A 30-cc balloon-type catheter, placed in the vagina, may press against the urethra sufficiently to control a patient's urine. The amount of inflation of the balloon is dependent on the anatomy of the specific patient.

6) An inflatable type balloon pessary may also be utilized in the vagina. Such pessaries are inflated by a rubber bulb with male-female type valve connections and various types of cutoff valves to retain the inflated air.

7) The "Edwards female incontinence device," designed by a British surgeon, Dr. L. E. Edwards, and available from surgical appliance houses,* consists of a

* and direct from the manufacturer, Chas. F. Thackray Ltd., London, Leeds, and Glasgow.

small ribbed pressure applicator, a steel spring, and a triangular supporting frame. The pressure applicator fits into the vagina and presses on the urethra so that the flow of urine is prevented.

8) Two or three pieces of facial tissue, twisted into a wedge-shaped cone and lubricated, may be pushed into the vagina in such a way as to exert pressure against the urethra and result in some measure of control in certain patients.

Unfortunately, many devices placed permanently in the vagina will, by virtue of their pressure, cause vaginal ulceration and are therefore unsatisfactory.

The use of absorbent materials with protective covers such as those mentioned for the use of male patients (EVER-SAFE, etc.) must be resorted to by some women—an unsatisfactory expedient at best for their incontinence problem.

The various types of operative procedures described in standard textbooks and the literature are recommended for specific instances. Denudation of the labia minora and sewing the labia together below the urethra may result in a vagina which will better retain balloon-type catheters or inflatable pessaries.

BLADDER SURGERY

Positioning

Supine Position

In performance of open bladder surgery, the patient is placed on the table in the supine position. The legs are separated as far as possible without sliding off the operating table. Adducting the legs facilitates any of several maneuvers which may be needed: (1) passage of an instrument transurethrally into the bladder; (2) rectal examination or elevation of the bladder neck by insertion of a finger into the rectum; (3) exertion of vaginal upward pressure with a finger in the vagina (especially in peformance of a Marshall-Marchetti-Krantz type of procedure); and (4) use of a sponge forceps in the vagina to elevate the bladder neck, etc.

Low Lithotomy Position to Facilitate Vaginal Examination or Exert Counterpressure During Bladder Neck Surgery

It is sometimes advantageous to place the patient in the low lithotomy position when one is doing bladder neck surgery, including suprapubic or retropubic prostatectomy. The thighs remain unflexed in a low position, but widely spread in the knee crutches so that the surgeon's assistant or a nurse assistant may take a position between the patient's thighs (see Fig. 39).

Counterpressure per vagina or urethral instrumentation can readily be done. Because of the dependent position of the extremity from knee to foot, elastic stockings for prevention of venous stasis are advisable.

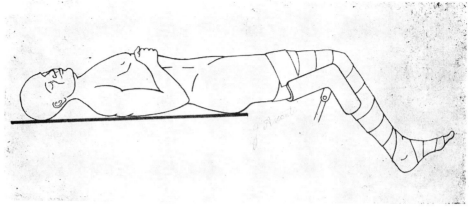

39. Positioning for bladder neck surgery
     A. Low lithotomy position

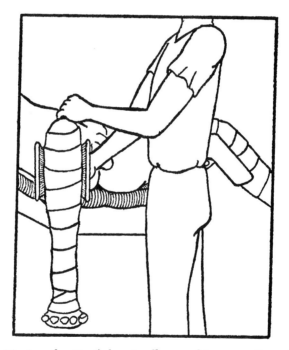

B. Positioning of patient's legs to allow working space for assistant

Use of Kidney Rest for Prostate and Bladder Neck Surgery

The patient's buttocks may be placed over the kidney rest in preparation for suprapubic or retropubic prostatectomy, bladder neck surgery, etc. By elevating the kidney rest, the bladder neck area is made more prominent and more readily accessible for performance of surgery in this area.

Incisions for Bladder Surgery

Commonly Used Incisions

The usual suprapubic incisions for bladder surgery are the vertical midline, the transverse, and the Pfannenstiel. For bladder neck surgery in females the transverse incision may be preferable. From the standpoint of cosmetic effect, so important to most women, the transverse incision is obviously preferred. For the male patient on whom bladder surgery is to be combined with hernia surgery, the transverse incision will afford exposure of the inguinal canal, but the hernia may also be approached from within the retroperitoneal space at the internal inguinal ring through a vertical midline incision.

On occasion it may be necessary to transect the recti muscles and/or the pyramidalis muscles close to the symphysis for more adequate and complete exposure. If muscle transection is done, repair (or muscle approximation) should be done preferably with interrupted suture.

Bladder Surgery Combined with Vasectomy

In males, a transverse incision often lends itself well to the additional performance of vasectomy. Separate scrotal incisions following the bladder surgery therefore are obviated.

Ligation of the vas deferens may also be done through a vertical midline incision, the vas deferens being found adherent to the peritoneum laterally.

Specialized Helpful Techniques

Facilitating Bladder Exposure

To aid bladder exposure (and of particular value where a secondary operation in the region of the bladder is done) the bladder may be filled either with air, saline, or water (the volume depending on the existing condition) before making the incision. This facilitates wiping (by blunt dissection with gauze on finger or stick sponge) the peritoneum from the bladder. The choice of medium is left to the operating surgeon. Air as the medium is more convenient, obviating the suction of fluid when the bladder is opened, but it should be avoided when dealing with a contracted bladder. Cracking of the mucosal barrier by distention can result in an air embolus.

Method for "Y-V Plasty" Pre-Bladder-Incision Marking

Prior to making the Y incision in contemplation of a Y-V plasty (or other type of plasty) one may use the electrosurgical unit to very lightly fulgurate the ends of both stems of the V aspect of the Y incision. This serves as a guide in making the required incision.

A marking dye such as methylene blue may also be used.

Opening of the Bladder

The bladder may be opened either transversely or vertically, depending on the procedure being performed. When one is doing a low suprapubic prostatectomy which may require extension of the incision into the bladder neck for better visualization of the prostatic capsule, a vertical incision is made. If one is contemplating an intravesical procedure, a transverse incision may be used. After a transverse incision is begun, fingers are inserted inside the bladder and retracted laterally to widen the bladder incision. This type of cystotomy is less apt to open vessels in the bladder wall.

Retraction of the Bladder Wall to Facilitate Exposure

Almost any type of retractor used in abdominal surgery may be utilized to keep the recti muscles separated and the wound open, but the Balfour or ring retractor is preferred. For better exposure within the bladder, one may use 3-0 mattress catgut suture through the bladder wall incisional edge on both sides, fixing the bladder wall incisional edge to the abdominal wall fascia in such a manner as to hold the bladder widely open. These sutures, tied loosely, may be left until the bladder procedure is terminated. As stated previously, the recti muscles at the symphysis may be divided if more exposure is needed.

Also, for retraction within the bladder, one may use malleable or Deaver retractors over lap sponges. "Stick sponges" provide good retraction. The assistant employs one in each lateral recess of the bladder, pushing backward (cephalad) and downward on the stick sponges.

If the Masson-Judd bladder retractor is utilized, the retractor is placed in the bladder and as the retractor is opened, the edges of the bladder are raised with an Allis clamp on each side, positioning the bladder edge over the top of the retractor until the latter is fully opened. The retractor will then remain entirely within the bladder—otherwise, it has a tendency to slip out of the bladder.

Extraperitonealization of the Bladder for Wider Bladder Manipulation

In performing a widespread procedure on a bladder which is difficult to mobilize, one may extraperitonealize the bladder and make it more readily workable for subtotal cystectomy, etc. The peritoneum is gauze-wiped off the bladder anteriorly as much as possible. At the region of the dome of the bladder, the peritoneum is usually very firmly attached to the bladder and, at times, may be removed only by sharp dissection. To circumvent sharp dissection and facilitate mobilization of the bladder, a transverse incision of the peritoneum is made in this area. The bladder is grasped with Allis clamps or Babcock forceps and pulled upward.

An incision is then made in the peritoneum, posterior and parallel to the

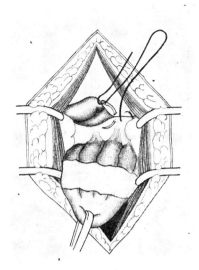

40. Cuff of peritoneum attached to extraperitonealized bladder

first transverse incision, over the bladder wall below the area of firm attachment of the peritoneum. The posterior pelvic peritoneum is swept off the bladder wall easily by blunt dissection, and the lateral ends of the posterior peritoneal incision are continued upward to meet the lateral ends of the anterior peritoneal incision. Following this the bladder is retracted or pulled out of the way and the peritoneum is closed with continuous fine catgut suture. A cuff of peritoneum (Fig. 40) remains attached to the now completely extraperitonealized bladder.

Traction for Better Visualization

A lesion deep in the bladder—a tumor, for example—may be better visualized and excised by placing black silk traction sutures through the bladder wall around the tumor. Allis forceps may be substituted for the traction sutures. Forceps would obviously not be applied to the tumor or in its vicinity.

Ureteral Orifice Location in Open Surgery on the Bladder

Urologists are familiar with the occasional case in which the search for the ureteral orifice through an opened bladder proves difficult, or often unsuccessful. This is most apt to occur in bladders previously operated upon, or when inflammation or tumor is present. If severe ureteral obstruction exists, indigo carmine will not help to identify the ureteral orifice. Also, with ureteral obstruction a discrete jet of indigo carmine may be absent, the dye material oozing diffusely through an edematous or tumorous area making ureteral orifice identification impossible.

The problem of identifying the orifice may be solved by exposing the ureter as it crosses the promontory. A urethral filiform can be passed downward into the bladder through a tiny ureterotomy. For sturdier ureteral intubation a woven follower may be attached to this filiform. A ureteral catheter may be substituted for the filiform and followers.

Making a Bladder Diverticulum More Accessible

A bladder diverticulum situated in the posterior or lateral wall near the trigone may be difficult to mobilize extravesically. Approaching the diverticulum transvesically simplifies the procedure. One or more of the following maneuvers may be helpful:

1) A finger may be inserted into the diverticular os and a circumferential incision made around the os. The finger acts as a guide to dissection and as a tractor while mobilizing the diverticulum.

2) The diverticulum may be packed with 1- or 2-inch gauze, converting a flaccid sac into a rigid structure and facilitating its dissection and mobilization.

3) The distal end of the sac may be grasped with an Allis clamp through the os and the sac pulled into the bladder lumen. The mucosa of the sac may be incised near the Allis clamp and the perivesical tissue pushed away.

4) Allis clamps may be placed around the os in conjunction with a finger in the sac.

A combined perivesical and transvesical approach is sometimes utilized, pushing the diverticulum toward the bladder with either a finger or a hemostat. The procedure of choice will depend on the size and location of the diverticulum. The surgeon must remember that either the peritoneum or ureter may be nearby.

Fulguration of Anterior Wall Bladder Tumors

Tumors located in the dome of the bladder, just at or near the air bubble, are at times difficult to resect transurethrally. The tumor moves away from the tip of the electrode or the resectoscope loop. Any one of the following aids may be helpful:

1) With very little fluid in the bladder, utilizing resectoscopic forceps (A.C. M.I.), one may grasp the tumor near its base and pull the tumor off with a quick pull of the resectoscopic sheath. The tumor may then be pulled out of the bladder with the cups of the blade closed. Alternatively, one may grasp the base of the tumor with this same forceps, and by utilizing the fulgurating current thoroughly fulgurate the base before pulling the tumor off. With fulguration of its base, the tumor becomes more rigid, so that the resectoscope loop may also be used more successfully in tumor removal.

2) One may have an assistant or the circulating nurse place a clenched fist on the patient's abdomen and push downward in the suprapubic area. This brings the tumor closer to the operating instrument. The bladder should be empty or only partially filled to facilitate this maneuver.

3) One may resect the tumor with the water inflow turned off so that the tumor does not slowly and gradually recede from the area of accessibility.

4) One may lower the head of the table so that the patient is lying at an angle of 45 degrees or in a deep Trendelenburg position. The irrigating fluid in the bladder may actually pull the anterior surface downward as the fluid fills the posterior vault and floor of the bladder. The dome is brought down to a more accessible area.

5) A double catheterizing cystoscope may be used with a fulgurating electrode on one side and a ureteral catheter on the other. A syringe and needle are attached to the catheter to suck out the air bubble. The lesion in the region of the former air bubble may now be much better visualized. This, too, by removing the air and gases produced during resection, minimizes the possibility of an intravesical explosion.

6) Cystoscopy done in a modified knee-chest or Kraske position (in a female patient) will also permit access to these difficult lesions of the dome. The lesions would now be on the equivalent of the floor area were the patient in the usual position.

7) A female patient may be placed face down on the cystoscopy table with legs supported by arm boards. This changes the position of the tumor from anterior to posterior.

Aid to Resection of Large Bladder Tumors

It is often difficult and time-consuming to resect the bulk of the tissue of a large, mushy bladder tumor. Frequent clearing of fulgurated tissue from the resectoscope loop is required. With the bladder filled only enough to allow free flow of irrigating fluid into the Ellik evacuator, one may try to suck up the bulk of the tumor into the evacuator, leaving only the base of the tumor to be resected.

Contrast Cystography Immediately Following Transurethral Resection of Bladder Tumor. Mucosal Water Barrier

In performing contrast cystograms immediately following transurethral resections of bladder tumors, one may demonstrate the opaque contrast material outside the bladder about 70 percent of the time. Extravasation of fluid also occurs following transurethral prostatectomy.* When bladder mucosa is incised, the water barrier is eliminated. Extravasation under these circumstances is not dependent on the grade of the tumor or the depth of the resection. One may see this perfusion of fluid through the wall of a normal bladder after incising only the mucosa.

Study of transvesical extravasation following the incision of the bladder mucosa leads to the following conclusions:

1) The bladder mucosa serves as a water barrier.

2) Under average fluid pressure conditions, from 200 to 400 ml of irrigating

---

* See *Perivesical Fluid Extravasation*, in Chapter Eight.

material is extravasated outside the bladder during the usual transurethral resection for bladder tumor.

3) Extravasated fluid must be taken into account as a previously unconsidered cause of polyhydration. If the surgery is prolonged, several liters of irrigating fluid may extravasate.

4) One must be concerned with the bladder fluid volume during transurethral resection of prostate and bladder tumors. The irrigating percolator should be marked off at 100-ml levels so that one does not overdistend the bladder beyond the point of 300 to 500 ml of fluid.

5) Irrigating water pressure should be kept to a minimum.

6) Malignant cells are carried directly outside the bladder, as well as being transmitted through the opened lymphatic and blood vessels. In most cases there must be enough host resistance to absorb and make innocuous these extravasated tumor cells. In some instances where perivesical tumor becomes evident, we can now account for the spread of tumor cells in this area.

7) The importance of the early fulguration of a bladder tumor base is evident.

Surgical Planes in Cystectomy and Radical Retropubic Prostatectomy. Use of Vein Stripper for Dissection

In performing cystectomy and/or radical retropubic prostatectomy, it is useful to divide the vas near the internal inguinal ring. This is done as soon as the prevesical space is opened. One may then follow the vas by finger dissection down to the ampulla and adjacent seminal vesicle, where a plane of dissection is developed between these structures and the rectum.

This facilitates subsequent freeing-up of the seminal vesicles posteriorly after the urethra is severed and the prostate is retracted upward.

Neither excessive bleeding nor damage to the ureter, bladder, or rectum occur with this "blind dissection." If there are lateral bands adherent to the vas which are hard to define with the finger, an external vein stripper slipped over the vas will facilitate freeing it from adjacent adhesions.

Tumorous nodes are easily palpated as the vas is dissected free. The finding of tumorous nodes emphasizes all the more the need for doing complete pelvic lymphadenectomy prior to the prostatoseminovesiculectomy.

The vas, being friable, may break off during dissection. Minimal pulling force is exerted to avoid this. Radical node dissection is done following mobilization of the prostate and seminal vesicles, though some urologists proceed with node dissection before this mobilization. The latter approach probably will become the technique of preference in cancer surgery.

The described surgical planes technique is very useful for both radical retropubic prostatectomy and cystectomy since it also leads one very quickly down to the region of the major blood supply to the prostate and bladder.

Aids in Anterior Cystourethropexy (Marshall-Marchetti-Krantz Procedure)

The urethrovesical suspension operation may be made easier by elevation of the urethra and bladder neck during the placing of the elevation sutures.

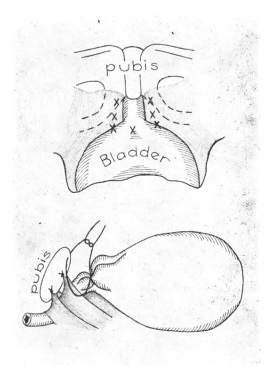

41. Modification of Marshall-Marchetti-Krantz procedure. Note suture placement.

This may be done in several ways. One may have the circulating nurse insert a sterile gloved finger into the previously prepared vagina and elevate the bladder neck and vagina on either side of the urethra. The surgeon then grasps the designated areas with an Allis clamp.

Instead of utilizing the assistance of the nurse, one may use a sponge forceps placed in the vagina at the time the patient is draped. Elevation of the forceps to the position desired is easily accomplished by the surgeon.

To locate the bladder neck one merely pulls down on the previously inserted balloon catheter. Elevating sutures are placed precisely and easily alongside the urethra in the exact location desired by the operator.

The authors, in doing their Marshall-Marchetti-Krantz procedure, place the sutures deeply into the midline of the underside of the symphysis fibrocartilage (sutures placed into the periosteum laterally to the central fibrocartilage will easily tear out when tied). All of the sutures placed in the midline tend to imbricate the urethra—this is an important deviation from the usual suture placement.

After two or three sutures have been placed through the endopelvic fascia on either side of the urethra below the bladder neck, a suture is placed approximately 5 mm proximal (bladder side of bladder neck) to the bladder neck at the 3, 12, and 9 o'clock positions. This suture is then cinched up tightly and tied, and is then also sutured to the underside of the fibrocartilage of the symphysis pubis.

This last-placed suture is a urethral lengthening suture (see Fig. 41). We therefore not only angulate the urethra but also lengthen the urethra by making the bladder neck more proximal. This has been found very helpful in ensuring the success of the procedure.

Use of Kollmann Dilator During Vesicourethroplasty

During anterior urethroplasty or Y-V plasty, difficulty may be encountered in isolating the distal end of the incision in the urethra. To minimize this problem one may pass the curved Kollmann dilator (without the rubber sheath) transurethrally before or after the bladder neck incision has been made. Gentle expansion of the blades of the dilator will open the urethra, clearly exposing the edge of the distal incision and holding it stable for accuracy in suture placement.

Watertight Closures in Urethral and Bladder Repair

To be certain of a watertight closure during urethral or bladder surgery (or even in surgery on the renal pelvis), one may inject indigo carmine with syringe and 25-gauge needle and observe the repair site to see if there is any escape of blue dye. This very readily will show any leakage. The needle site should be distant from the repair site so that the puncture site leak will not be confusing.

(See also aids to surgical correction of bladder fistulae at end of this chapter.)

Cystostomy Drainage

Suprapubic Cystostomy, Rapid and Simple Method

During urethroplasty or perineal surgery it is at times desirable to add cystostomy drainage. A rapid, technically simple, and usually safe technique for obtaining cystostomy drainage is as follows: A curved sound is passed through the perineal urethra into the distended bladder, and the external distal end of the instrument is depressed. A suprapubic incision is made over the palpable tip of the sound just above the symphysis. A suprapubic balloon catheter can then be drawn into the bladder after coupling the sound and catheter at the catheter drainage fenestra. The sound is withdrawn and disconnected from the catheter. The balloon catheter is withdrawn suprapubically to the desired position. When one is certain the balloon is in the bladder, it is inflated.

The bladder should always be overdistended with fluid in order to push away the intestinal loops which may be in that area. Bowel injury is more apt to occur if the patient has had previous perivesical injury, previous cystostomy, perivesical suprapubic extravasation, etc.

A convenient alternate procedure is to use the Lowsley curved prostatic retractor. The retractor is passed transurethrally and the anterior bladder wall is tented up to guide the suprapubic skin incision. After extending the incision through the tented abdominal wall, the retractor end is brought out suprapubically and the jaws are opened; thus a silk suture can be passed through the mechanism and attached to the tip of a Malecot catheter. After closing the jaws of the retractor, the catheter is drawn into the bladder and out through the perineum, where the silk suture is cut and removed and the Malecot catheter drawn back into the bladder.

It may be difficult to palpate the tip of the sound or the Lowsley prostatic retractor if the patient is obese and has a short suspensory ligament.

Special Perforated-Tip Sound for Rapid Simple Cystostomy

Several sounds of different sizes may have holes drilled transversely about 1 cm from the tip. When incision is made over the tip of such a sound for the rapid cystostomy just described, a silk suture may be tied to the sound through the hole and the other end tied to a balloon catheter. After withdrawal of the sound, suture, and catheter tip through the urethral meatus for separation, the catheter may be withdrawn suprapubically back to the bladder.

A Kollmann dilator may replace the perforated-tip sound in the above procedure. Alcock interlocking sounds may also be used.

Bladder Drainage with Intracath to Mobilize Ureter in Region Behind Bladder

Occasionally during abdominal surgery one must mobilize the ureter in the region behind the bladder. One may find the bladder inconveniently full due to failure to empty preoperatively or to the urine accumulated during surgery. The need for preparation and redraping may make catheterization difficult or time-consuming.

Aspiration with a large needle may be done (the Deseret 14 French or other similar intracath works very well for this). The intracath may be left in postoperatively and brought out through a stab wound. The same intracath also works very well for diversionary drainage of the renal pelvis.

Electrosurgical Bedside Suprapubic Cystostomy

Under local anesthesia one may make a small skin incision just above the symphysis in the midline. A small Bugbee tip electrode may be placed through the tip of a 16 French balloon-type catheter. By utilizing the electrosurgical cutting current, as well as the coagulating current, one can "fulgurate one's way" into the bladder with the balloon-type catheter following

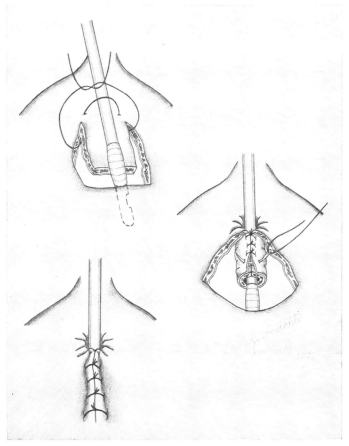

42. Bladder flap method of correcting leaking suprapubic cystostomy

and draped over the Bugbee tip electrode. The balloon is inflated. The flow of urine through the catheter heralds the entrance into the bladder, and the electrode is then withdrawn from inside the catheter. The hole made by the Bugbee tip electrode at the distal end of the catheter serves as an additional drainage opening.

Surgical Correction of Leaking Suprapubic Cystostomy

Though suprapubic cystostomy is often the most satisfactory method for long-term bladder drainage, urinary leakage around the suprapubic catheter is a frequently bothersome complication. This more often occurs in an elderly thin patient whose abdominal wall is atrophied to the degree that the combined thickness of bladder and abdominal walls may be less than a centimeter. Attempts at overfilling the balloon-type catheter, or the application of traction, are rarely successful in preventing leakage.

A method of surgical correction of this condition is suggested. A midline

suprapubic incision incorporating the sinus tract is made down to the bladder. The bladder is mobilized. A rectangular bladder flap is cut with its
base directed toward the bladder neck. This flap is then inverted down into
the bladder and sutured as a tube around a balloon-type catheter (Fig. 42).
The mucosa of this tube is on the outside of the flap, the exact opposite of
the Boari flap arrangement. The bladder tube is closed in two layers—a muscular layer of 2-0 chromic catgut and a mucosal layer of 4-0 or 5-0 plain
catgut. The bladder defect is closed either transversely or vertically. The
recti muscles and fascia are approximated or even inverted to create an
increase in abdominal wall thickness in the midline.

Drainage from the retropubic space out alongside the suprapubic tube
can be provided by a small Penrose drain for a few days.

The suprapubic sinus fashioned by this operation is at least one or two
inches in length, making leakage around the catheter most unlikely.

Anchoring Cystostomy Tubing

The plastic tubing placed in the bladder as an intracath must be tied in
to prevent its slipping out. Adhesive alone is not dependable.

A "stick tie" (suture ligature) may be taken into the skin with 2-0 black
silk suture. This is then looped several times around the cystostomy tubing

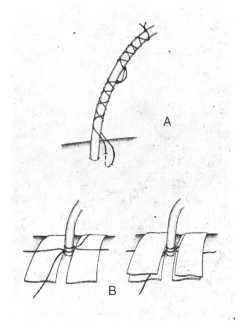

43. Anchoring cystostomy tubing
    A. Spiraled-suture and
       multiple-knot method
    B. Tied and taped-down method

and tied (Fig. 43A). Another knot is made above the area of this previous tie producing a loop of black silk suture. The suture is then again wrapped around the plastic tubing and triple-tied, and finally another knot is tied opposite the triple tie and around the plastic tubing. In this manner, the plastic tubing is tied in three separate areas by wrapping suture rather firmly around the plastic tubing.

Some men prefer to tie silk or cotton around the plastic tubing, leaving the ends long. Pieces of adhesive tape are applied to the skin, previously treated with tincture of benzoin, and the sutures are placed over the adhesive and covered with pieces of adhesive. Two such ties are placed around the plastic tubing and strapped to the skin in four quadrants; see Figure 43B. This is not as dependable as the method just previously described.

Retention anchoring discs are available with some of the manufactured percutaneous cystostomy sets.

Urethrovesical Drainage Tube

There are occasions in which an older, disoriented bedfast patient may require placement of a catheter into a small, shrunken bladder. One may utilize a Silastic tube of long length into which a number of holes have been cut. This tube may be passed through a simple cystostomy and out through the urethra. There is thus no balloon to irritate the bladder neck, and the patient does not tug persistently at the tube, as a rule. Such tubes may be easily irrigated.

The tube also may be readily changed by drawing a new tube through after tying it to the old one, or possibly placing a suture through the old and new tubes and then pulling them through.

One may mark this catheter so that the multiple openings are properly oriented inside the bladder. A black silk tie through the catheter may be used to mark the urethral meatus point or the abdominal skin site. The Silastic tubing may also be cut to such length that one will have at least 12 inches of tubing emerging from the cystostomy end and 12 inches of tubing emerging from the urethral end.

The tube may be anchored down to the abdomen in several places by the method illustrated in Figures 43A and B, or to the penis by the technique shown in Figure 48 (Chapter Seven).

Urinary Drainage Bags

There are presently on the market very satisfactory catheters of plastic or Silastic materials, with ingenious irrigation and closed drainage systems available to meet most urologic needs. These new products favor the reduction of urinary infection and its sequelae and contribute a great deal to patient comfort and safety.

Postoperative Retention

Acute Retention in the Postoperative Patient

Following surgery, especially gynecologic or rectal, a patient is frequently unable to void. Whether this is due to localized pain and secondary spasm, neurogenic dysfunction, sphincter spasm, hysterical reaction, neuropsychic reaction, or is secondary to anesthesia, the following aids are suggested:

1) Sitz baths, with the patient requested to void while sitting in warm water, may be effective.

2) A warm enema, with the patient requested to void while expelling fecal contents, may be tried.

3) Bethanechol chloride (Urecholine), 2.5 to 5 mg subcutaneously, will many times start the patient voiding spontaneously, but should be used cautiously because of severe side effects (see section under Neurogenic Bladder earlier in this chapter, regarding Urecholine test for neurogenic bladder).

4) Bladder instillation of one-half to one ounce of one percent *aqueous* mercurochrome or 1:1500 aqueous gentian violet will produce a chemical trigonitis which frequently will initiate voiding. These solutions should not be left in the bladder longer than 30 minutes because they will increase the severity of the chemical trigonitis to an excessive degree.

5) Filling the patient's bladder with sterile refrigerated ice water or saline (in a quantity of 100 to 200 ml) after the bladder has been completely emptied by catheterization, may be effective. The bladder is usually filled to the point where the patient has a desire to void and the catheter is then removed and the patient requested to void.

The last-described technique is often the most effective. This method and (4) are utilized in persistent retention cases. Often several catheterizations are necessary. Prolonged catheter drainage may on occasion be required. Once the voiding pattern has been started, the patient will usually be able to void freely thereafter.

"Y-Tube" Gradual Decompression

When gradual decompression of the bladder is desired in patients with acute retention, the following method is helpful.

A catheter, with the outflow clamped, is inserted transurethrally into the bladder and the balloon of the catheter is inflated. The outflow portion of the catheter is connected to plastic drainage tubing which, in turn, goes to a glass Y and then to drainage tubing and collection bottle. The glass Y is taped to an intravenous stand (see Fig. 44) at such a height that when the catheter outflow is opened, urine just reaches the junction of the Y. The height of the Y is then decreased periodically, depending on the rate of decompression desired.

It is essential that the upper limb of the Y be open; otherwise a siphon effect would be produced.

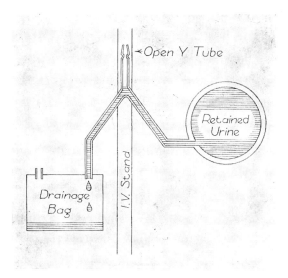

44. Y-tube device for gradual decompression of the bladder

Many urologists disregard the gradual decompression technique in acute retention patients. Following several instances of severe gross hematuria, acute renal shutdown, and profuse diuresis with severe sodium loss, the authors are inclined to use gradual decompression.

Blood Clots in the Bladder and Their Removal

Blood clots in the bladder may be evacuated by continuous or frequent irrigations. One sometimes finds a clot trapped within the lumen of the catheter, so that one can inject fluid into the bladder (preferably with a Toomey syringe) but fluid will not aspirate. It is obvious that the clot is serving as a ball valve within the lumen of the catheter. Vigorous injection and aspiration with 25 to 30 ml of sterile saline may dislodge the clot. This should be abandoned after two to three attempts, to prevent overdistention of the bladder.

Such a catheter must be replaced, but before doing so the catheter balloon should be deflated and the catheter passed further into the bladder. Frequently the problem is an accumulation of clots around the eye of the catheter rather than a clot within the catheter lumen. With the catheter in this higher position, evacuation of clots is often successful.

If a clot remains in the eye of the catheter and no drainage can be obtained, one may maintain suction on the catheter while removing it. By this method the obstructing clot is sucked out. One may then insert a new 24 French 30-ml balloon-type catheter and the process of irrigation is repeated, using preferably the Toomey syringe. To effectively evacuate clots, one must usually vigorously inject the irrigating fluid into the bladder to "stir

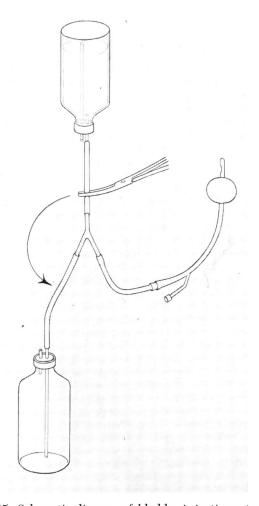

45. Schematic diagram of bladder irrigation setup

up" the clots and then vigorously aspirate. If necessary, again the catheter may be removed, maintaining suction to aspirate troublesome clots.

If the bleeding is so brisk that even with continuous irrigation and the above-described method of pulling the catheter out of the bladder, the clots still cannot be entirely removed, it may then be necessary to further aspirate the clots with a Toomey syringe via a resectoscope or cystoscope or a large, rigid urethral catheter. A large (24 French) Robinson catheter provides a lumen of more adequate size than that of a comparably sized balloon catheter. Often bleeding will continue until all the clots are removed.

In some instances, the patient must be taken back to the operating room and under anesthesia the clots are evacuated through a cystoscope or resectoscope. A search must be made for the bleeding site and this, if found, is fulgurated via resectoscope or Bugbee electrode through the cystoscope or panendoscope. More often than not, after evacuating the clots, bleeding sites are not seen, the bleeding subsiding spontaneously.

Some of the procedures described above may be done under intravenous meperidine (Demerol) amnesia, intravenous diazepam (Valium), methohexital sodium (Brevital), or other favored methods of analgesia. The urologist should always be aware that there is a limit to what the patient can tolerate, and should not hesitate to return the patient to the operating room to correct the problem.

Other means of irrigation may be used, as for example, the Asepto syringe, the Nesbit Young and Y-tube types of irrigation apparatus (see Fig. 45 for latter), the 30-ml syringe, etc. These methods, however, are usually not effective if a considerable number of clots have been allowed to accumulate in the bladder.

Very often the return flow may continue to be bloody, but the patient may have no active bleeding. This is usually due to the dissolution of the clots within the bladder. When all clots are removed, and if no bleeding is present, the return flow should be almost clear.

(See also *Control of Bladder Hemorrhage Due to Cytoxan Therapy, etc.,* in earlier part of this chapter.)

Suprapubic Catheterization for Retention and Avoidance of Indwelling Catheter

Numerous situations require suprapubic catheterization or trocar catheter aspirations of the bladder to obviate a transurethral inlying catheter.

Patients in retention who do not tolerate transurethral catheters; patients with impassable urethral stricture, prostatic hyperplasia, or impacted urethral stone; children from whom sterile urine specimens are needed, etc., are a few of the indicated reasons for suprapubic catheterization not previously mentioned under discussion of cystostomy in the *Bladder Surgery* section. Many gynecologists use suprapubic puncture catheterization on patients subjected to any type of pelvic surgery in whom they wish to avoid transurethral catheters. Gynecological surgeons often emplace the suprapubic catheter under vision, with the surgical wound open, at the time of pelvic surgery.

The method of placement of the catheter is as follows: under local, intravenous amnesia or general anesthesia, *with the bladder full,* a needle (the intracath type of needle and plastic catheter over or within the needle) is placed into the bladder by insertion immediately above the upper border of the symphysis in the midline and directed in a downward direction at an angle of 10 to 15 degrees. The needle is withdrawn after the plastic tubing is pushed well down into the bladder.

Due to the thickness of the abdominal wall, the intracath and plastic catheter over or within the needle may be too short. In such a situation, a disposable cystostomy set manufactured by Dow Corning (Silastic Cystocath) consisting of a long needle, Silastic tubing and a disc which is glued to the skin to fix the tubing, may prove valuable. Many comparable units made by other manufacturers are available.

Some urologists still prefer doing a trocar cystotomy. Trocars are available through which one may pass a balloon catheter. Some of the trocars are made with an open side so that a catheter may be passed and the trocar removed. The technique in these situations requires anesthesia and the making of a small skin incision followed by the insertion of the trocar.

One must always be cautious that the bladder is full when doing a trocar cystotomy, so that there is minimum danger of injury to large or small bowel. *Trocar puncture or needle puncture of the bladder is extremely hazardous in the previously operated-upon bladder.*

Intracath and Thoracocentesis Sets for Suprapubic Drainage

If an intracath type of needle with plastic tubing inside the needle is used, there frequently is slight leakage because the needle wound is larger than is the plastic tubing. Many suprapubic needles of the intracath type are available.

A satisfactory suprapubic cystostomy-type puncture placement may be made with a thoracocentesis set. This consists of a needle of about 12 French in caliber with plastic tubing on the outside of the shaft of the needle, so that one has a drainage lumen equivalent to that of a 16 French urethral catheter. The specially prepared cystostomy units available through most surgical supply companies may also be used.

Suprapubic Drainage Tubes for Long-Term Use

The Argyle trocar catheter has been utilized successfully for stricture patients in retention with blood clots within the bladder. The catheter can be easily passed suprapubically under local anesthesia and the clots may be readily evacuated. Although used primarily for chest suction drainage, this type of catheter is valuable for urologic use. The catheter is available in sizes 20 and 28 French.

BLADDER FISTULAE

Diagnosis and Localization

Vesicovaginal Fistulae

Loss of urine due to vesicovaginal fistula may often be confused with bladder incontinence due to other factors. At times, one may be able to see a vesicovaginal fistula on looking into the bladder with a cystoscope. One

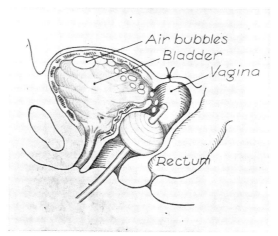

46. Use of air in bladder to demonstrate vesicovaginal fistula

may inject dye per catheter into the bladder and place a vaginal speculum sideways into the vagina (or use downward traction on the posterior lip of the speculum) and with the aid of the cystoscope and the light in the bladder, clearly see the fistulous opening in the vagina as fluid freely flows from the bladder into the vagina.

Dyes of various types may be employed. Indigo carmine, 5 ml in approximately 100 ml of water or saline, may be used. A like amount (100 ml) of boiled milk may be used. The latter is slightly more difficult to see but less bothersome in its staining characteristics than the dye material.

Demonstration of Tiny, Elusive Vesicovaginal and Colovesical Fistulae

A balloon catheter may be placed in the vagina and the balloon inflated to 30 to 40 ml in size. By pumping air into the vagina through the balloon catheter during cystoscopic examination, the opening or openings of very tiny fistulae in the bladder may be pinpointed (Fig. 46). This same technique may be used at surgery with the opened bladder partially filled with water.

Air pumped into the colon during cystoscopic examination will also occasionally demonstrate the opening of a colovesical fistula. It is easy to see the bubbles of air floating through the water and the site from which they emerge.

If barium flux is found in a centrifuged urine specimen in a patient after the administration of a liquid barium enema for lower bowel study, this too confirms the presence of a colovesical, colourethral, or coloureteral communication. Charcoal also may be given by mouth or by enema when this diagnosis is suspected. The presence of black flux in the bladder, on cystoscopic examination, or its presence in the urine, is of diagnostic significance.

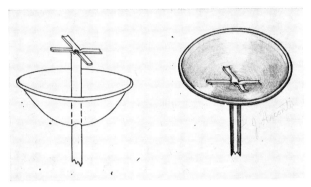

47. Modification of contraceptive diaphragm to serve as urine collection device

Diagnosis in Enterovesical Fistulae

To demonstrate the existence of an enterovesical fistula, one may use pyrvinium pamoate (Povan), a drug used for pinworm (Enterobius vermicularis) in children. This is a red dye and an effective antiparasitic. The dye is absorbed and remains within the gastrointestinal tract. Should there subsequently be any red dye mixed with the urine, there is obvious communication between the intestine and the bladder.

Treatment and Repair of Bladder Fistulae

Urine Collection Devices for Patients with Vesicovaginal Fistulae

The patient with a vesicovaginal fistula is an unhappy person because of being constantly wet with urine. Various methods of urine collection have been suggested:

1) Some patients will remain dry if one will anchor a urethral catheter connected to a leg bag. Others, however, will leak urine vaginally despite the catheter being in place.

2) Tampons changed at regular intervals may serve for some patients.

3) A new product devised for the menstruating patient can serve effectively for fistula patients. This is a plastic cup * worn just within the vagina. It is bell-shaped and has a small handle at the lowermost end. One may remove the handle and cut a small opening the size of an 18 French balloon-type catheter. The catheter may be passed through the appliance and the balloon of the catheter blown up to about 7 ml. This balloon fits very snugly in the bottom of the bell. The device is placed within the vagina by the patient, and the catheter may then be connected to a leg bag, or at night to bedside drainage. A leg bag worn at night will not be of adequate volume. Also, the patient may turn and lie atop the leg bag, leading to complications.

4) Another simple, inexpensive device to help keep the patient dry employs a standard contraceptive diaphragm. The patient should be measured for dia-

* Tassaway®, made by Tassette, Inc., 155 South Robertson Boulevard, Beverly Hills, California 90211.

phragm size. Rubber tubing of proper size to fit and reach the leg bag may be vulcanized to the diaphragm after the appropriate hole is cut in the middle of the diaphragm (Fig. 47). Urine then collects in the diaphragm and by means of the tubing passes into the leg bag (or to bedside drainage).

Retrograde Ureteropyelography in Patients with Vesicoureterovaginal Fistulae

Intravenous pyelography to investigate the upper urinary tract usually is done prior to vesicovaginal fistula repair. However, the occasional incidence of vesicovaginal fistula associated with an intramural ureterovaginal fistula may be overlooked. Because of this, one should do bulb ureteropyelograms prior to vesicovaginal fistula repair.

Transvesical Fulguration of Vesicovaginal Fistulae

When one is dealing with a very small vesicovaginal fistula, the tip of a conical small Bugbee electrode may by means of an operating cystoscope be inserted through the full length of the fistula and very LIGHTLY fulgurated. The fistula may be fulgurated vaginally, as well as urethrally.

Following fulguration, a balloon-type catheter may be inserted into the bladder and retained for a period of several weeks with the patient lying in bed in a position in which there is the least leakage. It may be necessary for the patient to lie on her abdomen to keep from leaking urine vaginally despite the presence of the catheter.

Convincing a patient of the necessity of remaining in bed for several weeks is generally most difficult. This fulguration method may make it possible for tiny fistulae to close in ambulatory patients in some cases. It frequently is necessary to lightly refulgurate a fistula of this type. Excessive granulation tissue noted vaginally at the sinus site should be coagulated or treated with a silver nitrate stick.

Surgical Position for Repair of Vesicovaginal Fistulae

Please refer to Chapter Seven, section entitled *Positioning the Female Patient on the Operating Table for Urethral Surgery.*

Retraction for Repair of Vesicovaginal Fistulae

In doing transvesical repair of a vesicovaginal fistula, the vagina is always prepared prior to surgery. Immediately after the "prep," one may thread through the vesicovaginal fistula (with the aid of vaginal forceps and speculum) 2-0 black silk which has been previously tied around either two folded 4- by 4-inch pieces of gauze or tied around and sutured through the bulb of a 2-oz Asepto syringe.

One may also use varied types of flat discs of approximately the same size through which silk suture may be tied, or a balloon-type catheter with the balloon distended to about 30 ml in size. When the bladder is opened, one grasps and pulls on the black silk suture. By utilizing pull on the suture tied around the larger vaginally placed object, the fistula area is raised. We have often seen situations in which the fistula has been elevated to the level of the abdominal skin. This greatly facilitates excision and repair of the fistula.

Chapter Seven

THE URETHRA AND ITS INSTRUMENTATION

A VOLUME COULD BE written covering the urethra and urethral instrumentation alone, with reference to "tricks of the trade," gadgets, and shortcuts in diagnostic, surgical, and therapeutic applications. There are many controversial aspects amongst these same subjects relating to the urethra. We shall try to avoid many of the questionable spheres.

DIAGNOSTIC FACTORS

Causes of Urinary Retention Directly Related to the Urethra

Acute urinary retention specifically related to the urethra may be due to any of the following: stricture, stones or other foreign bodies, diverticula, carcinoma, blood clots, or severe edema.

Neurogenic dysfunction, psychogenic dysfunction, sphincter spasm secondary to inflammation and infection of adjacent structures, specific drug action or sensitivity, foreign bodies in the rectum or vagina with spasm, or rectal and vaginal spasm *per se* due to numerous types of localized pathology, may all cause retention of urine.

Due to their location, lesions of the prostate, including prostatic hyperplasia, acute prostatitis, and prostatic carcinoma, intimately involve the urethra. These conditions are treated in Chapter Eight of this volume. Bladder pathology such as tumor fronds or blood clots may also cause acute retention. Other causes of acute retention are noted elsewhere in the book.

Examining the Urethra

Urethral and Vaginal Visualization in Children

Combining an infant Vest lens with the sheath ordinarily used for the infant resectoscope makes an excellent urethral observation instrument for children. The nasal speculum may also be used in a female child. The newer fiber optic infant cystourethroscopes are superb instruments for both inspection and instrumentation.

Urethral Caliber in Normal Female Children

The urethral caliber in normal female children has been well studied by Drs. Immergut, Culp, and Flocks. This warrants repetition here. The size of the urethra usually will calibrate the same as the size of the urethral meatus. If the meatus is smaller, meatotomy may be necessary.

Age in Years	Median Size (French)
0–4	14
5–9	16
10–14	20
15–20	26

The Otoscope as a Urethroscope

The meatus and distal urethra can and should be examined under vision through the Welch-Allyn otoscope. In this manner small papillomata often found within the urethral meatus in the region of the fossa navicularis, may be seen where otherwise they are often missed.

A fringe benefit of owning a Welch-Allyn otoscope is that it may be used as a light power source with incandescent-type cystoscopes. The two female terminals in the instrument will accommodate the male terminals of the cystoscopic light cord. The batteries must be fully charged to provide 3 volts.

One may also use the nasal speculum and otoscope for inspection of the floor of the distal female urethra when looking for dilated ducts. An acutely bent fine probe and a binocular loupe may be helpful aids under these circumstances.

When using the ostoscope either in the urethra or in any other portion of the anatomy, one must be very careful not to use an electrode through the metal fenestrum of the otoscope because of the danger of shorting out. More recent instruments are provided with plastic specula.

COMMON URETHRAL PROBLEMS
Urethritis

Nonspecific Urethritis

Nonspecific anterior urethritis in the male patient is very frequently encountered. The three-glass urine test is most helpful in localizing the portion of urethra* involved. Cultures fail to reveal the presence of the gonococcus or other specific organism. Search for Trichomonas or Monilia very often also is unsuccessful.

Obtaining a history that the patient's sex partner does have a vaginal discharge which seems to be irritating to the penis following intercourse should make one suspicious of Trichomonas or Monilia.

Treatment: Failing to demonstrate a specific pathogen, a "shotgun" type of combined medication has proven helpful in a majority of these cases. The male patient is administered at least 1,600,000 units of penicillin G by mouth four times per day for ten days. The patient and sex partner

---

* See description of three-glass urine test in *Urinalysis, Points of Emphasis*, Chapter Two.

must take metronidazole (Flagyl) tablets by mouth. The male patient, in addition, must take an oxytetracycline. It is surprising to note the extremely high success rate in response to this triple type of "shotgun" regime. A patient with Monilia may be adversely affected by this therapy; close supervision is therefore required so that the regimen is discontinued if symptoms worsen.

Should the above treatment fail, a 3 percent Achromycin ® (tetracycline hydrochloride) ointment injected with a 5-ml plain-tipped syringe weekly for a period of two to five weeks has proven successful. About 90 percent of patients experience relief of the urethral discharge. The 3 percent Achromycin ointment may prove as successful in the male patient as is the nitrofurazone (Furacin) suppository in the treatment of the female.

The "Urethral Syndrome" in Women

The urethra is the site of multiple and varied complaints in female patients and these are due to a variety of conditions. Therapeutic modalities include urethral dilatation, internal urethrotomy, bladder irrigation, fulguration of polypoid structures at the bladder neck, fulguration of the granular tissue in the proximal half of the urethra, fulguration and incision of (or unroofing of) periurethral and Skene's glands, repair of unsuspected and undiagnosed urethral diverticula, removal of suburethral fibrotic tissue, estrogen cream treatment and/or oral estrogens for post-menopausal atrophic urethritis, etc.

Atrophic Urethritis

Characteristically, in atrophic urethritis, urinalyses are consistently normal. Patients with this complaint respond to estrogen therapy but only when given to the point of saturation. Patients with cicatricial atrophic post-menopausal urethritis must indefinitely continue the use of an estrogen cream, even in minimal quantities, in order to remain free of symptomatology.

Urethral caruncles very often will disappear following the adequate application of an estrogen cream.

Incompletely Ruptured Hymenal Ring Syndrome: Treatment

Occasionally one sees a patient who gives a history of dyspareunia, severe urge to void immediately after sexual intercourse, chronic vaginitis and lack of orgasm. Some of these patients will show a relative introversion of the urethral meatus into the vagina, like that of a relative hypospadias. This is best demonstrated by pushing downward on the posterior vaginal outlet with the examining fingers at the 5 and 7 o'clock positions.

This condition, described in the literature by some writers as the incompletely ruptured hymenal ring, will often respond dramatically to merely incising this hymenal ring on either side of the urethra. A small radial incision is made bilaterally just lateral to the urethral meatus in the introitus. The mucosa is spread widely with hemostats and a thickened, rounded tissue is encountered. This hymenal ring is grasped with an Allis clamp and a wedge is excised bilaterally. Figure-of-eight 3-0 chromic sutures are used to close the incision and to control bleeding.

The urethra then remains unchanged in its direction when downward pressure is thereafter exerted at the 5 and 7 o'clock positions.

Occasionally in a woman with relative hypospadias a hood of mucosa is seen covering the superior portion of the urethral meatus when downward pressure is applied at 5 and 7 o'clock. This hood may help to milk contaminants into the urethra during intercourse, and should either be excised or slit and closed transversely.

Additional Effective Procedures for Female Urethral Syndrome

For patients who complain of typical urethral syndrome symptoms the fulguration of infected paraurethral and Skene's glands, as well as the posterior urethra and trigone when indicated, often results in complete cure.

A fine-tip electrode is used to fulgurate and destroy paraurethral ducts and glands. Whenever possible, visible ducts should be unroofed by insertion of the electrode to the full depth of the duct, exposing the duct throughout its entire length. This promotes healing from the bottom up and results ultimately in complete obliteration of the duct by scar.

Protuberant infected granulomatous meatal tissue is also thoroughly fulgurated.

Very light fulguration of the entire trigone follows for the pseudomembranous trigonitis. Edematous tabs (pseudopolypi) and hillocks of the mucosa at the vesical neck and proximal half of the urethra are lightly fulgurated. This coagulation must be very superficial, destroying only the chronically altered mucous membrane. If the coagulation is carried too deeply, postoperative scarring, hemorrhage, acute retention, etc., may occur.

An 18 or 20 French catheter is left indwelling for 48 hours. The day following the removal of the catheter the patient may be discharged from the hospital. Healing requires six to eight weeks, during which time symptoms of mild chronic cystitis are expected to appear and gradually subside; mild hematuria may occur for three to four weeks and the patient should be so advised.

During the ensuing year an attack of acute cystitis may alert one to the fact that an infected duct was overlooked at the time of the original procedure. Ablation of the residual duct may be done in the outpatient department or in the office under local anesthesia.

The effectiveness of the above-described technique is ascribed by some urologists to its psychotherapeutic effect. Others feel that it is of questionable value—they believe the patient would not dare disaffirm its effectiveness out of fear of going through the whole cycle again.

Further Considerations Regarding the Female Urethral Syndrome

Whatever feelings the urologist may have regarding the etiology of this problem, patients deserve a trial of carefully considered treatment after careful and complete urologic evaluation. The complaints of these patients should not be considered psychogenic in origin simply because of the lack of abnormalities in the urine or of overt pathologic findings.

Emotional stress or allergy may predispose the patient to daytime frequency of urination. A compulsive liquid intake should be considered, especially in the neurotic or alcoholic patient and those on a reducing diet. Intermittent attacks of oliguria followed by polyuria should lead one to suspect psychocyclic edema. Nocturia without positive urologic findings may be due to habit, fretful sleep, allergy, early cardiac failure or late-night refreshments.

Some urologists believe the urethral syndrome to be the result of submucosal fibrosis in the urethra due to chronic infection which produces no overt pathologic findings but subtle changes in the physiology of micturition. Urethral dilations which break up this fibrosis, iron out the urethra, and disrupt epithelial pockets are widely used. Furacin in acute cases and phenol, glycerine or silver nitrate in chronic cases appear to cause the urothelium to revert to a more normal pattern. The very nervous patient or the patient with so-called congestive syndrome responds to hot sitz baths and the use of tranquilizers.

The urethral syndrome offers many imponderables. The conscientious urologist who carefully studies each of his patients with these complaints and lets them know that he cares enough to try multiple approaches to the problem will be rewarded with rare loyalty and gratitude.

Atrophy of the Prostatic Urethra in the Aged

Urethroscopy in some aged male patients shows an extremely tight, white, dry, avascular and fibrous sheath-like prostatic urethra devoid of any glandular tissue. This finding may also follow transurethral prostatectomy. These older patients have symptoms of prostatism that bring them to the urologist but on cystoscopy there is very little or no prostatic hyperplasia evident.

Any resection in these cases is too much resection and will result in atrophy of the meager glandular tissue. Better results are obtained in these patients with estrogen-androgen therapy, reassurance, occasional dilatation of the urethra with a Kollmann dilator, and antispasmodics when obstruction is not a major factor.

A detailed explanation to the referring physician to discourage transurethral resection for this type of patient is indicated.

Narrowing at the Meatus—Meatotomy

Narrowing of the terminal urethra is most common. Meatotomy, therefore, should be done freely. The narrowing may be just within the meatus, at the fossa navicularis. To remedy this in male patients, one needs merely, after local or general anesthesia, to place a straight clamp (one blade within the urethra and one on the outside of the urethra) on the frenal aspect of the glans penis. This may be left on for a period of 6 to 10 minutes for hemostasis. The incision is then made in the clamped area.

One may elect to place a suture at the lower end of the meatotomy wound, tying an absorbable suture into a number of knots; this knot will lie between the cut edges to hold them open. One may instead place sutures slightly lateral to the midline (one suture on each side) to keep the meatus open.

Mucosa-to-mucosa approximation with several sutures will prevent secondary meatal stenosis. Alternatively, the crushed cut edges may be treated with electrocautery, silver nitrate stick, or gold leaf, to prevent this stenosis.

Maintaining Patency After Meatotomy

The meatus should be opened from time to time manually (the patient or parent is instructed to do so before each voiding) and a sulfisoxazole diolamine (Gantrisin) ophthalmic ointment or polymyxin-B bacitracin (Polysporin) ophthalmic ointment is applied at least three times daily. The opthalmic tip allows for easier application of the ointment. This affords antisepsis in addition to lubricating the edges; there is thus less chance of the meatotomy sealing over.

If frequent meatal dilation seems indicated during the healing phase, urethral meatal dilators are available to the patient at surgical supply houses. Alternatively, one may give a catheter plug, plastic golf tee, or tapered plastic needle container to the patient or parent with the instruction to lubricate this with the antiseptic ointment and pass it into the meatus three times daily. When the cut edges have been sutured as described in the foregoing paragraphs, healing takes place *per primam*—it is not necessary to depend on repeated meatal dilations to prevent secondary stenosis.

Use of a Cotton Cone in the Meatus to Maintain Patency

The following method is a most practical one. One may take an applicator stick and by rolling cotton on it form a cone approximately 4 to 5 cm in length. The most proximal portion in relation to the urethra should be small, to allow placing it in the meatus. The cotton cone is lubricated well with petrolatum and forced into the urethra tightly enough so that it will remain there. The cotton is then held with the finger and the applicator stick removed.

The patient wears this or a replacement cone 24 hours a day for at least one week. He is shown how to make the cone and how to fit it into the urethra so that he does not injure himself or make the procedure too painful to carry out. Follow-up calibration of the urethra is necessary, as is dilation on rare occasion.

Maintaining Urethral Meatotomy Caliber in Male Children

In boys, a single suture of 5-0 Dermalon ® or nylon at the inferior margin of a meatotomy incision with five or six knots is left in position for five or six weeks until compete healing has occurred. This stitch discourages healing from the inferior margin of the incision. The stitch also marks the limit of the opening; thus the parent may more easily maintain the wide meatus. Even though their intentions are good, mothers will not spread open the incision as often or as adequately as necessary. The single stitch may be removed after complete healing.

(See also *Convenient Dilators for Patient Self-Use*, in Chapter One.)

Urethral Stricture

Obstruction in the anterior urethra usually is due to urethral stricture. One common cause of this problem is iatrogenic. The occurrence of stricture secondary to the previous use of bacteriostatic catheters has been fairly well established. Latex catheters covered with Teflon ® or Silastic catheters are much less apt to create strictures than are latex or red rubber catheters.

Another iatrogenic cause of stricture may be the performance of transurethral prostatectomy through a resectoscope sheath too large for the patient's urethra. Inflammation secondary to mucosal abrasion with too large a sheath, even going on to pressure necrosis, is said to be the main cause of strictures at the end of the penis and the fossa navicularis.

Other iatrogenic causes of stricture are trauma and burns of the urethra secondary to short circuits of the electrosurgical unit.

Noniatrogenic strictures generally result from specific and nonspecific urethritis.

Prevention of Postoperative Stricture

Some urologists feel that prior to transurethral prostatectomy one should use a bougie-à-boule to size 30 to calibrate the urethra. If the bougie-à-boule "hangs up" either at the meatus or anywhere in the anterior urethra, a cut through this narrowing should be made with the Otis or Maisonneuve urethrotome to size 32 French.

It is believed by many that the urethrotome is as important for the resectionist as is the balloon catheter. Postoperative strictures seem to be relatively few in those instances in which the urethrotome is used for areas of narrowing, as determined by the bougie-a-boule.

Meatotomy is frequently done dorsally rather than ventrally. This incision, though more vascular, seems to provide better healing with less likelihood of scar formation and can be done with a scalpel or urethrotome.

When transurethral resection of the prostate is indicated, perineal urethrostomy must occasionally be done when dealing with severe anterior strictures. The stricture may otherwise be aggravated.

Treatment of Urethral Stricture with Steroids

A urethral stricture readily located and palpable in the penile portion of the urethra may be treated by direct injection of a steroid in the dosage of 1 to 2 ml every several days for three to four doses. The response desired is like that of injection of a keloid with steroid medication; results with strictures are not as satisfactory.

A flexible needle may be utilized through the endoscope for deeply situated strictures.

Dilation should usually be done in conjunction with this treatment.

Stricture in Female Children

A bougie-a-boule should be utilized to determine the presence of urethral stricture in little girls, and also the presence of a "Lyon's ring." This concentric cicatricial ring, located just within the urethral meatus, was originally described by Dr. Richard Lyons of Berkeley, California.

The ring often will not be demonstrated when using ordinary sounds in dilating the urethra, but it will very definitely be evident with the use of a bougie-a-boule. By gently withdrawing the bougie-à-boule, if this is of sufficiently large size, the constricting ring will be everted out beyond the urethral meatus. With a scalpel, an incision is made at the 12 o'clock position. One may then utilize a slightly larger bougie-a-boule and cut still deeper. Additional incisions may be made on either side of the midline if one is not sufficient.

One may also use a urethrotome to cut the constricting area.

Should bleeding be troublesome, pinpoint fulguration may be done to effect hemostasis, though pressure is usually adequate.

Lubrication of the Urethra Prior to Instrumentation

Adequate lubrication of the urethra before any instrumentation attempt is exceedingly important. One may place the tip of a sterilized tube of anesthetic lubricating jelly at the meatus and squeeze the tube contents into the urethra. Another means consists of the use of a 10-cc non-Luer-lock syringe filled with lubricating jelly; the tip is placed within the urethral meatus and the syringe barrel is then emplaced for injection of the lubricant. One may do the same with an Asepto syringe.

The Becton-Dickinson tip No. 470-K is a small stainless-steel tip which fits any size ordinary piston syringe; this may be sterilized and attached to the syringe to inject solutions or lubrication into the urethra.

Additional Lubrication Prior to 'Scope Introduction

Some urologists prefer the use of mineral oil to lubricate the sheath of the resectoscope prior to introducing it into the urethra. The instrument seems to slide more easily, though the amount of oil used is not enough to make one's hand slippery or to impair vision. Other men use Vaseline on the resectoscope sheath.

Both substances should be used sparingly on the resectoscope sheath, since both will conduct current and serious burn damage may result if arcs from the current of the electrosurgical unit leap across the resectoscope to the glans penis due to collection of oil or Vaseline on the glans. Vaseline in particular may wipe off somewhat and collect in this manner.

Use of Filiforms and Followers for Urethral Strictures in Male Patients

For patients in acute retention due to urethral stricture, the use of filiforms and followers is indicated. Should there be difficulty in passing a filiform into the bladder, the passage of multiple filiforms (up to five or six of them) may eventually result in successful passage of one filiform into the bladder.

A filiform with a spiral tip may pass more readily than the straight-tip filiform. Pulling on the penis straight upward and rotating the filiform both clockwise and counterclockwise while passing it slowly and gently will sometimes allow passage.

After passing a spiral-tip filiform as far as possible without undue pushing, one may pass beside it a second filiform. If this too fails to reach the bladder, one may pass alongside these a third, fourth, fifth, or sixth filiform to hopefully overcome the stricture.

It may be helpful to grasp the end of the filiform with the sterile gloved finger and squeeze the tip with the fingernail, *so that a very slight angulation is made at the end of the filiform for a distance of 1 to 2 mm.* This maneuver may allow the filiform to slide through the stricture.

When all else fails, and before the field becomes bloody, one may try to visualize with a panendoscope the area of stricture and under vision pass a filiform.

Direct-Vision Passage of Filiforms by Use of a Panendoscope

Endoscopy may be of value when it is impossible to introduce a filiform into the bladder. A No. 20 or 24 French panendoscope is passed under anesthesia, using great care not to traumatize the urethra. Bleeding may occur from too vigorous manipulation with filiforms or passage of the panendoscope, and it then becomes impossible to "look one's way in."

With the panendoscope in place and the irrigating fluid flowing rapidly, the opening through the stricture may be visualized. A filiform may be passed under vision through the stricture. The panendoscope is removed as the filiform is pushed farther into the urethra. Care must be exercised that withdrawal of the panendoscope sheath does not also pull out the filiform.

Woven or steel (Le Fort) followers are then passed. If unsuccessful, other filiforms might pass alongside the one already placed. The filiforms may then be tied in place and left inlying for four to seven days.

If one is unable to pass any instrument, cystostomy is indicated. After several days, when the acute inflammatory aspect of the urethral trauma has subsided, one may then again attempt to do direct-vision instrumentation as a first choice before instrumentation by filiforms.

Infection is frequently present when the patient with a severe stricture is initially seen. Chemotherapy usually makes easier a second attempt at overcoming the strictured area.

Methods of Anchoring Filiforms or Catheters

If the patient has a long foreskin and is apt to develop a paraphimosis by having the foreskin pulled back, one may proceed thus: an area of penis, pubic area, and abdomen up to the umbilicus is shaved the width of the safety razor. This shaved area is then sponged with tincture of benzoin compound. Tincture of benzoin is also placed circumferentially on the skin just proximal to the corona of the glans.

When the benzoin has become "sticky," a one-inch-wide piece of adhesive is placed in the shaven path from the coronal sulcus to the umbilicus. A piece of one-inch-wide adhesive is also circumferentially placed loosely around the penis over the tincture of benzoin, just behind the corona. Braided suture* is looped over another such piece of adhesive, as shown in Figure 48. This is placed circularly around the penis over the first layer of adhesive. The loops extend slightly beyond the urethral meatus. At least six equally spaced loops should be so placed that they span the complete penile circumference. The catheter or filiform may buckle and slip out between widely spaced loops.

Similar suture material is passed through each one of these loops in suc-

---

* Spools of heavy black button or carpet thread purchased in any notions or department or variety store also serve this purpose.

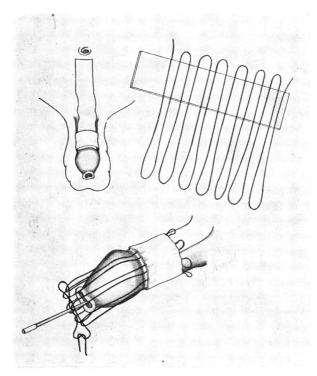

48. Anchoring filiform or nonballoon catheter

cession and then tied with a triple knot snugly around the filiform or catheter.

With circumcised patients, one may eliminate the tape running from the
coronal sulcus to the umbilicus but otherwise proceed as described. The
adhesive in circumcised patients usually will not slip off over the corona.
Therefore the adhesive strip lengthwise from the penis to the abdomen is
unnecessary.

The described procedure provides reliable anchoring with relatively little
slippage.

Varied Materials Utilized to Tie in Filiforms and Catheters

Common string may be substituted for braided suture or carpet and button thread for anchoring a catheter, providing more holding surface between the string and catheter. The larger caliber of the string precludes its
use with filiforms.

Umbilical tape or adhesive strips also may be subsituted for the above-
mentioned materials when anchoring a catheter in the manner just described. Whatever material is used for the loops, fixing them close to the
urethral meatus with an adequate number of loops is necessary to prevent
the catheter from slipping out between them.

When adhesive tape is used instead of the loops the anchoring is not certain, since the adhesive becomes wet from urethral discharge and/or urine.

Manufactured Appliance for Anchoring Catheter

Rubberized appliances are marketed which fit around the penis behind the coronal sulcus. An opening is provided through which the catheter or filiform may be passed. These devices are not too satisfactory since the filiform slips through the opening in the device.

Suture Through Glans Penis to Anchor Catheter or Filiform

Some urologists take a suture through the glans penis and then tie the suture on to the filiform or catheter. Because of the pain to the patient whenever there is movement, this is not recommended as the method of choice. The suture may slough, too, permitting the filiform or catheter to fall out.

The suture through the glans will find greatest acceptance among urologists whose patients may be uncooperative by pulling out the filiform.

Further Dilation of Stricture

An indwelling filiform (or filiforms) acts as a dilator. After two days, additional filiforms usually may be passed into the bladder around the anchored filiform(s). If a number of filiforms have been indwelling, it may be possible to remove them and pass and anchor a small balloon-type catheter. This is dependent on the size to which the urethra has been dilated following placement of the filiforms.

Frequently, when a single filiform is passed and left in for four to seven days, small followers will easily pass. After adequate urethral lubrication a No. 10 to 12 French catheter can be passed and anchored. If a balloon-type catheter is successfully passed, progressive dilation may be accomplished by reinserting larger catheters every two to five days up to 22 to 24 French.

Black Silk Voided as Aid to Future Dilation of Stricture

In instances of severe urethral injury with long-standing scar and impassable stricture, and where one is anxious to maintain continuity, it may sometimes be possible to run 2-0 or 3-0 black suture down the suprapubic sinus tract when changing catheters, with the old catheter removed and the new not yet inserted. Sufficient length* of suture is passed into the bladder so that when the patient voids after clamping the cystostomy tube, the black silk passes into the urethra and out through the meatus.

When the black silk passes out through the meatus, it is tied to a filiform or sutured to a small, sturdy catheter. The suprapubic balloon catheter is

---

* Passing too much suture into the bladder will result in the suture coiling up in a "ball" proximal to the stricture.

either deflated or completely removed and the black silk is pulled out supra-pubically. The filiform or catheter is led into the bladder transurethrally. By not disturbing the black silk, larger catheters or followers later may be passed transurethrally, using the same silk as a guide after first removing the smaller indwelling catheter, filiform, etc. One may seesaw back and forth in this manner for some period of time. After each manipulation the suprapubic catheter is replaced.

The sterility of the ends of silk must be maintained so that contamination and consequent infection will not take place. Catheters are best fixed at their tip to the black suture. Several inches of black silk should precede the catheter into the urethra. The silk is well lubricated before being pulled back into the urethra.

This trick of the trade may also be used at the time of open cystostomy when all attempts at passage up or down the urethra have failed. The silk is again passed out the abdominal wound alongside the cystostomy catheter.

Control of Bleeding from a Bulbous Urethral Stricture

Bleeding from a bulbous urethral stricture which has been dilated in the office or hospital outpatient department can many times be controlled by the patient using perineal pressure. Two-finger pressure is maintained in the perineum for a period of at least ten minutes. A frantic telephone call may sometimes be obviated.

There are infrequent instances in which a patient with a severely bleeding post-instrumentation urethra must be subjected to fulguration.

Severe Urethral Strictures with Diverticula

The Johanson urethroplasty has been utilized very successfully in cases of severe urethral stricture. Strictures associated with diverticula may also be handled by the Johanson method. Subsequent to the first-stage urethroplasty, the diverticular cavities may diminish to the point where they may be hardly identifiable. The Turner-Warwick approach has also been a favorite operation for stricture in male patients.

Internal Urethrotomy in Treatment of Urethral Strictures: Indication

The rationale for performance of internal urethrotomy, and the method by which it should be done, have been long debated. The pendulum has swung back and forth over the years on these questions. Its moderate recent gain in popularity would indicate there is a definite place for this procedure in present-day urology.

One definite indication for it would appear to be in conjunction with transurethral resection of the prostate. The resectoscope sheath must move to and fro through the urethra *throughout* the operative procedure. If this is not accomplished one can expect aggravation of a preexisting stricture or the development of a stricture in an otherwise normal urethra. The incidence of stricture after transurethral prostatectomy has been reported as from 10 to 20 percent.

Many cases of stricture result from ischemic necrosis or abrasion with associated inflammation because the No. 28 French resectoscope sheath may be tight within the urethra. Current leak with burn by electrosurgical machine malfunction, shorting-out due to resectoscope or loop current leak, poor grounding, etc., in addition to specific or nonspecific catheter urethritis, also account for some strictures. Bladder neck contractures occur also following prostate surgery.

Internal urethrotomy is often done when the No. 28 French McCarthy resectoscope sheath is not readily passed or when it does not have a free to-and-fro movement after passage even though its insertion was easy. Areas of urethral narrowing are determined easily by means of bougie-à-boule calibration. Passage of a sound of equivalent size will often cause this narrowing to be overlooked.

When the urethral channel is considered inadequate, the operator has the option of performing an internal urethrotomy or of using a smaller sheath (24 or 26 French). The size of the prostate will guide the operator's decision since more tissue can be removed with the large resectoscope loop.

Some urologists use the urethrotome routinely with transurethral resection (32 or 34 French), passing the blade through the entire length of the urethra. Using this procedure, these urologists have reported a much lower incidence of stricture.

Methods Employed in Internal Urethrotomy

Urethrotomy may be done with several different instruments and by different methods. It should be preceded by urethrography, and this should be repeated several months after the corrective procedure. If an incision is necessary in the fossa navicularis, the Otis or Maisonneuve urethrotome is used, but incision can also be done with a scalpel. Some urologists prefer the Riba urethrotome, though this electrical urethrotome is usually employed for a deeper lesion.

URETHROTOMY WITH THE STRAIGHT-MODEL URETHROTOME. The urethrotome is placed in the urethra in the closed position beyond the area of stricture. It is utilized anyplace in the anterior urethra. The calibration dial of the urethrotome is opened to 34 to 36 French, and the cutting blade of the urethrotome is withdrawn.

In most cases the urethrotome is placed in such position that the knife blade will make the cut at exactly 12 o'clock. With this position the incision is assumed to be in the fibrous septum between the corpora cavernosa, thereby minimizing bleeding. Bleeding is often profuse. Many urologists, therefore, are not too specific as to the position of the incision. The 11 and 1 o'clock positions are often utilized.

With the wearing of Silastic catheters over longer periods of time after internal urethrotomy, recurrence of stenoses should be less than reported in previous years.

Internal urethrotomy with the Otis urethrotome is common practice by many urologists for meatal or distal urethral stenoses in young girls and older women.

ELECTROSURGICAL URETHROTOMY. Some urologists prefer to do internal urethrotomy using electrosurgical means, employing a tip electrode. A No. 24 French resectoscope sheath is passed into the well-lubricated urethra to the strictured area. Then under direct vision, with the working element of the resectoscope, the stricture is cut with a Moulder knife electrode at the 12 o'clock position. As a rule, the resectoscope sheath will then pass into the bladder easily.

If the strictured area is insufficiently cut at the 12 o'clock position, further cuts may need to be made at the 10 and 2 o'clock positions. If the cuts are made slowly and deliberately, bleeding is usually minimal. If significant bleeding does occur, the bleeding points may be fulgurated with the same electrosurgical unit.

URETHROTOMY WITH THE RIBA ELECTROURETHROTOME. This instrument is of considerable value and its use warrants reevaluation. The flexible-shaft urethrotome, with provisions for attaching a standard filiform tip to pass through a urethral stricture, has a wire cutting loop which may be varied in size from 12 to 30 French. The urethrotome is readily passed through most urethral strictures, the loop opened, the electrical current applied, and the stricture then cut up to 30 French in size as the instrument is withdrawn with the loop in the dorsal midline portion of the urethra. A No. 24 French balloon-type silicone-coated or Silastic catheter may be inserted into the bladder and left indwelling. Hemostasis is obtained by compression of the urethra by the indwelling catheter.

Catheterization After Urethrotomy

If the indwelling catheter is not left in place long enough, the stricture will recur. In previous years this happened very often and for this reason the electrosurgical internal urethrotomy and "cold knife" internal urethrotomy as methods of treating strictures lost a good deal of appeal.

A No. 24 French balloon-type silicone-coated or Silastic catheter inserted after urethrotomy and left in place for four to six weeks keeps the area open while healing is progressing. The complications of infection, extravasation, or serious hemorrhage are minimal. The incidence of stricture recurrence is moderate when handled in this manner.

External Urethrotomy

A urethral sound may be passed to the bulbous urethra and an incision made directly over the sound. The cut edges of skin, subcutaneous tissues, and urethra may all be grasped with an Allis forceps on either side. A transverse or vertical incision into the urethra may also be made over the tip of the sound. It is helpful in this latter case to gently grasp the proximal cut edge of the urethra with Kelly clamps.

Perineal Urethrotomy

INDICATIONS FOR EXTERNAL PERINEAL URETHROTOMY. In doing transurethral resection, if dilation is difficult or if after dilation the resectoscope sheath is bound at the meatus and along several areas of the urethra, perineal urethrotomy is indicated.

The elderly debilitated male with a difficult stricture requiring repeated dilation might benefit by a permanent perineal urethrostomy. This could be accomplished using the same technique utilized in a first-stage Johanson urethroplasty for a bulbous urethral stricture.

TECHNIQUE IN EXTERNAL PERINEAL URETHROTOMY. A simple method of doing a perineal urethrotomy follows: a long-beaked resectoscope sheath is inserted into the urethra with a Timberlake obturator in place. The obturator is removed and the sheath is held so that the tip with its oblique fenestra is palpable through the perineum 2 to 3 cm behind the scrotum.

A vertical incision is made over the palpable fenestra of the sheath through the skin and deeper tissues, exposing the instrument. The sheath tip is then pushed through the perineal skin incision. A second resectoscope sheath (of the same size or next size smaller) with the Timberlake obturator in place is guided into the bulbous urethra by placing the protruding angled end of the obturator into the oblique fenestra of the sheath which is protruding from the urethrotomy. As the second sheath enters the urethra, the sheath in the penile urethra is gradually withdrawn. The tip of the second sheath can easily be guided with its obturator through the membranous urethra into the bladder. The original perineal vertical incision must be generous enough to permit this intra- and extra-manipulation of the obturator end.

Following the endoscopic resection, the urethrotomy site is not closed. A small strip of iodoform gauze is packed into the opening and left in place. After three days the pack is removed. This packing prevents hematoma formation beneath the skin edges. Although the patient may lose a few drops of urine from the urethrotomy site for a day or so, it invariably closes. Most urologists use large folded abdominal pads over the urethrotomy site with pressure-type adhesive if there is mild bleeding.

INSTRUMENTS FOR PERINEAL URETHROTOMY. A clamp which is useful for the

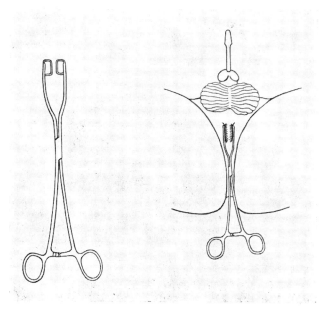

49. Perineal urethrotomy clamp and
its use in immobilizing perineal
tissues around urethral sound

anchoring of a sound in the perineum during urethrotomy is one called
"Pucker's hallux forceps." The instrument resembles a large towel forceps
with beads to stop deep penetration of the sharp points.

Kyril B. Conger [*] described a clamp devised to tighten the perineal
tissues overlying a sound in the urethra. Perineal urethrotomy is facilitated
by the use of this instrument (Fig. 49).

AIDING EXPOSURE IN PERINEAL URETHROTOMY. When performing perineal
urethrotomy, one may make a transverse incision across the urethra after
the urethra has been exposed. The lower lip of the urethra (bladder side)
may be grasped with mosquito clamps and this lower lip may then be
bivalved. The distal aspect of the urethra is held by clamps, affording better exposure for subsequent passage of instruments into the bladder.

Bladder Neck Contracture

Common Modalities of Treatment

Following prostatectomy, whether transurethral or open surgical, contracture of the bladder neck is a not uncommon occurrence. It is discon-
certing when, during the performance of cystoscopy on a postoperative
patient, a bladder neck is viewed which is barely large enough to admit a

[*] Kyril B. Conger. "New Clamp For Use in Perineal Urethrostomy," *Journal of Urology,* Vol.
90 No. 2 (August, 1963), p. 242.

No. 4 French filiform. Small-caliber bladder necks may be treated by transurethral resection of the entire circumference of the bladder neck, or the urethrotome may be used to make cuts at the bladder neck (invariably at 12, 3, 6, and 9 o'clock).

Incisions should be made so that one can very easily pass a Kollmann dilator and open it to a 45 French caliber without feeling any constriction of the bladder neck.

Alternative Treatment

Some urologists feel that the recurrence of bladder neck contracture is less common after use of the punctate cutting electrode, Moulder knife, or the Bugbee electrode. Multiple incisions at the bladder neck are required with all the above.

Healing of the bladder neck in the wide-open position is the secret for success. Unfortunately, the bladder neck will contract in many instances after the above procedure, so that in some cases open surgery of the bladder neck with Y-V plasty must be done.

Ensuring Success of Multiple-Incision Contracture Treatments

Frequent bladder neck dilatations, at least once per week for six to eight weeks, or the long wearing of a 24 French silicone-coated or non-irritating plastic catheter for six to eight weeks will help to ensure success of the treatments just described.

Repair of Bladder Neck Contracture Concomitant with Ureteral Reimplantation

A certain number of young male patients require ureteral reimplantation. During surgery some of these patients are found to also have tight bladder necks. The formal Y-V plasty may be done, or a modified procedure may be used. A longitudinal incision may be made through the prostatic capsule and prostatic tissue down to, but not through, the urethral mucosa and left wide open. This is, in principle, the same as the Ramstedt operation for pyloric stenosis.

This type of widening of the bladder neck serves as a good alternative to the formal Y-V plasty. A posterior wedge resection of the bladder neck can be added to the procedure if a wider bladder neck is desired.

Maneuver for Dilating Vesicle Neck

While the Kollmann dilator is the instrument of choice for dilating the bladder neck, a healing bladder neck may be dilated by rather forcibly pushing a sound from side to side. Patients with a very small urethra may often be dilated successfully in this manner.

Vesicle Neck and Urethral Dilators for Women

When urological instruments are not available, the Hegar cervical dilators function well for bladder neck and urethral dilation of the female patient. All desired sizes are available.

Transurethral Management of Post-Resection Vesicle Neck Fibrosis

Cicatricial contracture of the bladder neck may follow transurethral prostatectomy. In such instances, it may be difficult to blindly pass filiforms into the bladder. The following technique may be helpful.

By use of a panendoscope the contracted bladder neck is visualized. A filiform, via the operating element of the panendoscope, is passed into the bladder. The operating instrument is removed, followed by removal of the panendoscope sheath. Because of the length of the filiform, it may be necessary to apply perineal pressure over the filiform after partially removing the endoscopic sheath. This may keep the filiform from coming out with the sheath. Additional length to the filiform may be obtained by attaching a follower small enough to pass through the operating instrument.

Once the bladder neck is dilated to the desired size, the operator may elect from any of the previously described procedures to correct the contracture.

Following transurethral prostatic resection in those selected cases where bladder neck contracture is anticipated, it is the custom of the authors to make incisions at 3, 6, and 9 o'clock. Secondary bladder neck contracture is most likely to occur in those cases where there is no intravesical protrusion of the prostate, the hyperplasia being confined to the prostatic urethra, or in the "tight" prostatic urethra and bladder neck due to long-standing prostatic inflammation. In both of these situations resection of the bladder neck still leaves one with a relatively small bladder neck which can easily contract significantly.

LESS COMMON URETHRAL PATHOLOGY

Foreign Body in the Male Urethra

If urethral obstruction is not due to tumor or stricture, a stone or foreign body may be present. One must attempt to remove this by using either a foreign body forceps through a panendoscope or, in some instances, it may be possible to place a stone forceps within the urethra to remove the object. If the object is too large, or if wedged, one may be required to make an incision directly over the foreign body and thus remove it.

At times, a hemostat passed through the urethral meatus may be used to remove a foreign body or stone. This may also be done under vision by using a No. 16 French panendoscope and passing a small hemostat alongside the endoscope. This presupposes that the object to be removed is lodged not far from the urethral meatus.

Frequently a stone is lodged just within the urethral meatus which is "relatively stenotic." Dilating the meatus, which usually pushes the stone back up the urethra, often results in spontaneous passage of the stone on the next voiding.

The great variety of the foreign bodies lost in the urethra makes description of their removal impossible in this book.

Office Treatment of Calculi
Arrested in the Male Urethra

An occasional bladder or kidney stone may become arrested in the urethra during passage from the bladder to the external urinary meatus. A filiform may be passed beyond the calculus and then the Johnson stone basket threaded on to the filiform and passed up the urethra beyond the stone. The calculus will engage and may be withdrawn under local anesthesia or Brevital amnesia in the office. This obviates doing external urethrotomy.

In lieu of the stone basket, the loop catheter may be utilized. The catheter is passed into the bladder, a loop is made, and the looped catheter is slowly withdrawn. Alternatively, a small balloon catheter may be inserted and the balloon blown up with 2 to 4 ml of water and then slowly withdrawn. A stone may be "delivered" in this manner on occasion.

Urethral Condylomata

Condylomata acuminata usually are readily handled by excision, fulguration, circumcision, and meatotomy. Upon occasion, recurrence of these tumors may be rapid and persistent. Involvement proximal to the fossa navicularis is uncommon and usually is single, but may recur following fulguration. Possible involvement of the entire urethra may be a difficult problem. Vesical involvement is an extremely serious problem and often may be cured only by cystectomy.

In the event urethral recurrences are multiple and persistent, the Johanson urethroplasty has been utilized with success. When the urethra seems to have a normal appearance following the first stage of the Johanson procedure, then the second stage of the urethroplasty may be done. In many instances in which this approach has been utilized, the condylomata have not recurred.

Thiotepa and colchicine have been used for intraurethral lesions with some success.

Carcinoma of the Urethra

Carcinoma of the urethra may also simulate a stricture. One may be able to pass a panendoscope and look into the urethra to see if the typical fungating appearance of a carcinoma is or is not present. Biopsy should be taken freely in suspicious instances. In addition to the usual modes of biopsy, the ureteral stone basket may be used as already described for ureteral tumors.

Possible Urethral Involvement in Carcinoma of the Glans Penis

In instances of carcinoma of the glans penis, inspection of the urethra *per se* does not suffice to disprove the presence of disease in the urethra. It cannot be stressed too emphatically that sections should be done to ensure that there is no cancer in the urethra, if the treatment planned is less than radical.

Female Urethral Diverticula

Identification of Urethral Diverticula

Urethral diverticula are seen more frequently of late due to increased awareness on the part of urologists. Identification of the diverticula, however, can be a difficult and frustrating task. For better preoperative localization of a diverticulum in females, one may take urethrograms utilizing the Trattner double-balloon urethrographic catheter. Even with this instrument there usually is leakage of contrast material at the urethral meatus.

The authors have found the following method helpful in visualizing these diverticula. One may tie off the drainage opening (the eye) in a No. 16 French balloon catheter distal to the balloon with 3-0 silk suture. A fenestra is made with scissors in the catheter immediately proximal to the balloon. Care must be used that the opening is made on the side of the catheter opposite the balloon filling lumen.

The catheter is then passed, the balloon blown up with about 8 to 10 ml of water, and the catheter put on tension as the contrast material is injected through the catheter. One finger is utilized to maintain pressure at the urethral meatus to keep the contrast material from running out of the urethra. Anterior, posterior, and lateral views are then taken by injection.

Unfortunately, the above technique does result in undue X-ray exposure to the urologist. If one must employ this technique often, a special shielded gauntlet should be used to protect the hand and forearm.

Alternative methods employ oil contrast material or mixed equal parts of contrast material and lubricating jelly injected by means of blunt-tip Asepto syringes or non-Luer-lock disposable syringes. A viscous material is less apt to pass through the often tiny diverticular os.

Surgical Treatment of Female Urethral Diverticula

When the diverticulum is identified, a Dourmashkin olive-tip ureteral catheter with inflatable balloon is passed into the diverticulum. The balloon is distended to facilitate dissection. An inverted "U" incision is utilized, the base of the U nearest the urethral meatus. In this manner a flap of anterior vaginal wall is turned back to approach the diverticulum.

When the incision is closed, a staggered closure is accomplished. This minimizes the possibility of a secondary urethrovaginal fistula.

Other standard methods of repair of urethral diverticula are well described elsewhere. It is important to stress the need of search for the presence of multiple or additional small diverticula which continue to plague the patient in the postoperative period.

The method of surgical treatment by vaginal incision into the diverticulum, phenolizing its lining, and packing of the diverticulum with iodoform gauze as the area granulates in solidly, is also to be considered. A successful refinement of this is vaginal incision into the diverticulum, phenolizing the lining, packing with Gelfoam and closing of the diverticulum and vaginal mucosa.

ADDITIONAL AIDS TO URETHRAL SURGERY AND INSTRUMENTATION

Orientation

Aid to Passage of Sound Prior to Additional Instrumentation

With an anesthetized patient in the lithotomy position, it may be difficult to pass a sound easily. A false passage may be produced if the procedure is not discontinued. The patient's legs may be placed flat on the table to facilitate instrument passage. After adequate dilation of the urethra, a cystoscope, resectoscope, or other instrument in use will readily pass after the patient has again been placed in the regular lithotomy position. This change-of-position maneuver may be very useful and time-saving.

Before taking the patient down from the lithotomy position, successful passage of the sound may also be accomplished using a finger rectally to guide the sound through the membranous and prostatic urethra. This maneuver is particularly helpful in the male child.

Positioning the Female Patient on the Operating Table for Urethral Surgery

The patient may be placed on the operating table on her abdomen.

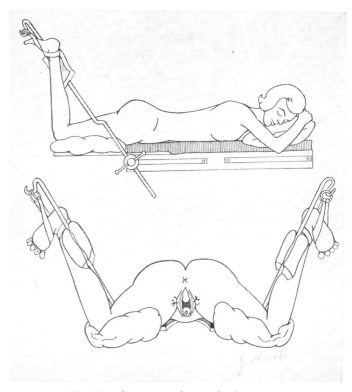

50. Female position for urethral surgery

The symphysis is placed over the end of the table with the tail gate down. The usual intravenous arm boards are placed under the table pad, extending parallel with the table to support each thigh to the knee. Pillows may be placed under the legs on the arm boards. The lower extremities are flexed at the knee and each foot is tied to a leg brace.

The labia are held apart with adhesive tape or by a suture to each thigh. A retractor is utilized to raise the vaginal floor by pulling it upward. The underside of the urethra is widely and completely exposed in this position, as illustrated in Figure 50.

Care must be taken to completely shield the extremities from the metal leg braces to prevent grounding out in using the electrosurgical unit.

Dressing for Post-Instrumentation Urethral Bleeding in Male Patients

A dressing of cotton balls, facial tissues, and ultra-thin clear plastic cling-type paper such as "Saran Wrap" or "Glad® Wrap" may be used when there is bleeding from the meatus following instrumentation. One may use three to four cotton balls within a piece of facial tissue. The cotton balls are placed over the urethral meatus, and the tissue wrapped around the penis to include the cotton balls. The inside of the tissue may

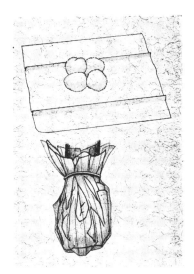

51. Simple dressing for post-instrumentation bleeding in male patients

be reinforced with an opened-up 4- by 4-inch gauze. A piece of plastic wrap is then wrapped around the tissue and the entire penis. This is held loosely on the penis by a rubber band (see Fig. 51).

Should there be any leakage or drainage through the dressing, the plastic wrap will maintain the drainage within itself, avoiding the soiling of the patient's clothing. The plastic wrap is nonallergenic and has been found quite satisfactory. Small plastic sandwich bags, easily obtainable in food markets, may be used in the same manner, as may other types of thin plastic material.

Catheterization

Aids to Catheterization: Anesthesia and Prelubrication

When a patient is in acute retention, catherization is first attempted with a soft Robinson catheter (or Coudé-tip Tiemann catheter) or a balloon-type catheter. Instrumentation is facilitated if topical local anesthesia is instilled into the urethra and the patient is then sedated with 25 to 100 mg of meperidine hydrochloride (Demerol) intravenously or intramuscularly. Any other appropriate narcotic may be utilized. Intravenous diazepam (Valium), 5 mg, or sodium methohexital (Brevital) to the amnesia level (described at length in Chapter One) are also effective.

Prelubrication is essential. One may cold-sterilize an unopened tube of lubricating jelly, insert the tip of the tube into the meatus, and inject 10 to 15 ml of jelly into the urethra; or one may remove the bulb of an Asepto syringe or the plunger of a 10- or 20-ml syringe, fill the syringe with the lubricant, place the tip of the syringe within the meatus, and inject the lubricating jelly into the urethra.

Instead of lubricating jelly one may use lidocaine (Xylocaine) jelly for both lubrication and anesthesia. Xylocaine viscous, used for gastric or esophogeal topical anesthesia, previously autoclaved for sterility may be used. This is far less expensive than the lidocaine jelly.

Improvised Stylet for Balloon-Type Catheter

If unable to pass a balloon-type urethral catheter in the absence of a stylet or mandrin, a wire coat hanger may be used to devise such an instrument. It is safer to use a ureteral catheter with a wire stylet, which may be passed inside of a well-lubricated balloon catheter. The wire stylet may be fixed to the catheter with a hemostat on the drainage lumen. With this arrangement the end of the catheter can be fashioned into a Coudé tip.

The novice is warned against the use of a wire stylet. It is best left to those with considerable manipulative experience. The ureteral catheter splinting device, sometimes used with two wires for better rigidity, is much safer in the hands of the beginner. The inexperienced should use the technique described immediately below before using any splinted catheter and, if unsuccessful, then use the ureteral splinting device. If this fails, call for help. Too vigorous urethral manipulation by the novice has frequently led to unnecessary emergent open surgery.

A disposable flexible stylet based on the above principle may soon be on the market.

Coudé-Tip Catheter in Prostatic Hyperplasia

In patients with prostatic hyperplasia a Robinson or balloon-type catheter often cannot be readily passed. The Coudé-tip Tiemann catheter may here be employed. The No. 16 French Coudé-tip catheter will readily pass over the hypertrophied middle lobe of the prostate. Following the emptying of the bladder a latex balloon-type catheter is then often easily introduced into the decompressed bladder. Coudé-tip balloon catheters are available. If a Coudé-tip catheter cannot be passed, a urethral stricture must be suspected. Dilation may be necessary.
(See additional aids to catheterization in Chapter Eight.)

Urethral Catheter for Infants

The plastic premature or infant feeding tube is an excellent substitute for a urethral catheter for an infant. Additional holes should be cut in this catheter to ensure better drainage. These holes may be cut with a fine scissors or burnt into the catheter with a heated needle.

Long-Term Constant Drainage per Urethra

A small-gauge plastic catheter passed per urethra can provide excellent constant drainage. The Gibbon catheter, an extremely long catheter designed for use with a British drainage bottle, in sizes 8 or 10 French, has served well in cases of chronic retention. Pediatric feeding tubes may also serve the same purpose. The newly available plastic catheters will also improve this situation.

Aid to Maintenance of Sterility in Treatment of Retention Catheter Patients

Recent attention has been justifiably directed toward urethral catheterization and catheter drainage as a contributory cause of urinary tract infections. The education of medical and nursing personnel in the care of the catheter has been inadequate and underemphasized. Much importance is placed on the sterile insertion of urethral catheters. Little concern is shown for the distal end of the catheter once it is inserted.

When a catheter is connected to a disposable plastic drainage tube, the cap which maintains sterility during packaging is often discarded. Therefore, the plastic drainage tube tip which fits into the catheter becomes grossly contaminated. When a patient's bed is changed and the catheter disconnected, the plastic drainage tubing often falls to the floor. The nursing aide, without hesitancy, often reconnects the drainage tube without proper sterilization.

To circumvent this break in sterile technique, the end of the plastic tubing must be immersed, on disconnection, in a test tube fastened to the patient's bed with adhesive tape (see Fig. 52). The test tube is filled with aqueous activitated dealdehyde (Cidex).

Until such time as all manufacturers of disposable plastic tubing provide a more permanent means of protecting the sterility of this tubing, this idea may be useful. The attachment of a Cidex-filled test tube to the patient's bed, with instruction to nursing and paramedical personnel to be sure that the plastic tip which fits into the catheter must be placed in the Cidex-filled test tube, will help ensure the sterility of the system.

Emphasis should be placed on treating the open end of the catheter like an open wound, covering it with sterile gauze which is held on by adhesive tape or rubber band. A sterile connection point on hooking up to a leg bag must also be emphasized. Leg bags are best used only while the patient is ambulatory. Too often the one-way valve in the disposable bag is defective. It is a common sight to see a patient resting in bed with thighs flexed, the urine literally draining back into the bladder from the bag.

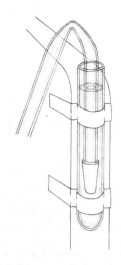

52. Bedside test tube and solution to ensure sterility of catheter drainage tubing

Prevention of Irritation and Infection from Indwelling Urethral Catheter

Some patients do not tolerate any type of indwelling urethral catheter. This may be true whether the catheter be red rubber, latex, or silicone-coated. Many of these patients develop a severe urethritis around the catheter with later severe stricture formation.

A successful means of coping with this problem is to wrap Kling dressing around the penis and catheter and keep this dressing continuously moist with hexylresorcinol (ST-37). Approximately eight to ten loops of Kling are wound around the catheter-penis junction. The patient is instructed to keep this dressing moistened with the ST-37 which is kept at the bedside. ST-37 reduces surface tension and consequently has a thinning effect on the mucoid discharge in patients sensitive to the catheter. The solution is drawn up into the space between the catheter and the urethra by capillary action.

In females, the catheter and urethral meatus are washed at least twice daily with pHisoHex®. The incidence of urethritis in both males and females is dramatically reduced by use of the preparations mentioned. One may also apply a cream-like application of Neosporin® or neomycin-like type of antibiotic to the catheter and urethral meatus about twice to three times daily. The dressing is changed at this time for male patients.

Retention of Balloon Catheter

Difficulties in Deflating Balloon Catheters

After passing a balloon catheter into the bladder, the balloon of the catheter can be inflated with ease. On attempting to remove the catheter, however, one finds occasionally that the balloon will not deflate.

In some instances a tiny piece of excess rubber (a manufacturing defect) may act as a ball valve, allowing fluid to be injected into the balloon to distend it but preventing fluid from running out to deflate it. More often the portion of the inflating lumen within the balloon is compressed by the pressure of the balloon due to defective manufacturing. A tiny piece of lint or cotton or other foreign body (which may have gotten into the filling fluid at the time the balloon was first distended) may be caught within the stem of the balloon. Crush of the catheter during insertion by the hemostat, to prevent catheter drainage, may at the same time seal off the inflating arm of the catheter.

Distending the Balloon with Fluid to Point of Rupture

A 5-ml latex balloon will hold up to 85 to 90 ml of fluid before the balloon will rupture. This small-sized balloon may very easily be distended within the bladder to this volume or slightly more to cause it to rupture. When it is necessary to rupture the balloon, the patient should be forewarned that there will be a "pop" as the balloon ruptures.

Deflating Latex Balloons of Larger Size

A 30-ml bag will hold up to 225 ml of fluid before rupturing. The 75-ml bag (utilized on rare occasions in patients subjected to open prostatectomy) may be filled up to 1325 ml before the balloon will rupture. Obviously, these larger amounts of fluid would not be tolerated by the patient. It is necessary to use other means to deflate these balloons.

The catheter may be transected just beyond the meatus, first grasping the drainage lumen *wall only* to prevent slippage of the catheter back into the urethra. If there was obstruction in the filling stem in the severed section, the balloon will empty. If not, a wire ureteral stylet is passed through the inflating lumen down to the inside of the balloon. The stylet may overcome the problem and the balloon will deflate.

Dissolution of Balloon

One may first partially fill the bladder with sterile water or saline and then inject into the filling stem of the balloon 0.5 ml of ether, xylol (xylene), or chloroform. These agents will dissolve the balloon, but at body temperature markedly expand (in the gas form) and usually rupture the balloon before dissolving it. For this reason, these agents may be dangerous with the larger balloons. Sterile water or saline will dilute their effect on the bladder. The bladder should immediately be irrigated free of all of the agent.

If the balloon is not intact after deflation (this should always be carefully checked when the catheter is removed), a piece of rubber may remain within the bladder. Fragments frequently may be flushed out with an endoscopic sheath and the Ellik evacuator. Also, with a cystoscope and a cystoscopic rongeur or alligator forceps, fragments can be removed from the bladder. With the bladder incompletely filled, the loose rubber may be easily seen. When the bladder has been filled with fluid, the rubber particle may be difficult to see as it usually floats on top of the irrigating solution and may be lost in the air bubble in the bladder. The fragment may be hiding in a diverticulum, if one is present. One may defer instrumentation and await the patient voiding out the rubber. One of our patients voided a portion of his balloon catheter some ten months later. However, the fragment may act as a stone nidus if not eventually passed.

Mineral Oil to Deflate Catheter Balloon

Another method for deflation is to inject mineral oil into the balloon. This is best done with a 10-ml syringe utilizing a 20-gauge needle. With a 5-ml balloon, 5 ml of oil is sufficient; with a 30-ml balloon, 10 ml of oil is required. In ten to fifteen minutes, one should attempt removal of the catheter. If it does not come out easily, ten more minutes of waiting are required. The bag is usually ruptured (torn) by the oil, but does not fragment.

Other Methods of Rupturing Balloon

One may distend the balloon to a size as large as the patient will tolerate. Using a 22- to 25-gauge spinal needle with its stylet, the balloon may be punctured suprapubically or perineally (percutaneously).

One may also take a whistle-tip ureteral catheter with its stylet and pass this alongside the urethral catheter until one meets the obstruction of the balloon, and then push the wire stylet (preferably with its tip sharpened in advance) out beyond the whistle-tip opening of the catheter and puncture the balloon. A Bugbee electrode may be passed until an obstruction is met (invariably the balloon), and then a short burst of electrofulguration may be given to cause rupture of the balloon.

In the female, it is a very simple matter to pass a needle alongside the catheter to rupture the balloon.

Chapter Eight

THE PROSTATE

DIAGNOSTIC CONSIDERATIONS

Introduction

FEW INTERNAL ORGANS lend themselves to diagnostic procedures, palpation, and expression of contents as does the prostate gland. The prostate's location is also advantageous for needle biopsy either via the perineum or transrectally.

Biopsy of the Prostate

Those who advocate the transrectal approach for prostatic needle biopsy contend that one may more reliably do a biopsy on the suspicious nodule by placement directly over it. With the perineal biopsy, the interposed tissue makes palpation of the needle (transrectally) more difficult. With a small nodule, the operator feels less confident that the needle has entered the lesion in question.

The authors routinely prescribe the use of a broad-spectrum antibiotic for five days after any needle biopsy of the prostate.

Improved Method for Transrectal Biopsy

In the performance of transrectal biopsy care should be taken to puncture the rectum only at the intended site of biopsy. One may place a sterile glove on one's hand and over the index finger place the biopsy needle. Another sterile glove (or sterile finger cot) is then pulled on over the biopsy needle. The needle thus lies betwen two sterile gloves. When the nodule in the prostate is palpated, the needle is pushed through the outer sterile glove. Needle contact with other areas of the rectum is eliminated, reducing the possibility of infection.

Disposable Needle for Prostatic Biopsy

Biopsy of the prostate may be very satisfactorily done with the disposable "Tru-Cut ®" biopsy needle (Travenol Laboratories). The needle is manufactured in lengths of 4½ and 6 inches.

Many other brands of biopsy needles are available, among them the Vim-Silverman, the Franklin modification of the Vim-Silverman, the Hutchings, the Turkel, and the Biegeleisen.

The advantages of the Tru-Cut needle are said to be its lighter weight, improved adherence of needle to tissue, slightly larger size of specimen core, and extreme sharpness. Many urologists claim a higher success rate in obtaining specimens by use of this needle.

Though some physicians report that they reuse the needle to make it possible to reduce the cost to the patient, the authors feel that the crucial nature of biopsy procedures should not be compromised by the loss of flexibility and keenness inherent in reutilization of an instrument such as a biopsy needle, particularly one which is marketed as disposable. Too much depends upon the results of a biopsy to permit such false economies.

PATHOLOGY OF THE PROSTATE

Prostatitis

Phenylbutazone (Butazolidin) for Prostatitis (and Epididymitis)

Phenylbutazone (Butazolidin) has been used to accelerate the resolution of induration in instances of acute epididymitis. It also has been found valuable in the treatment of acute prostatitis, used in conjunction with proper antibacterial medications. The usual dosage is 100 mg two or three times daily for one to two weeks, and then one time daily for the next one to two weeks.

The medication has anti-inflammatory and antipyretic actions, as well as analgesic and uricosuric properties.

Phenylbutazone must not be used in children or the very aged because of its toxicity. The physician must watch for signs and symptoms that suggest intestinal ulceration or hemorrhage, skin reactions, and blood picture changes.

As with all other medications, one should become acquainted with the dangers of the use of phenylbutazone before prescribing it.

Variable Therapeutic Modalities for Chronic Prostatitis

Urologists do not always agree on the efficacy of prostate massage, dilation with such instruments as the Kollmann dilator, sitz baths, choice of oral anti-infective drugs, estrogen therapy, etc., in the treatment of chronic prostatitis. The following information may be of some value in deciding on the treatment of choice:

Prostatic Massage: Some patients with vague complaints of pain in the low back, rectal, perineal, or groin area felt to be related to chronic prostatitis, report definite relief with prostatic massage. A trial of weekly massage for three to four treatments is probably justified. Massage should be gentle but firm; undue pressure serves no purpose and is painful. Massage is sometimes an excellent means of suggesting to the examiner that the patient's complaints are psychogenic. Such a patient appears to benefit unreasonably from the treatment and often has to be "talked out" of continual massages.

The occasional patient with a "boggy" prostate containing an excessive amount of fluid may experience some relief of symptoms.

Many patients with chronic prostatitis will periodically have subacute episodes with aggravation of symptoms. When these occur, chemotherapy should first be instituted for a few days before considering massage. Failure to do this may lead to the complication of acute epididymitis.

ANTI-INFECTIVE DRUGS: In approximately 50 percent of cases a causative organism cannot be isolated. Almost any anti-infective drug seems to give at least partial symptomatic relief as long as the patient remains on medication. It is probably best to avoid such nonspecific drug therapy when dealing with the patient with mild symptoms. For patients with frequent episodes of increased symptomatology, low daily doses for several months usually eliminate or minimize "flare-up" symptoms.

Kanamycin, in 0.5-gm doses every five days, for three to five doses, has been found particularly helpful in alleviating chronic symptoms.

ESTROGENS: Daily estrogens, for example, 1.25 mg Premarin® for ten to twelve days, has been very effective for many patients. If relief is not complete, the therapy may be repeated again in one to three months.

DILATION: The patient with long-standing chronic prostatitis may develop sufficient fibrosis to cause some stenosis of the prostatic urethra and bladder neck. This stenosis tends to aggravate the existing chronic inflammation. When more conservative therapy fails to relieve the patient's symptoms, Kollmann dilation of the area may provide relief. This is best preceded by a broad-spectrum antibiotic for a few days to prevent the occurrence of secondary epididymitis.

RECTAL HEAT: Symptomatic relief can be provided by way of rectal heat with instruments such as the Aquamatic-K® connection to the Sissner prostatic cooler. This eliminates the debilitating effect (to some patients) of hot sitz baths.

Granulomatous Prostatitis

Corticosteroids have been reported effective in aiding resolution of the hard prostatic nodules displayed in true granulomatous prostatitis. One of us saw rapid subsidence of an enormous prostate, proven by biopsy to be due to granulomatous prostatitis, in a 23-year-old man with severe obstructive symptoms. The patient had a marked eosinophilia, and one year earlier had been hospitalized with eosinophilic pneumonia.

Biopsy is almost invariably necessary to differentiate carcinoma from granulomatous prostatitis.

TABLE V
ESTIMATING PROSTATIC
ENLARGEMENT

Endoscopic Findings

Gland Size	Findings on Rectal Palpation	Intraurethral Lateral	Intraurethral Middle or Dorsal Portion of Laterals	Intravesical Middle or Dorsal Portion of Laterals	Approximate Amount of Tissue to Be Removed
Normal	No protrusion into rectal lumen	Concave lateral prostatic urethral walls	1–2 cm between veru and prostatic border	Does not cover trigone	Up to 10 gm (average normal weight 20+ gm)
Grade I	Encroaches 0–1 cm into rectal lumen	Lateral lobes bulge inward but do not touch in midline	2–3 cm between veru and prostatic border	Covers up to one-half of trigone	Up to 15 gm
Grade II	Encroaches 1–2 cm into rectal lumen	Lateral lobes touch in midline	3–4 cm between veru and prostatic border	Covers from one-half to all of trigone	15 to 50 gm
Grade III	Encroaches 2–3 cm into rectal lumen	Lateral lobes touch in midline for 2–3 cm	4–5 cm between veru and prostatic border	Covers more than trigone	50 to 125 gm
Grade IV	Encroaches more than 3 cm into rectal lumen	Lateral lobes touch in midline more than 3 cm	More than 5 cm between veru and prostatic border	Extends up into fundus	More than 125 gm

Prostatic Hyperplasia

Criteria for Judging the Size of Prostatic Enlargement

Table V presents criteria contributed by Roger Barnes, M.D., for the estimation of prostate size. These standards are generally well accepted.

Employment of Larger Size Catheters in Prostatic Hyperplasia

On occasion, it may be difficult to pass a No. 16 or 18 French Coudé-tip Tiemann catheter, yet a No. 22 or 24 French will pass with little effort. This is possible because the larger catheter will wedge the lateral lobes apart and pass successfully whereas the smaller catheter may be caught under the lateral lobes. It is obvious from this fact and from previous sections on urethral catheterization (in Chapter Seven) that a No. 22 or 24 French Coudé-tip Tiemann catheter is a very valuable instrument to have at hand.

Because of the above same circumstances, the operator may be unable to pass a small metal sound, though a large one will "drop in."

Use of Van Buren Sound to Aid Passage of Balloon Catheter in Prostatic Hyperplasia

In the presence of prostatic hyperplasia, a straight-tip balloon catheter may be indicated but may not pass. Having evacuated the bladder (with Coudé-tip Tiemann catheter) and established that hyperplasia is the only obstructive disease present, the following may be attempted:

A No. 22 or 24 French Van Buren sound is passed into the already anesthetized urethra and left in place. After a few minutes the sound is removed and quickly followed by a straight balloon catheter which often passes into the bladder. The explanation for this is that the lobes of the prostate are wedged apart and held out of the way long enough to quickly insert a straight catheter. Coudé-tip Tiemann balloon catheters often are passed easily without the use of a sound.

Alternatives to this technique include use of the wire-reinforced ureteral stylet or wire catheter guide discussed in Chapter Seven.

Mention should be made that quite often a straight catheter will pass merely by simply evacuating the distended bladder, even though it had previously met with obstruction. Bladder distention apparently alters the prostatic position within the pelvis. This hypothesis is suggested by the observation that the prostate is quite prominent on rectal examination prior to evacuation of the bladder but protrudes far less into the rectum after evacuation.

(See also extensive discussions of catheter passage following prostatectomy in subsequent sections of this chapter.)

Carcinoma of Prostate

Treatment for Patients with Prostatic Carcinoma

Changing concepts dictate the treatment of carcinoma of the prostate. Urologists differ in their methodology. The recent literature and textbooks are referred to for standardized therapy.

It is imperative that a tissue diagnosis be made before instituting any therapy. This is done either on the surgical specimen or the needle biopsy specimen. Classifications of prostatic carcinoma are many and varied; a simplified version is utilized here.

The stage I carcinoma may require radical surgery, with additional therapy begun if progression of the disease becomes apparent. Stage II carcinomas, when low-grade and localized to the prostate in healthy young men, should also be considered for radical surgery. Stage II and III high-grade tumors should be considered for cobalt irradiation.

If estrogens are used, the acceptable dose of diethylstilbestrol should be so small as to minimize cardiovascular complications. Small doses of estrogen (1 mg daily) are as effective as larger doses (100 mg daily) of the same medication.

Urologists still disagree as to whether orchiectomy need be done early or late or at all in the treatment of prostatic carcinoma. At the time of this writing, early orchiectomy is favored by many writers.

For patients with localized metastases from carcinoma of the prostate, the following modalities have been used: (1) large doses of polyestradiol phosphate by frequent injection, (2) localized cobalt therapy, (3) radio-active phosphorus (sodium P^{32} phosphate) treatment preceded by testosterone or parathyroid hormone for a few days, (4) vinblastine (Velban) intravenously, (5) orchiectomy, (6) adrenalectomy, (7) hypophysectomy, and (8) chordotomy.

In recent years, sodium fluoride has been utilized in the dosage of one 25-mg capsule four times per day. It has been postulated that this aids the increase in deposition of calcium and phosphorus in bony structures, sometimes relieving pain due to bony metastasis. Dramatic response has been reported in some cases.

Intermittent Estrogen Therapy

In treating carcinoma of the prostate, some urologists advocate the withholding of estrogen therapy until there is symptomatic need of this treatment, or advancement of the disease as shown by rectal palpation. Minimal dosage schedule is advocated (1 mg per day of stilbestrol, for example) until regression is apparent, and then treatment is stopped. It is felt that intermittent use of estrogens may prolong the effectiveness and lessen complications and side effects. Orchiectomy is done also when the need arises. Radiation therapy to the breast should be done prior to beginning estrogen therapy to prevent the "tender breast."

Intractable Pain in Carcinoma of the Prostate: Overcoming Ineffectiveness of Estrogen

Patients in whom estrogen therapy seems to have lost effectiveness may be given intramuscular testosterone in the form of Testosterone Cypionate, 100 mg daily, for about 15 days. Beginning on the fifth day of this drug administration, the patient may be treated with a daily dose of 2 millicuries of radioactive phosphorus (sodium P^{32} phosphate), given intravenously, for five days, for a total dosage of 10 millicuries. Following this treatment, on the eleventh day estrogen therapy may then be resumed.

Mention should be made of reports that the resumption of estrogens after sodium P^{32} phosphate leads to a high incidence of cerebrovascular accidents and phlebothrombosis with emboli; this possibility must be "traded off" with the possible advantages of the treatment and most carefully considered.

Because testosterone may stimulate the growth of prostatic carcinoma, fresh parathyroid has been substituted for testosterone in preparation of the patient for selective pickup of radiophosphorus by the bone tumors. Parathormone acts upon bone and renal tubules. Calcium and phosphates are mobilized from the bone and the threshold of renal tubules for excretion of calcium is lowered. Hypercalcemia and hypophosphatemia result. The urinary excretion of calcium and phosphorus is increased. Upon withdrawal of the parathormone for 24 hours, radiophosphorus will be sought out by the bone, reducing total body irradiation.

Radiophosphorus must be given over a protracted period until the patient's tolerance levels are reached to achieve a good effect. The ill effects seen with testosterone and sodium P^{32} phosphate are not noted.

Preliminary reports, using this method of therapy, have been very encouraging.[*]

PROSTATE SURGERY

Special Problems Related to Prostate Surgery

Surgery Scheduling Should Include Arrangements for Postoperative Care

The most disturbing aspects of postoperative care in prostatectomy patients are those of bleeding and catheter care. The elderly male patient is often sensitive to catheter manipulation by female nurses. The authors find also that nurses in intensive care units, though they may have excellent training in almost all types of serious illness, are inexperienced in the care of prostatectomized patients.

The authors, therefore, have for years used the services of former military service-trained corpsmen who are especially trained as "catheter technicians." Depending on the volume of prostate surgery performed, some hospitals have set up "Post-Prostatectomy Units" or "Urology Units" in which catheter technicians are employed on a 24-hour basis especially for the post-prostatectomy patients. These technicians may be licensed vocational nurses. A few may be registered male nurses.

A post-prostatectomy patient entrusted to the care of these technicians for the first 24 hours after surgery has an excellent start to an uneventful postoperative course. Postoperative nursing care for the patient is arranged for at the time he is scheduled for surgery.

Unfortunately, the specially trained nurse or the above-described Urol-

---

[*] E. C. Tong and P. Finkelstein, "Treatment of Prostatic Bone Metastases With Parathormone and Radioactive Phosphorus," *Journal of Urology*, 109:71 (1973).

Preoperative Orders

The following routine orders will apply to all our patients in your hospital for surgery:

1. Routine blood.
2. Routine urine.
*3. Type and cross-match for two units of blood.
*4. Bleeding and clotting time, platelet count.
*5. Prothrombin time and partial thromboplastin time.
6. Regular diet.
7. Cleansing enema HS (soap suds, saline, etc.).
8. Nothing per os after midnight.
9. Routine chest film.
10. Anesthesiologist to order preoperative medication.
11. Diabetic patients to have blood sugar on afternoon of admission and fasting blood sugar in morning prior to surgery.
12. Shave and prep. for

  a. All prostate, scrotal, and bladder surgery (except cystoscopy where no prep. is necessary): suprapubic area, perineum, and scrotum.
  b. All kidney or ureteral surgery: right or left flank and abdomen.
  c. All cystoscopic procedures: no prep.

*For all scrotal, penile, and cystoscopic procedures (except TUR prostate and TUR bladder) omit orders 3, 4, and 5.

When there is to be any deviation from the above orders we shall so notify you.

_____ M.D.

53. Sample form: preoperative hospital orders, all urologic surgery

ogy Units may not be available. Careful attention to hemostasis at the time of surgery remains the final answer to an uneventful postoperative course.

Preparation for Possible Bleeding Problems

The performance of routine blood counts and smears, platelet counts, prothrombin time and partial thromboplastin time, will make known in advance of surgery most bleeding problems that may be encountered in a given patient. Therefore, this type of blood workup should be done on all patients subjected to prostatectomy.

POSTOPERATIVE ORDERS

FOLLOW THOSE ORDERS DENOTED BY CIRCLE
DELETE THOSE ORDERS DENOTED BY X

1. Two units of fresh whole blood <u>available at all times</u>.
2. _____<u>diet</u>.
3. I.V._____.
4. Dangle at bedside tonight.
5. Ambulate with leg bag b.i.d. starting first postoperative day.
6. Meperidine (Demerol)____mg. I.M. q 3 to 4 hrs. prn pain.
7. Dihydromorphinone (Dilaudid) gr.____I.M. q 3 to 4 hrs. prn pain.
8. _____ @ h.s. prn sleep, repeat ____ times.
9. Sodium cephalothin (Keflin) 500 mg. I.V. push Q6H.
10. Cephaloridine (Loridine) 500 mg. I.M. q 8 hr. x 3 days.
11. Cephalexin (Keflex) 500 mg. q.i.d. x ____ days.
12. Diazepam (Valium) 5 mg. I.M. or P.O. q ____hrs. prn restlessness.
13. Dimenhydrinate (Dramamine) 50 mg. I.M. q 4 to 6 hrs. prn nausea.
14. Bucladin® tab+ sublingually q 4 to 6 hrs. prn nausea.
15. Perphenazine (Trilafon) 5 mg. I.M. q 4 to 6 hrs. prn nausea.
16. Mineral oil 1 oz. (30 ml.) b.i.d. starting first postoperative day, may mix with orange juice.
17. Connect catheter to Nesbit-Young closed irrigation system.
18. Connect catheter to through-and-through irrigation drainage system.
19. Irrigate catheter with sterile normal saline to maintain drainage pink to straw in color and transparent in appearance. Amount and frequency of irrigation should be determined by amount of bleeding, if any. DO NOT IRRIGATE IF BLEEDING IS MINIMAL.
20. Use Toomey or suitable piston syringe to aspirate clots, if present.
21. DO NOT CLAMP CATHETER.
22. Have sterile container filled with aqueous activated glutaraldehyde (Cidex) solution taped to bed, to be used for soaking disconnected drainage tube connection end.
23. Blood pressure and pulse q 15 min. until stable, then q.i.d.
24. Massage legs and encourage deep breathing frequently (_____) on day of surgery.
25. Intake and output hourly first four hours, then q 4 hrs. for first 24 hrs., then routine intake and output. NOTIFY DOCTOR if large volume fluid output first four hours.
26. Apply Cortisporin® ointment into urethral meatus and wrap penis and adjacent catheter with Kling® roll gauze daily. Keep gauze moist with ST-37.
27. Intermittent positive pressure breathing with normal saline t.i.d. for three days.
28. Private duty male nurses for first 24 hrs; arranged by attending physician.

_____ M.D.

54. Sample form: postoperative hospital orders for patients following prostate surgery

A careful history preoperatively should include direct questioning of the patient regarding bleeding problems with any previous surgery and the presence of a "bleeder" in the family.

All contemplated prostatectomy patients should be preoperatively typed and cross-matched and have available in surgery at least two units of blood, even though seldom used. If additional blood is not readily available on demand, additional units should be typed and cross-matched in advance.

Orders for Surgical Patients

Preoperative and Postoperative Orders to Hospitals

Figures 53 and 54 are examples of order sheets sent to the Director of Nurses at hospitals where patients are to be admitted for surgery; these forms have proved most helpful. The postoperative orders are updated constantly to include new instructions and drug orders thought to be advantageous in light of new advances.

Instructions to Patients Regarding Prostate Surgery After-Care

It is advisable to give the patient about to undergo prostate surgery a printed list of instructions (see sample form, Fig. 55) as to his conduct and management after he leaves the hospital. This should preferably be given as part of his preoperative explanation. Informed consent should be obtained at the same time (see *Informed Consent: Use of Audiovisual Aids* in Chapter One).

The instructions should explain to the patient that he should not become alarmed because of bleeding, without blood clots. A common explanation utilized for clarity is that two drops of ink is very little but may look like a lot when dropped into a quart of water. A bladder full of urine with several drops of blood in it may likewise have the appearance of a severely bloody urine. The patient should be told that when there are more than four to six blood clots in the urine with one voiding session, then bleeding is of greater than expected volume, and he must report to the physician immediately. When there are only occasional small clots found in the urine, the patient is reassured that this is not to be viewed with alarm.

The patient is advised also as to bowel function, activity, forcing of fluids, diet, walking, automobile driving, and sexual behavior. He should also be instructed as to the use of postoperative medications for a period of six to eight weeks. He is advised that this period of time will elapse before complete healing will have taken place.

The patient is instructed to report to the physician should there be decrease in the size of the stream, suggesting the presence of a meatal or bladder neck stricture in formation. The possibility of testicular swelling, with development of epididymitis, is also explained. He is told that there may be the presence of pyuria for a period of six to eight weeks or longer, and that his referring physician need not become alarmed about this and begin to place the patient on varied antibiotics in an attempt to clear the pyuria.

INSTRUCTIONS TO PATIENT FOLLOWING PROSTATE SURGERY

There are several important things you should know and understand about your prostate surgery. The following information has been prepared to explain what can be expected after surgery, and to answer the commonly asked questions.

In all cases of prostate surgery, a tube (catheter) is left in the natural channel for several days. After the catheter is removed you may experience some burning on urination and/or a frequent desire to empty the bladder and/or some discomfort at the time of urinating. These symptoms usually disappear within a few weeks.

A certain amount of bleeding in the urine is a common occurrence after the removal of the catheter, and is no cause for concern. The appearance of a small amount of blood at the beginning or end of urination is common and will usually clear by itself. On emptying the bladder, the urine may appear bloody throughout; this may be coffee-colored, or may be brighter red. A very small amount of blood present in the bladder will cause this discoloration and, again, this is no cause for concern. If there is more serious bleeding, the urine will appear bright red and soft clots will be present, appearing like small pieces of liver. Should more than 5 to 6 clots be present in a single voiding, your urologist must be contacted immediately at any time, day or night.

Your urine may be cloudy for several weeks after surgery and for this reason you must take the prescribed medication for a period of 6 to 8 weeks postoperatively. The cloudiness will clear as the prostate area continues to heal.

You are encouraged to drink at least 8 glasses of fluids per day. This may be water, tea, milk, etc. You should avoid alcoholic beverages and spicy foods until healing is complete — usually a period of 6 to 8 weeks. You may be up and about within the limits of comfort.

Should there be difficulty in beginning the urinary stream, try to void while sitting in a bathtub filled with warm or hot water. After voiding, rebathe by tub or shower. Should there be some urinary dribbling, exercise the control muscle by starting the urination, then shutting off the stream for a few seconds, and then allow full voiding again. Continue this stop-start exercise with each urination, over many weeks if necessary, until the control improves.

Following prostate surgery, you should refrain from sexual activity for at least 3 or 4 weeks. Do not be alarmed if no fluid appears on ejaculation. Speak to the doctor for an explanation of this.

Avoid strenuous exercises and straining. Use mineral oil or Milk of Magnesia if necessary for bowel movements. You may drive a car approximately 14 days after surgery.

When you arrive home from the hospital, call our office for future appointments and report your condition.

Call us concerning any questions you may have.

55. Sample of form given to prostate surgery patient regarding his postoperative care

These postoperative instructions will markedly decrease the number of telephone calls from patients in the postoperative phase.

Most patients about to undergo prostatectomy have many questions. *Life After Fifty: The Prostate Age* * is a valuable book which answers

---

* Henry M. Weyrauch, M.D., *Life After Fifty: The Prostate Age* (Los Angeles, Ward-Ritchie Press, 1967).

these questions in language written especially for the layman. One of us (J.S.A.) loans this book to his patients, who are invariably delighted with the author's witty, authoritative approach to diagnosis, treatment, and postoperative care. Several such books must be kept on hand, as the wives and close friends of the patients find the book equally delightful. These books are always eventually returned by the patient during the postoperative office visits, with a little reminding.

Transurethral Resection of the Prostate

Placement of Resection Equipment

During transurethral prostatectomy, difficulty is encountered with the placement of the irrigating tubing, electroresection cords, and instrument lighting cords. Numerous brackets, slings, and suspension devices have been utilized to help with this problem. The following simple solution is preferred by one of us:

For freer movement of the resectoscope, it is desirable to have cords and tubing connect to the resectoscope from the same side. A small tunnel is formed from the sterile draping, the roof of the tunnel being secured with a towel clip. The cords and irrigation tube come through the tunnel, which has been located preferably in the region of the lateral aspects of the patient's groin. This tunnel may be located on either the right or left side of the patient, depending on the location of the electrocautery, light and water sources. The tubing and cords are made long enough to provide slack and eliminate any pull (refer to Fig. 6 in Chapter One, as well as the additional suggestions included in *Devices for Holding Cystoscopy Cords, Tubing, etc.* in the first chapter).

Assuring Proper Function of Resectoscope: Care and Maintenance of Cystoscope, Resectoscope, Panendoscope, etc.

It is recommended that one read the booklets of cystoscopic instrument manufacturing companies, in which the structure and mechanical details of urologic instruments are described. One should also fully understand the *care* of such instruments—this should not be entrusted entirely to operating room personnel. One hears occasionally of a resectoscope and associated elements such as loops being placed in an autoclave by a well-meaning nurse!

Electrosurgical Units

Electrosurgical units (tube cutting, spark gap, transistor) have specific factors characteristic of the type of machine. The following must be checked to assure proper functioning of the resectoscope. *There will be poor cutting (or no cutting) if:*

1) *Spark gaps (in such machines) are not in adjustment.* Gaps should be on adjustment before each operation.

2) *Spark gap facings are carbonized or pitted.* Over long periods of use, the tungsten gap facings will grow "peaks and valleys" which interfere with proper adjustment of the gaps and cause uneven firing. If not too worn, such gaps may be cleaned satisfactorily with abrasive strips. It is better to replace them to be certain of new-machine performance. Regular changing of the cutting-gap assembly in such machines, every 18 months, is suggested. The newer transistorized units eliminate this problem.

3) *Cords are old, with insulation cracked, or strands of copper conductor broken.* It is possible to have breaks of wire strands inside the insulation which will reduce the cutting power even though the higher voltage coagulating power seems to be satisfactory. A continuity test on these cords may reveal breaks, but a more certain way is to stretch them by pulling. If the wire strands inside are broken, the rubber insulation will stretch or possibly break.

4) *Poor ground continuity from the patient to a true ground exists.* In the case of metal cabinet machines, grounding is accomplished from the patient plate through the patient cord, the metal cabinet, on through the third (ground) wire in the electrical supply cable to a true ground. Be certain this third wire is connected to a true ground. If it is attached to the metal wall receptacle box, which is invariably so with explosion-proof plugs, it must be ascertained that there is B-X cable or pipe in the walls to which this box is attached.

It is also possible that ground continuity might be interrupted because there is a break or corrosion at the point where the tab is riveted (or connected by other means) to the patient plate or grounding plate. This can be checked by the use of an ohmmeter, which is an indispensable piece of equipment for every cystoscopy room. *Every nurse or technician working in a cystoscopy room or in surgery where electrosurgical equipment is in use must be familiar with the method of using an ohmmeter to check continuity of electrical wires.*

Poorly grounded, old-style (malleable) plates are certainly taboo in this day and age of electrosurgical units. Every surgical suite should use grounding plates for electrosurgical units of sufficient size to allow a *safety factor* in the event there is short-circuiting of current. *This factor should not exceed 1.5 watts per square centimeter of patient-plate surface area, or 9.675 watts per square inch.*

The power wattage of the electrosurgical unit employed in usual cutting and coagulation should be known. Personnel should be critically aware that the indifferent electrode or grounding plate must be of adequate size for a 100 percent safety factor. The plate must be entirely under the patient where complete contact is made; the plate and wire connection must be adequate and secure. All points of electrical contact must be complete. Avoidance of "hills and valleys" type of indifferent electrode contact must be avoided. The buttocks usually serves as an excellent area of contact.

The body surface must be covered in areas of contact with the metal of the operating table to avoid accidental burns by grounding-out.

5) *Voltage is too low.* Electrosurgical units are manufactured to operate on 110 to 120 volts in the United States. Any voltage drop will reduce the cutting power in proportion. A loss of more than 10 volts will supply too little power for underwater cutting. VOLTAGE SHOULD *ALWAYS* BE TESTED UNDER LOAD. The power company will test line voltage for you if a voltmeter is not

available. Most operating room supervisors will overlook this aspect of function of the operating suite, as will most urologists.

It is again stressed that monitoring of the electrical equipment must be frequently performed. An inexpensive combination home and automobile "VOM" meter can be purchased to measure both voltage and resistance (ohms).

6) *Foot pedal contact is faulty.* Good contact at the terminal is necessary.

Resectoscope

With the resecting instrument itself, there will be poor function if:

1) *There is corrosion of the insulation of the wire loop.* Sterilizing solutions such as Cidex may cause corrosion of the insulating material. The wire shorts out and overheats the entire loop (stem, etc.). This heat is transmitted to all metal parts of the electrosurgical unit, which becomes a "hot rod."

Such damage is invisible. Possible conductivity of current to other metal parts of the resectoscope must be determined with an ohmmeter. If any "short circuiting" is measured on the meter, the loop should be discarded.

It is essential that cutting loops be sterilized with gas to avoid corrosion, and that they be checked with an ohmmeter prior to sterilization. It is recommended that they be packaged in pairs.

2) *Other cutting loop problems exist.* If a metal sheath is used, the loop must not come in contact with the *metal.* Such an occurrence could cause urethral burns or burns to the operator. With poor insulation on either side of the cutting loop (worn plastic insulators) contact with the lens may occur, producing metal burns around the lens, or a spark may fly from the resectoscope to the operator's nose or eye.

3) *Resectoscope blocks are burned out.* The proximal end of the resectoscope cutting loop must be pushed as far into the block as it will go before tightening the screw lock. One must guard against possible bending of the wire terminal at the proximal end of the loop. Poor contact can result in burning out of the block.

4) *Light bulb burns out.* This can be the result of an arcing from the nearby loop if the surgeon fails to remove his foot from the treadle at the precise moment that the loop completes its excursion through the tissue and sheath. The surgeon should develop complete coordination between hand and foot so that he is off the footswitch as soon as the loop is through the tissue. Such arcing can further be aggravated by too high a power setting or too slow a cut.

5) *Sheaths are charred.* If the lower edge of the beak of the sheath has been charred or foreshortened, tissue will not be cut off cleanly. Numerous incompletely resected tags of tissue result. Charring can be caused as a result of arcing from the loop (as described above). Arcing is encouraged if bits of tissue are left adhering to the loop.

6) *Incandescent light is dim.* This may result from a worn incandescent light, a poor contact of the fine wire terminal on the bulb, or seepage of water into the socket. Application of the wax furnished by the manufacturer to the thread of the bulb after partially screwing it into the socket will keep moisture out. After the wax is applied, the bulb is tightly seated on the socket.

7) *Poor electrical contacts exist.* Poor contact of the electrosurgical unit cord to the resectoscope terminal can cause malfunction. A loose fit is the usual explanation for this malfunction but there can also be a break in continuity be-

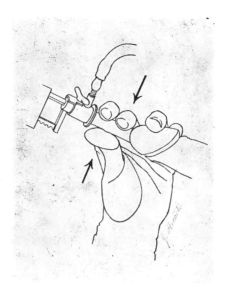

56. Aid to efficient cutting of prostatic tissue during resection

tween the cord and its male terminal. With a No. 16 knife blade one may make tighter the female terminal of the resectoscope, or a large hemostat may be used to bend the male terminal of the electrosurgical cord slightly so that a tighter fit with the resectoscope is obtained.

Errors in Technique

Additional miscellaneous causes of malfunction during resection include:

1) *Improper pressure against tissue.* At the start of the operation, the bulging prostate forces itself into the fenestrum of the sheath. After a few cuts of tissue are taken it becomes necessary to apply pressure on the instrument to accomplish this. It no longer is a bulging gland after a few cuts and does not "push" its way into the window of the sheath. Unless the tissue is forced into the fenestrum, it is not possible for the loop to cut through.

The bite of tissue may be taken by pressure of the index finger and forefinger on the ventral aspect of the sheath, and by slightly less upward pressure of the thumb from the dorsal aspect. A "fulcrum effect" is thus accomplished (see Fig. 56).

2) *Power setting too high, and cutting done too slowly.* In the presence of these two conditions, the tissue tends to overcoagulate and a cumulative wall of coagulum is built up which becomes increasingly difficult to cut through.

Lens System

VISUAL CLARITY OF LENS SYSTEM. There is often a good deal of difficulty with vision through the cystoscopic lens. The lens can be readily cleaned as follows: an applicator stick is cut or broken on a bias. The oblique tip that results is dipped in vinegar and the tip is then rubbed over the lens. This may be wiped with a 3- by 3-inch or 4- by 4-inch gauze square which has been opened up to form one layer. One may also wipe the eyepiece of the telescope with vinegar. Poor vision may at times be secondary to water leaking in behind the lens because of a break in the cement. In this case, repair must be effected.

SPLIT IMAGES OF RESECTOSCOPE OR CYSTOSCOPE LENSES. If the entire field has been decreased, there may be a bend in the sheath and/or bending of the telescope. By looking through the telescope and slightly bending it one direction or another, one may be able to regain a normal field. The slight bending of the telescope will serve to indicate the proper direction of bend required. Inspection may then reveal the location of the abnormal bend. Improper seating (bending) of the telescope within the sheath or insulating block will also split the image.

Concerning Resectoscope Sheaths and Loops

The No. 28 (blue) resectoscope loop may be used with the 26 French *fiberglass* sheath. This combination provides the best loop size with a smaller sheath.

To determine why the 26 French metal sheath will not accommodate the 28 French loop, and to compare the actual internal and external diameters of metal and fiberglass sheaths, the following measurements were made:

Sheath Size (French)	Sheath Material	External Diameter (mm)	Internal Diameter (mm)	External Diameter (French scale)	Sheath Wall Thickness (mm)
26	Metal	8.428	7.120	25.28	0.65
26	Fiberglass	8.783	7.569	26.34	0.60
28	Metal	9.685	8.052	29.05	0.81
28	Fiberglass	9.550	8.026	28.65	0.76

It is apparent that the wall of the 26 French fiberglass sheath is a little thinner and the external diameter a little larger than that of the 26 French metal sheath, accounting for the greater internal diameter of the former.

Since the 26 French fiberglass sheath accommodates the 28 loop, there appears to be no advantage to using the 28 French fiberglass sheath unless the operator wishes to cut extra large pieces of tissue (as described later in this chapter: see *Aid to Satisfactory Cutting with the Resectoscope Loop*).

Technique: Aids in Transurethral Resection of the Prostate

The actual techniques of prostatic resection are well covered in standard textbooks especially written in regard to this subject. The practical aids which follow are suggestions which may not be found in such works.

PRELUBRICATION. As the operation proceeds, free movement of the sheath diminishes frequently when using K-Y® jelly, the jelly being either washed or milked out of the urethra. The authors have found that Vaseline clings to the sheath throughout the operation. A thin coat is applied to the sheath. K-Y jelly is applied to the obturator tip only to facilitate introduction.

One must be aware of the possibility of arcing at the urethral meatus, the Vaseline acting as a conductor. Too generous an application of Vaseline will sometimes also result in the passage of "Vaseline balls" postoperatively. Vaseline collecting at the meatus must be wiped away.

As previously mentioned, internal urethrotomy aids in free movement of the sheath within the urethra.

FACILITATING PASSAGE OF RESECTOSCOPE SHEATH. Even with adequate preliminary dilation of the urethra, one occasionally finds that the sheath will not pass. This may be remedied by passing the sheath, with obturator inserted, beyond the fossa navicularis or as far in as the sheath will easily pass. The obturator is removed and the resectoscope inserted, completing the passage under vision.

If this proves impossible, the sheath is left within the unobstructed portion of the urethra and a No. 14 or 16 French Tiemann catheter is used as a guide to finish the pass. The distal flare end of the catheter is cut off and the catheter passed through the resectoscope sheath to its distal point of obstruction and then on into the bladder. The distal end of the catheter is grasped with a hemostat, so that it may not accidentally be passed completely into the bladder. Both the catheter and sheath are advanced, rather than merely pushing the sheath over the stationary catheter. The catheter is then removed.

PASSING THE RESECTOSCOPE SHEATH WHEN ANGULATION AT THE VESICLE NECK IS PRESENT. The already indwelling catheter (if less than 20 French in size) or a 14 French Robinson catheter, attached to a Timberlake obturator, may be employed to overcome this problem. The obturator must be at least one size smaller than the resectoscope sheath.

A ⅛-inch hole is drilled in the tip of the Timberlake obturator about ⅜ inch from the end. The desired obturator and sheath are assembled. The indwelling catheter is cut off proximal to the funnel portion and seated over the obturator tip. The cut catheter can then be sutured to the Timberlake obturator though the hole in the tip, using No. 0 chromic or silk suture. The diameter of the catheter at the site of the obturator tip must be less than the internal diameter of the resectoscope sheath.

The sheath with assembled obturator is then passed, being guided into place by the already present catheter. When in place, the obturator is withdrawn, pulling the catheter with it.

The knot must be securely tied so that the suture does not become dislodged when the obturator is withdrawn through the sheath. Should the catheter be left behind in the bladder, it may be readily extracted using either the Alcock forceps to pull the catheter through the resecto-scope sheath or the Bodner resectoscopic utility forceps applied to the working element of the resectoscope.

PREVENTING ERECTION DURING PROSTATECTOMY. Whatever the type of anesthesia employed during transurethral resection, some patients will develop an erection, making manipulation of the resectoscope difficult. Erections will subside if one wraps wet 4- by 4-inch gauze (cooled with ice water) around the base of the penis. A nurse may pour additional ice water on the gauze from time to time to maintain the penis in a flaccid non-erectile state.

Curare-like substances, muscle relaxants, sympathetic and parasympa-thetic blocking agents, and the inducing of deeper sleep with added intravenous barbiturates or inhalation anesthetic agents have not been effective in decreasing erections. Methocarbamol (Robaxin) and metaxa-lone (Skelaxin) have been utilized with questionable success.

The exact physiology causing these erections is unknown to the authors.

NECESSITY FOR MEATOTOMY. It may be necessary to do a urethral me-atotomy to allow the passage of a 28 French resectoscope sheath. As previously mentioned, most meatotomies are done by first placing a straight hemostat on the frenal end of the meatus for ten minutes to control hemo-stasis and then cutting the crushed area with scissors or scalpel. Various other methods of meatotomy may be utilized, including cutting with the electrosurgical unit, and dorsal or ventral incision with the Otis urethro-tome. (See also the section on Penis in Chapter Nine.)

AVOIDANCE OF OBTURATOR NERVE STIMULATION EFFECT. When one re-sects close to the capsule, in the region of 10 to 11, or 1 to 2 o'clock, the obturator nerve is stimulated and the patient's leg will jump in the stirrup. This is most apt to occur with current "shorting out." Therefore, the loop of the resectoscope should be immediately replaced. The pa-tient's legs should preferably be tied down in the stirrups with stock-inette tied loosely over the stirrup.

Troublesome nerve stimulation can be eliminated by injection of 20 ml of a 0.5 percent Xylocaine hydrochloride solution lateral to the prostate and seminal vesicle. The solution diffuses into the deep pelvic area, block-ing the obturator nerve.

MANAGEMENT OF EXTRAVASATION. When a gradual climb in blood pres-sure is noted during performance of transurethral prostatectomy and there is slowly increasing abdominal distention and abdominal muscular rigidity, perivesical fluid extravasation is obviously present.

One of the major advantages of spinal anesthesia is the early recogni-tion of extravasation. With general anesthesia the signs just described become apparent only with larger amounts of extravasated fluid. Under low spinal anesthesia it is noted early that the patient becomes restless and usually complains of abdominal or back pain. Nausea and vomiting frequently occur. When extravasation is recognized, early discontinuation of the operative procedure with catheter drainage will frequently suffice. Whenever there is doubt in the operator's mind about the adequacy of catheter drainage only, suprapubic perivesical drainage should be instituted.

A suprapubic incision is made just above the symphysis for a distance of about 3 to 5 cm. The rectus fascia is opened and with the blunt end of the scalpel handle the recti muscles are spread, permitting insertion of a finger down behind the symphysis. On occasion the cold irrigating fluid can be detected by the inserted finger if the amount of fluid has been excessive. Penrose drains should be placed deeply on the left and right sides of the space of Retzius.

The drains are usually removed within twenty-four hours. The areas through which extravasation takes place rapidly seal off. The patient's postoperative recovery is rapid, and hospitalization is not lengthened by this drainage maneuver. Morbidity is usually minimal. This small incision through the rectus fascia and insertion of Penrose drains often requires less than three to five minutes to perform.

Perivesical Fluid Extravasation. By doing contrast cystograms followed by emptying of the bladder and air cystograms, it can be shown in about 70 percent of instances that when the bladder-mucosal water barrier is cut following resection for a bladder tumor, fluid extravasates through the bladder to the area between the bladder and the reflected peritoneum.

Fluid extravasation also occurs in transurethral prostatectomy, so that a minimal fluid volume of about 300 ml may be found outside of the resected prostatic bed. In most instances the patient will absorb this fluid with relatively little difficulty. There are times, however, in which more extensive extravasation occurs, requiring suprapubic drainage as described.

Aid to Satisfactory Cutting with the Resectoscope Loop. In performing transurethral prostatectomy, the resecting loop may be widened to obtain larger pieces of resected tissue if this is desired by the operator. It must be remembered that when the loop is pulled laterally to widen it, there is a shortening of the loop in the vertical direction. As a result, the loop at the end of its excursion may not meet the lower edge of the sheath fenestra. This will result in an incomplete resection of tissue, with the resected piece of tissue still attached to the prostate at one end.

To avoid this, the flexible stems of the loop must be bent down at the same time the loop is widened (as in Fig. 57). Test runs of the loop through the fenestra before inserting the sheath transurethrally will determine the degree of bending necessary. A shearing effect of the

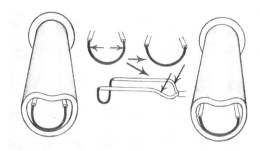

57. Suggested method of bending resectoscope loop for efficiency in resection.

loop on the sheath is necessary. The effect is analogous to the shearing, or lack of shearing, effect of the two blades of a scissors.

CLEANING LOOP OF RESECTOSCOPE DURING TRANSURETHRAL SURGERY. In the course of performing transurethral prostatectomy, and even more so when resecting bladder tumors, the resectoscope loop may not cut cleanly and burned tissue remains on the loop. To clean the wire of the loop, it may be very lightly brushed against the bristles of a small sterile hand scrub brush resting on the patient's abdomen. A piece of gauze or a small sterile tooth brush may be used for the same purpose.

REMOVAL OF PROSTATIC CALCULI UNDER RADIOGRAPHIC CONTROL. The difficulty of complete eradication of minute prostatic calculi transurethrally has led some urologists to recommend open prostatectomy. These calculi may, however, be successfully removed by the transurethral method. Their removal is very important. Residual prostatic calculi account for much chronic infection and chronic prostatitis.

The peripheral location of these calculi near or impacted in the prostatic capsule is common knowledge. Often single or multiple stones will lie in small pockets which are actually capsular diverticula. These calculi are occasionally left behind. One should not forget to seek out these hidden calculi. A flat plate of the pelvis while the patient is still on the cystoscopy table will often reveal the presence of residual stones. Further resection is done to remove the remaining calculi and X-rays are repeated to ensure their removal. Freedom from postoperative symptomatology makes this added effort worthwhile.

Irrigation During Transurethral Resection of the Prostate

USE OF PROPER SOLUTION FOR IRRIGATION. It is of course necessary, in electrosurgical cutting and coagulating under water, to use an irrigating solution which is free of electrolytes. Most sterile tap water, because of the electrolytes contained therein, will seriously hamper the cutting and coagulating function of the electrosurgical unit. Distilled water may be utilized as the irrigating fluid but there is the danger of water absorption and hemolysis with the use of a hypotonic irrigating solution.

Common irrigating solutions used are glycine, 5 percent glucose in distilled water, urea, Sorbitol ® (Baxter Laboratories' trade name for 3.3% sorbitol), Cytal ® (Cutter Laboratories' trade name for an almost identical sorbitol product), and 3.5 to 5 percent mannitol obtainable under the trade name of Resectosol ® (McGaw Laboratories).

Urological personnel should understand the importance of using one of the above recommended solutions. Nurses and orderlies have been known to refill the irrigator with whatever water is handy and available at the time. This problem is nonexistent when disposable irrigating units are utilized.

MANNITOL SOLUTION AS AN IRRIGANT. Mannitol in 3.5 and 5 percent solution serves well as an irrigant for transurethral prostatectomy. It has been used as the irrigant of choice by one of us (H.B.) for prostatic re-section in over 1,000 cases. Because mannitol is an obligatory diuretic (excreted as a 5 percent solution, with concentration of 3.3 percent or greater being hypertonic), it stimulates the rapid output of fluids systemically absorbed through venous sinuses. Since it is not metabolized, this phase of any possible complication is also eliminated.

When one uses 500 ml of 15 to 20 percent mannitol (with 60 MEQ of sodium as sodium chloride) intravenously during the approximate hour of the transurethral prostatectomy, any small volume of washed-in fluids is stimulated to rapid excretion. Since small amounts of sodium chloride are pulled out with excreted mannitol, it has been determined that sodium as a 0.12 percent solution should be replaced in the plasma. Therefore, following the surgery, patients may be given a liter of 5 percent mannitol, 5 percent glucose, and 0.12 percent sodium chloride at the rate of 1 liter per eight hours, intravenously. With this regimen, a self-adjusting system for maintaining electrolytes and a built-in diuretic irrigating system is maintained. There is no increased excretion of potassium ions.

INTRAVENOUS OSMOLAR DIURETIC DURING TRANSURETHRAL PROSTATEC-TOMY. Because of better vision with water, some urologists continue to avoid the use of irrigating solutions. The use of 4 percent urea as an intravenous osmolar diuretic or 15 to 20 percent mannitol given intravenously seems to afford some protective value from the standpoint of possible hemolysis.

When the operation is started and completed with one of the isotonic solutions there is no disturbance in vision. When the operator begins with sterile water and then switches to an isotonic or hypertonic solution, he notes a change of clarity.

USE OF NONHEMOLYTIC IRRIGATING SOLUTIONS BY NEOPHYTE UROLO-GISTS. The following quotation seems particularly worthy of repetition here: "A statistical analysis of more than 20,000 transurethral resections done during a 20-year period provided data which we believe firmly support the thesis that the use of nonhemolytic irrigating solutions protects the patient and significantly reduces postoperative morbidity and mortality rates. It is our opinion that the use of nonhemolytic solutions is mandatory for urologic residents who are learning the operation and for others with relative inexperience with the operation. We advise their use by all resectionists." *

TRANSURETHRAL RESECTION REACTION. In instances of dilutional hyponatremia water overload syndrome during transurethral prostatectomy, furosemide (Lasix) in 40 to 80 mg dosage intravenously is most helpful. Caution must be exercised to prevent sodium and potassium loss. In some instances as much as 200 to 300 ml of 5 percent sodium chloride must be administered. Potassium must also be maintained.

Central venous pressure measurements will very early indicate oncoming reactions due to fluid overload and sodium loss. Some transurethral resectionists use furosemide routinely.

REFRIGERATED IRRIGATING SOLUTION. In the recent past, refrigerated irrigating solutions (from 37 to 40°F) have been used for resection. This seems to better control the bleeding during the procedure, but on return to the recovery room bleeding in alarming amounts often begins with reversion to normal body temperature. Most urologists no longer use iced solutions.

Continuation of the cold irrigating solution over a period of several hours and then gradual increase in the temperature of the solution, until finally room temperature is reached, could possibly be of value. Overall body temperature as well as rectal (prostatic) temperature should be monitored. The use of this procedure is, for the most part, not considered a satisfactory substitute for good hemostasis at the time of surgery.

CONTROL OF IRRIGATING FLUID IN THE BLADDER DURING TRANSURETHRAL PROSTATECTOMY. One may assume that approximately 400 to 450 ml of fluid will run into the bladder during a period of 30 to 70 seconds. During this time period the average urologist takes about ten bites of tissue.

To begin with, the irrigating fluid flows in more rapidly than 10 ml/second. As the bladder fills, the intravesical pressure increases, and the fluid flows in more slowly. Many urologists will continue cutting tissue until, as the result of the increased intravesical pressure, there is slowing down of the inflow to almost zero. The slowdown of inflowing irrigating solution is easily identified. Vision becomes impaired because blood is no longer being freely washed into the bladder from the lens site.

* John L. Emmett, Jas. H. Gilbaugh, Jr., and Peter McLean, "Fluid Absorption During Transurethral Resection: Comparison of Mortality and Morbidity After Irrigation With Water and Nonhemolytic Solutions," *Journal of Urology* 101:884 (1969).

If vision remains poor after emptying the bladder, the fluid inflow rate should be checked. One must consider also possible lightening of anesthesia with the patient bearing down to increase intravesical pressure, or even possible extravasation of fluid.

The bladders of some patients will distend up to 600 and 700 ml. The resectionist is then able to resect more tissue than he would in the bladder of average capacity. When bladder capacity is diminished, the bladder must be emptied more frequently and consequently a good deal of time is wasted in filling and emptying the bladder.

In order not to overdistend the bladder and to minimize high pressures during the course of irrigation, especially when many venous sinuses are open, the urologist of long experience, having predetermined the filling time, may during the latter part of the resection count off in seconds and empty the bladder at a stipulated time. By so doing, the irrigating solution may be shut off before the visual field is obscured by blood, indicating a high vesical pressure. For example, if the urologist has determined that it takes about 50 seconds of filling before the medium becomes cloudy, he may then count to 40 seconds and empty the bladder.

Additionally, urologists of long experience advocate turning on the water inflow only when cutting and coagulating are taking place, shutting off the inflow when these operations stop (some urologists do the exact opposite). This enables working a longer time without the necessity of emptying the bladder.

Control of Bleeding in Prostatic Surgery

BLEEDING DURING TRANSURETHRAL PROSTATECTOMY. Routine preoperative blood studies (mentioned in the beginning of this section) will forewarn the urologist of any bleeding tendencies in a patient. The fulguration of bleeding vessels may be done during or at the end of transurethral prostatic resection. Though one may fulgurate a particular spurting vessel, it may be necessary to cut through this vessel on two to three deeper levels, necessitating repetitive fulguration of the same vessel. For this reason the authors tend to defer fulguration of bleeders until near the end of the resection or at least until deep resection has been accomplished in the area of the arterial bleeder. If bleeding is such that vision is disturbed, some of the spurting vessels must be fulgurated long before the end of the resection is approached.

Drawing the resectoscope outward to the region of the verumontanum and cutting down slightly on the irrigating flowrate, nearing the end of the prostatectomy, may better demonstrate spurting vessels. These vessels then may be approached and fulgurated more readily.

SLOW CUTTING OR "BLENDED CURRENT" FOR BLEEDING CONTROL. At the beginning of a transurethral prostatectomy, one may make the initial cuts very slowly, especially in the 4 to 5 and 7 to 8 o'clock positions where the prostatic arteries enter. The cutting current, when used in a slow movement, will have some coagulating effect so as to control bleeding. Some resectionists will use the blended current (cut and coagulation) at this phase of the resection to control or minimize bleeding. Still other operators utilize the blended current for the entire transurethral prostatectomy.

Theoretically, the use of the blended current for complete resections causes greater postoperative slough and greater risk of secondary hemorrhage. This is probably more theoretical than true when the coagulating setting on the electrosurgical unit is *mild to moderate*. The decision to use a straight cutting current or a blended current will depend primarily on the vascularity of the particular prostate being operated upon. The operator may start with a straight cutting current and convert to a blended current if bleeding becomes troublesome. The postoperative care available to the patient will also dictate the type of current to be used. If specially trained personnel are not available, the operator would be wise to use the blended current.

RETROGRADE CUTTING AT VERUMONTANUM AREA. Tissue at the apex, especially just lateral to the verumontanum area, may be cut in retrograde fashion to ensure against accidental sphincter damage. Since bleeding is usually profuse at these points, the blended-current or slow-cutting technique may be used. If the tissue is not completely cut off, "standard bites" will remove these loose chips.

BLEEDING VESSEL HIDDEN BY SMALL KNOB OF TISSUE. There are times when it may be necessary to further resect a knob of tissue in order to visualize a bleeding vessel located behind this tissue.

VENOUS SINUS BLEEDING. One should not attempt repeated fulguration of venous oozing, especially from sinuses. This will quickly clear after the resectoscope has been removed and the catheter put in place. Once the operator stops inflating the prostatic capsule with irrigating solution, the capsule collapses and the veins will shortly stop bleeding. The catheter being smaller than the resectoscope sheath also contributes to capsule collapse.

Some urologists apply light traction on the bladder neck to prevent the entrance of subsequent irrigating fluid into the capsule. The balloon of the retention catheter should be inflated sufficiently to prevent it from being pulled into the prostatic fossa (this opens venous sinuses). Those who subscribe to traction return their patients to the recovery room with catheter either taped to the thigh on light traction, or with an opened wet sponge around the shaft of the catheter with a half knot at the urethral meatus and with the catheter on light traction. This light traction is applied for four to six hours.

If too much traction is applied with the opened sponge technique, pressure necrosis occurs at the meatus, with a resulting meatal stricture.

When traction is utilized, there is always some oozing of blood out the urethral meatus around the catheter. If bleeding is adequately controlled this amounts to less than 50 to 100 ml over a period of several hours. To avoid a frantic call from the nurse not familiar with this occurrence, she should be advised of this and she in turn can advise the apprehensive patient.

Other urologists disagree with the use of traction except for intravesical bladder neck bleeding areas. They use traction rarely, feeling that irrigation alone will suffice for venous or sinus bleeding, and that arterial bleeding will not be controlled by traction. Some urologists do not even use balloon catheters.

VENOUS SINUS BLEEDING EASILY CONTROLLED; ARTERIAL BLEEDING PERSISTS. Following transurethral resection, one should spend 3 to 5 minutes in irrigating the bladder. From 50 to 75 ml of irrigating fluid may be instilled into the bladder, and the bladder then allowed to empty. Frequently a profusely bloody drainage will clear to a very light pink color with this few minutes of irrigation. If the drainage remains severely bloody, then in all probability the bleeding is arterial and one should immediately replace the resectoscope and seek out the arterial bleeders which need fulguration.

Irrigation Following Transurethral Resection of the Prostate

THREE-WAY BALLOON-TYPE CATHETER FOLLOWING PROSTATECTOMY. Many resectionists use the three-way irrigating catheter following transurethral prostatectomy. Usually sterile saline is used to irrigate the bladder at the rate of 20 drops per minute, and is allowed to drain continuously. This constant type of irrigation will prevent the formation of blood clots.

The three-way catheter has become popular with nursing personnel. The ease with which new bottles of irrigating solution may be added (avoiding confrontation with the Asepto or Toomey syringe) and the simplicity of irrigation are great aids to the nursing staff.

The occasional patient with severe bleeding (invariably arterial) may require being taken back to surgery for additional fulguration.

METERED IRRIGATION METHOD USING THREE-WAY BALLOON-TYPE CATHETER. The irrigation method illustrated in Figure 58 has been found excellent for use with post-prostatectomy patients during the postoperative bleeding phase. A 24 French, 30-ml bag, three-way balloon catheter, preferably plastic or silicone-coated, may be anchored. A meter for measurement of intravenous irrigating fluid is adapted to the apparatus. The meter is adjusted so that irrigating fluid is administered at the rate of 100 to 150 ml per hour. A second reservoir (rarely needed) is provided for more copious irrigation.

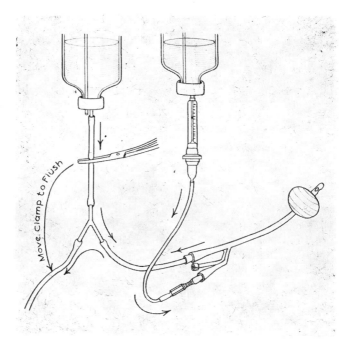

58. Metered irrigation system for use with three-way balloon catheter

The meter illustrated is the McGaw ® meter. With its use the flow will automatically stop if bladder pressure rises. Vastly improved post-prostatectomy irrigation is afforded by use of this method; minimal nursing care is required.

ORDERS TO NURSING STAFF FOR USE OF NESBIT-YOUNG (Y-TUBE) TYPE OF IRRIGATING APPARATUS. Personnel concerned with the post-prostatectomy patient may overdistend the bladder with irrigating fluid. They should therefore be instructed that when using Nesbit-Young apparatus, fluid is allowed to flow into the bladder only while one counts 5 seconds. In 5 seconds there will be approximately 50 ml of fluid in the bladder. The inflow is then cut off as the outflow is opened so that the bladder will empty.

When smaller-than-usual plastic tubing is employed, filling time takes approximately 8 seconds. The urologist should ascertain the proper number of seconds required and so instruct his personnel.

Nursing personnel may prefer to note fluid volume markings on the irrigating jar, but it is less distracting to count out the seconds and limit the bladder filling for each irrigation as above described.

Urethral Catheterization Following Transurethral Prostatectomy

CHOICE OF CATHETER FOLLOWING TRANSURETHRAL RESECTION. Some urologists prefer the Tiemann (or Coudé-tip) 22 or 24 French catheter to the balloon type of catheter following transurethral prostatectomy. These surgeons feel that the more rigid Tiemann catheter allows for better evacuation of clots in the presence of active bleeding. Another advantage is the larger lumen of a Tiemann catheter when compared to a balloon catheter of comparable size. The Tiemann catheter is more readily passed than the balloon catheter. The Coudé tip easily overrides the posterior lip of the bladder neck and does not as a rule tend to pass subtrigonally.

The inflated bag of the balloon catheter prevents contraction of the prostatic capsule if the balloon slips down into the prostatic urethra. Occasionally when the balloon is in the prostatic fossa the tip of the balloon catheter becomes lodged under the trigone, with subsequent poor drainage.

The disadvantage of the Tiemann catheter is inability to apply traction. It too may become lodged under the trigone if it slips down into the urethra.

The Tiemann catheter must be modified by cutting extra holes near the tip to promote free drainage and aspiration of clots.

FACILITATING PASSAGE OF A BALLOON CATHETER AFTER PROSTATECTOMY. If urethral trauma occurred prior to or during the insertion of the resectoscope sheath, it may be impossible to insert a balloon catheter at the end of the operative procedure. It is occasionally possible to insert a balloon catheter by first passing a small ureteral catheter (No. 4 French). The tip of the balloon catheter is then cut. The ureteral catheter is threaded inside the balloon catheter, exiting through the distal end of the urethral catheter. The ureteral catheter is of sufficient length so that the entire combination may be advanced until the balloon catheter is in the bladder. The balloon of the catheter is then inflated and the ureteral catheter removed.

FURTHER FACILITATING PASSAGE OF A BALLOON CATHETER. Frequently the straight balloon catheter will hold up at the bladder neck after transurethral resection of the prostate due to the deeply resected posterior fossa. There will be a relatively high bladder neck in such a situation. If the resection has been thin at this vesicocapsular junction the operator can easily push the end of the catheter through the junction subtrigonally. Irrigation will result in extravasation. The surgeon can anticipate this problem by inspecting the area in question before removal of the resectoscope.

In such a situation the surgeon may resort to a curved splinting device. The urethral catheter with an indwelling stylet (described in Chapter Seven) or a wire stylet may be used to guide the balloon catheter. Care must be taken when using the relatively rigid wire stylet, but it can be safely utilized if the catheter is guided along the anterior wall of the prostatic capsule avoiding the posterior bladder neck area. The curved tip of the catheter with stylet indwelling will help to ensure safe passage over the posterior bladder neck.

PUNCH CYSTOTOMY AS AID TO PASSING BALLOON-TYPE CATHETER. After the bladder has been filled with irrigating solution, a punch cystotomy with a large-bore needle may be done and the bladder sufficiently filled so that with suprapubic pressure exerted by the circulating nurse the patient develops a full urethral stream. The catheter is then usually passed easily into the bladder against the full voiding stream, after which the bag on the catheter can be safely inflated.

ADDITIONAL AIDS IN POST-RESECTION PASSAGE OF BALLOON CATHETER. Incision with the knife electrode at 5, 6, and 7 o'clock is advised as a routine at the end of a transurethral prostatectomy. Incisions at 3 and 9 o'clock are also frequently done. These incisions will often minimize the posterior bladder neck elevation in addition to discouraging bladder neck contractures.

With the urethra well lubricated, a continuous twisting motion of the catheter will allow it to override an obstructing posterior lip. Should the tip tend to go to the subtrigonal area, the continual advancement and rotation of the catheter allows the tip to "flip" over the prominent posterior lip.

A urethral catheter stylet or mandrin may be bent to a curve like that of a sound or Coudé-tipped catheter and used as an aid to passage of a catheter.

A large Tiemann catheter as previously described may also be used.

ANOTHER MEANS OF PASSAGE OF BALLOON-TYPE CATHETER. When all of the previously described methods of passing a catheter into the bladder have failed, the resectoscope may be reintroduced into the bladder under vision. If incisions at the 5, 6, and 7 o'clock positions are inadequate, they must be done to a deeper level. Incisions may also be done at the 3 and 9 o'clock positions. The resectoscope sheath is left in place.

Then an 18 to 20 French Coudé (Tiemann) catheter is prepared by cutting off the flare end. Several additional drainage eyes are cut with scissors. The catheter, well lubricated, is passed through the resectoscope sheath into the bladder. The distal end of the catheter is pushed as far as possible into the bladder with a hemostat as the resectoscope sheath is removed. Pressure must be applied perineally after partially removing the resectoscope sheath to hold the catheter in place while the sheath is totally removed, since the catheter disappears into the sheath during removal of the sheath through the penile urethra.

As an alternative to the above, a 20 French balloon catheter may be utilized (through the 28F resectoscope sheath), though its drainage lumen is not as large as a Coudé catheter of comparable size. This may be inserted through the resectoscope sheath, and the filling stem tied almost flush with the main shaft of the catheter with No. 0 or 1 black silk, after filling the balloon to 30 ml. The inflating arm is best pulled and put on stretch (thinned out) while being tied.

The inflating arm of the catheter should then be cut off, leaving a 1- to 2-mm projecting end. The distal flare end of the catheter is also cut so that it will go through the resectoscope sheath. The sheath is then removed. The inflated balloon prevents the catheter from slipping out.

A catheter larger than 20 French in size cannot be utilized in this manner.

Satisfactory bladder drainage cannot be accomplished in the presence of appreciable bleeding using this technique with a smaller catheter.

Anchoring of Tiemann catheters may be done with adhesive and black silk in the manner described under *Methods of Anchoring Filiforms or Catheters* in Chapter Seven. The reader is again reminded that more than one hole for drainage must be made in the Tiemann catheter—these are manufactured with a single drainage eye.

DETECTION OF LEAK OF BALLOON IN CATHETER. The addition of several drops of indigo carmine to the solution used to inflate the balloon gives one a very quick indication of leakage when blue-stained urine appears.

Suprapubic and Retropubic Prostatectomy

Operative Exposure of Prostate Facilitated by Kidney Lift

Use of the kidney lift to elevate the pelvis, previously mentioned, is especially advantageous in performing retropubic prostatectomy, suprapubic transvesical prostatectomy, cystectomy, and open resection with fulguration of tumors near the bladder neck. This is particularly helpful when operating on an obese patient. If a kidney lift is not available on a specific operating table, a sand bag or rolled-up turkish towel may be substituted.

The patient is placed on the table so that the upper border of the symphysis is over the upper border of the kidney rest. Raising the kidney rest elevates the prostate and opens up the pelvis so that enucleation is easier.

There may be an occasional transient mild drop in blood pressure with elevation of the kidney rest, which will usually be corrected on lowering the kidney rest.

Suprapubic Midline or Transverse Incision

For suprapubic or retropubic prostatectomy, one may use either a suprapubic midline incision, a transverse incision, or a Pfannenstiel incision. To eliminate an asymmetrical incision, some gynecologists have adopted the use of a plastic or steel template which is placed on the abdomen in the immediate suprapubic area.

In older patients, one is less apt to have herniation when the transverse incision is used.

Incision for Cystotomy, Midline or Transverse

In opening the bladder during suprapubic prostatectomy, either a vertical or a transverse incision may be used. Some urologists claim that the transverse incision will heal more readily. Many surgeons will make a low bladder incision and extend this into the bladder neck area and even into the bladder neck and prostatic urethra. This offers better exposure of the prostatic fossa after enucleation of the prostate. Bleeders are more easily seen and controlled. One will in actuality be performing a combination retropubic and suprapubic prostatectomy incision. The vertical incision lends itself best to this combined approach.

Care must be taken not to tear the distal end of the incision during enucleation of the prostate. Because of possible damage to the external sphincter if the prostatic capsule is torn distally many urologists prefer a transverse incision over the prostatic capsule (retropubically). Bleeding from the pericapsular veins may also be a disadvantage should tearing occur with the vertical incision. A suture at the distal end of the incision may be a safety factor.

Bladder Retraction

(Please refer to *Retraction of the Bladder Wall to Facilitate Exposure* and subsequent sections in Chapter Six.)

Treatment of the Posterior Lip of the Bladder Neck

Following enucleation of a prostatic adenoma, there is a sharp fall-off of the entire posterior lip of the bladder neck and prostatic capsule into the urethra, making it difficult to pass a catheter or any other urethral instrument. One may facilitate passage by taking a mattress suture through the posterior bladder neck at 6 o'clock, pulling the bladder mucosa down into the prostatic urethra and suturing it to the posterior prostatic capsule. This makes a smoother, more gradual sloping of the posterior lip of the bladder neck. The bladder neck surface also heals more rapidly by use of this aid.

Alternatively, one may treat the bladder neck in the fashion described below.

Prevention of Bladder Neck Contracture in Case of Thickened Bladder Neck

Often a thickened bladder neck is present, most apparent posteriorly. One frequently may eliminate this by placing hemostatic clamps at 5 and 7 o'clock and then removing a wedge of tissue in the form of a "V" between these two clamps. The area grasped by the clamps is sutured with figure-of-eight sutures to control bleeding and a mattress-type suture may be taken at 6 o'clock to again pull the bladder neck down to the midprostatic urethra as described above. This procedure serves to prevent bladder neck contracture and promotes more rapid healing.

Control of Bleeding Prior to Enucleation

The main arterial supply to the prostate originates from a branch (prostatic artery) of the inferior vesical artery bilaterally. These arteries, one on each side, enter the prostate near the bladder junction. One may estimate their location as they enter the prostatic capsule as being just below the bladder neck on the lateral and slightly posterior surface of the capsule.

When doing a retropubic prostatectomy, sutures are placed around the visible periprostatic veins above and below the intended transverse incision in the prostatic capsule. Control of the arterial bleeding is almost always assured by placing two sutures on each side through the full thickness of the prostatic capsule in the area described above. These two sutures on each side are placed to form a "V" with the vertex pointing laterally. When the transverse incision is made, each end of the incision extends laterally down to the open part of the V.

In addition to providing arterial hemostatic control, these sutures help to prevent tearing of the capsule laterally with extension posteriorly into the area of the rectum. In placing these arterial sutures, the operator must take care not to go too far posteriorly and creep up on the bladder lest he involve the ureter. Also, once the desired position is chosen and the suture inserted, the suture sweep through the capsule must be completed. Partially inserting the needle and withdrawing it because of undesirable position can lead to copious bleeding.

Lesser bleeding encountered during the transverse prostatic capsular incision is easily controlled as encountered with catgut No. 0 chromic suture ligatures or the electrosurgical unit.

When performing a suprapubic prostatectomy, wherever the cystotomy incision is located, these same lateral prostatic sutures may be utilized to prevent subsequent arterial bleeding after enucleation of the prostate. Hemostatic sutures through the periprostatic veins may also be of value but are of lesser importance.

Enucleation of the Prostate

Enucleation of the prostate suprapubically is usually most easily accomplished by breaking through the prostatic mucosa anteriorly between the lateral lobes. Almost any point within the urethra or bladder may be used where a cleavage plane seems apparent.

For the intravesical prostate, the mucosa at the junction of the prostate and bladder may be incised with a scalpel or electrosurgical unit (preferred) circumferentially around the adenoma. A slow blended current is used with the electrosurgical unit.

If this method is not utilized, the irregular torn edge of the bladder mucosa should be cleanly trimmed after enucleation.

Packing the Prostatic Fossa After Enucleation

Following enucleation of a prostate, it is common practice to pack the prostatic fossa with 1- or 2-inch hot vaginal rolls or other type of packing in an attempt to control bleeding. This idea of a hot pack after enucleation has

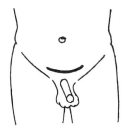

59. Low transverse incision for vasectomy with suprapubic or retropubic prostatectomy

been passed down from resident physician to resident physician. The heat applied is more apt to open vessels than to stimulate small vessels to contract. It is therefore suggested that the packing be moistened with cool water or saline rather than with hot fluid.

The packing is left in place for a period of 6 to 10 minutes and then gradually removed. Arterial bleeders are controlled as they are uncovered. Venous bleeders within the prostatic fossa are generally ignored but if located around the bladder neck they may be controlled by electrocoagulation or suture ligatures of chromic catgut.

Following the placement of a transurethral catheter, Oxycel ®, Gelfoam ® or Surgicel ® is utilized by some surgeons in the prostatic fossa as the balloon of the catheter is pulled down against the bladder neck. Avoidance of use of these foreign substances is preferable. If utilized, most of the substance may be removed several days postoperatively by irrigation with 5 percent sodium bicarbonate solution.

Time-Saving Vasectomy with Suprapubic or Retropubic Prostatectomy

With the Pfannenstiel or transverse incision, the vas deferens may be approached through the operative incision rather than making separate scrotal incisions. After prostatic enucleation, vasectomy is performed, utilizing the waiting time necessary for proper prostatic packing. The lower edge of the skin incision laterally is retracted outward and downward and the external inguinal ring is identified. The cord is held with Babcock forceps. The vas is isolated from the cord structures and a section of the vas deferens is excised. Both ends are ligated with 2-0 or 3-0 chromic suture. The procedure is performed bilaterally.

Some surgeons prefer to perform the vasectomy portion of the procedure after making the Pfannenstiel or transverse incision before proceeding with enucleation of the prostate suprapubically or retropubically.

Figure 59 illustrates the low, slightly curved, transverse suprapubic incision commonly used for the combined procedure. This incision makes both external rings easily accessible by retraction of the lower skin flaps. With the vertical midline incision as well as the transverse incision, the vas deferens may also be quickly isolated bilaterally "from within" the pelvis. The vas deferens is found near the internal inguinal ring closely adherent to the peritoneum.

Bladder Neck Bleeding

Bleeding of the bladder neck invariably seems to arise from vessels at 5 and 7 o'clock. Immediately after enucleation of the prostate, placement of a figure-of-eight suture at these points will often effect hemostasis. Preliminary placement of sutures through the prostatic capsule laterally as previously described frequently minimizes arterial bleeding near or around the bladder neck.

Circumferential Bladder Neck Suture for Control of Bleeding

A circumferential suture of 2-0 Tevdek or other such nonabsorbable slippery type of suture material may be placed around the bladder neck in purse-string-like fashion. The suture is brought out through the bladder neck and abdominal wall and tied over a bolster on the skin. A transurethral catheter is inserted into the bladder and traction is applied to the purse-string suture, "snugging up" the bladder neck around the catheter. As soon as hemostasis is obtained in the postoperative phase, the purse-string suture is removed. The purse-string temporary closure of the bladder neck confines bleeding to the prostatic fossa; the bladder remains relatively free of blood.

Urologists who utilize this method are most happy with their results. Reports of bladder neck contractures resulting from long-term use of this technique are supposedly rare. The authors question the rarity of bladder neck contracture due to this technique.

Intravesical Media for Easy Bladder Identification and Manipulation

Very often several hundred milliliters of water is instilled into the bladder prior to prostatectomy to raise the bladder into easy view after the recti muscles are retracted. This helps to lift the peritoneum up out of the way and facilitates reflecting the peritoneum off the bladder. The most common medium used for this purpose is sterile water or saline.

Some urologists instead use several hundred cubic centimeters of air. When the bladder is opened there is no need to drain bladder fluid. If good judgment is used, an air embolus as described in the literature should not be feared. A contracted, friable bladder would present a real risk. Usually, about 150 to 200 cc of air is introduced via a large calibrated syringe.

Packing of Prostatic Fossa for Hemostasis: Secondary Removal

On rare occasions, even with good arterial control of bleeding, there will be excessive oozing of blood from the prostatic fossa. This is most likely to occur following enucleation of a very large prostatic adenoma where a large "raw" surface area or rigid prostatic capsule remains. A patient who has had previous repeated severe bouts of prostatitis may have a markedly thickened capsule. Such a capsule will have many large bleeding venous sinuses that do not contract down. Electrocoagulation under these circumstances is futile. Packing of the prostatic fossa offers the simplest solution.

Gauze is packed into the prostatic fossa and brought out through the bladder wall, preferably sufficiently far from the bladder neck to assure good primary healing of the bladder neck if it was incised initially (cystotomy). The gauze is packed in a snug fashion but *not tightly*. If the original approach was retropubic, using a transverse prostatic capsular incision, it is best to do a cystotomy and pack through this incision to allow primary closure of the prostatic transverse incision.

The gauze is brought out through the abdominal incision, closing the wound loosely around the gauze. The gauze should be brought out as low as possible, to hopefully prevent an incisional hernia. Retention sutures are utilized in the closure of the abdominal wound, in addition to fascial and skin sutures.

The packing is removed under heavy sedation or, preferably, in the operating room two to five days postoperatively.

In addition to the direct hemostatic effect of the gauze against the bleeding capsule, the gauze acts as a wick. Blood runs up the moist wick, preventing the accumulation of excessive clots in the bladder. Bladder drainage is accomplished with a large balloon (30 French, 5-ml bag) cystostomy catheter. It is preferable to also insert a urethral balloon catheter into the bladder (20 or 22 French, 30-ml bag) prior to packing the fossa. This eliminates the need for later insertion after removal of the packing, a procedure which may at times be extremely difficult.

Postoperative wound and urinary tract infections should be anticipated with this procedure and treated appropriately.

With modern-day wide exposure of the prostatic fossa either retropubically or with a combined vesical-retropubic approach, packing is a poor substitute for the control of arterial bleeding. If adequate control has not been obtained, one can anticipate the necessity of returning the patient to the operating room for further search of elusive arterial bleeders.

Having failed to control arterial bleeding by all other means, including bilateral ligation of the hypogastric arteries, tight packing of the prostatic fossa must be done as a last desperate attempt to secure hemostasis.

Control of Bleeding in Prostatic Fossa by Transurethral Route

There will be the occasional open surgical case where the operator is unable to directly control the arterial bleeding. Bleeding in the prostatic fossa may be controlled by the use of a resectoscope passed transurethrally. The patient may be placed in stirrups prior to the prostatectomy so that he may be prepared for the passage of the resectoscope if needed. By passing the resectoscope and maintaining continuous suction above, the resectionist can very readily and quickly see spurting vessels and fulgurate them sufficiently to control bleeding. When he has finished, the transurethral catheter is placed.

To save time, the trained assistant surgeon may close the open surgical wound while the resectionist is controlling arterial bleeding transurethrally. *Some urologists, working as teams, control bleeding in this manner as a routine following prostatic enucleation.*

Ligation of Hypogastric Vessels for Control of Bleeding

Occasionally a hypogastric artery on one or both sides may be tied off to control bleeding from the prostatic fossa. This is to be utilized only as a last-resort means of controlling bleeding. One may tie off such a vessel in continuity, or one may doubly tie the vessel and divide it. The authors have also utilized large blood vessel clips to very readily tie off the hypogastric vessels.

Safety Measure for Retention of Catheter in Radical Retropubic Prostatectomy

Upon completion of the radical removal of the prostate, and prior to the anastomosis of the remaining bladder to the urethral stump, a cystostomy is created using a 24-French 5-ml balloon-type catheter. This is joined to the urethral 30-ml bag balloon catheter by suture material at the tips. With both balloons inflated, it is difficult for either catheter to become dislodged from the urinary tract even if one balloon were to be inadvertently deflated. This also resists the efforts of the patient to dislodge either catheter to some degree.

On the seventh or eighth postoperative day, traction placed on the deflated suprapubic tube permits its removal after the suture is visualized and cut at the incision site. The remaining urethral 30-ml bag balloon-type catheter retracts again into the bladder. The cystostomy closes spontaneously. The 30-ml balloon-type urethral catheter is removed when the anastomosis is intact and suprapubic drainage has ceased.

Bladder Neck Retraction After Radical Retropubic Prostatectomy

The "new" bladder neck following radical retropubic prostatectomy is sutured to the urethral stump. It is necessary to decrease by suture the wide lumen of the resected bladder opening. To prevent bladder neck retraction from the urethral junction, some urologists prefer to use several reinforcing or stay sutures. This may be easily accomplished by placing long 14- or 18-

gauge spinal needles percutaneously through the perineum and urogenital diaphragm. Traction sutures from the bladder neck area are passed through these needles. Having removed the needles, the sutures are tied in the perineum over bolsters.

This procedure is not intended to replace the production of a bladder tubular flap to bridge the gap between bladder and membranous urethra, nor the procedure of a transverse bladder wall incision closed vertically for the same purpose. Instead, it may supplement these procedures.

Traction on Urethral Catheter Following Suprapubic Prostatectomy

There are several ways to apply traction on a urethral catheter following suprapubic prostatectomy. The catheter may be tied to a metal frame which fits up against and around the penis and perineal area, or traction may be applied to the catheter which is taped to the thigh, using multiple single overlapping pieces of tape. A long string and a 1-lb weight may be tied to the catheter filling arm and led over a pulley at the foot of the bed as with orthopedic traction.

A simple alternative method is to open up a 4- by 4-inch gauze square, wet it, put the catheter on pull and then tie the gauze to the catheter with a single loop. The glans penis is retracted to prevent its inclusion in the gauze tie. The wet gauze does not slip on the catheter. Tension may be adjusted by grasping the catheter on both sides of the gauze tie and stretching the catheter (thinning it out) while an assistant pushes the gauze away from the penis. The tied gauze loop must not constrict the catheter lumen. As previously mentioned in this chapter, pressure necrosis with resulting stricture formation can occur at the meatus with undue or prolonged traction against the meatus and glans penis.

Balloon Capacity

As previously noted,* a 30-ml latex balloon-type catheter may be blown up to 225 ml before the balloon will rupture. When such a catheter is used after enucleation in a patient with a large bladder neck, the balloon may be inflated to 60, 75, 100 ml or even larger without fear of rupturing.

Cystostomy Drainage Catheters After Open Prostatectomy

Various catheters are utilized by urologic surgeons for cystostomy drainage. The Pezzer, four-wing Malecot, straight red rubber or balloon-type catheters are commonly used, either directly through the bladder and wound or through stab wounds of the bladder and abdominal wall. At the same time, 20 to 24 French balloon-type catheters with 30-ml or larger bags, are left transurethrally.

The use of two suprapubic tubes with no catheter transurethrally is described below.

---

* *Deflating Latex Balloons of Larger Size*, Chapter Seven

"Double-Barrel" Cystostomy

Following suprapubic or retropubic prostatectomy, two suprapubic catheters may be left in place, preferably being brought out via stab wounds. These are used for continuous irrigation in the immediate postoperative period. When bleeding is well controlled, one of these catheters may be removed. The second catheter is allowed to drain for approximately five more days and then is removed.

The suprapubic cystostomy wound usually heals without difficulty. Urethral catheterization or instrumentation under these circumstances is unnecessary. The incidence of postoperative chills and fever secondary to urethral instrumentation is by this means eliminated. The possibility of urethral stricture secondary to urethritis from the catheter is also avoided.

Closure of Suprapubic Midline Incision

During closure of a midline suprapubic incision, the recti muscles very often are loosely approximated with 2-0 chromic sutures. This may or may not have a tendency to prevent diastasis. Rectus muscle sutures may be reinforced by first taking a tuck in the underside of the rectus fascia on one side. The suture is then continued through the rectus muscle on each side and to the underside of the rectus fascia on the opposite side (see Fig. 60).

By loosely tying these structures together, the actual grasping of the fascia is more apt to hold the rectus muscle in approximation. The strain and stress is placed on the fascia rather than on the muscle. There will be relatively little muscle atrophy. The fascia is closed separately in another layer.

Protection Against Inadvertent Removal of Suprapubic Catheter: Facilitating the Passage of Catheter in Difficult-to-Catheterize Urethra

As the result of stricture or previous manipulation, false passages may have developed in the urethra. It may be necessary to have some type of aid to insert a catheter transurethrally into the patient's bladder following prostatectomy.

A No. 10 or 12 French Tiemann or Robinson catheter may be passed in a retrograde fashion through the bladder neck and out the urethral meatus.

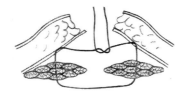

60.   Method of suturing fascia to hold recti muscles in
approximation on closing supra-pubic midline incision

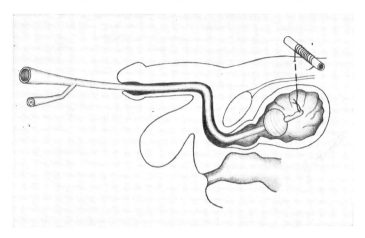

61. Method of aiding reinsertion of catheters into difficult-to-catheterize urethra

Heavy black silk is tied on to the end of this catheter emerging from the meatus. The other end of this black silk is tied or sutured to the end of a balloon-type catheter. When the red rubber catheter is withdrawn suprapubically, the balloon catheter follows it into the bladder. The balloon is inflated.

In the presence of serious injury to the urethra, it may be desirable to leave a guide in place for future urethral catheterization. The suture on the balloon catheter is left about 18 inches long and brought out through a stab wound in the abdomen (see Fig. 61). The excess suture is tied and wound around tubing or a tongue blade and secured to the abdominal wall. When it is necessary to change the urethral catheter, the old indwelling catheter is removed, first unwinding the black silk suture. The suture is removed from the old catheter and tied to the new catheter; it is then pulled at its suprapubic exit, guiding the new catheter into the bladder.

By keeping this suture tied to each successive catheter, one may continue this technique indefinitely.

Leaving the guide in place and fixed to the abdominal wall also prevents the catheter from falling out should the balloon deflate inadvertently.

Should an accessory suprapubic cystostomy catheter be inadvertently removed in the postoperative course, the silk suture guide may be used for the insertion of larger urethral catheters to maintain good bladder drainage.

Postoperative Care

Inability to Void Following Transurethral Prostatectomy

A patient may not be able to void following transurethral resection of the prostate for any one of a number of reasons, among which are the following: (1) blood clot, (2) residual prostatic tissue or loose chips, (3) Vaseline ball, (4) undetected calculi, (5) fecal impaction, (6) collapse of capsule into the posterior urethra, (7) edema of the prostatic urethra, (8) urethral sphincter spasm, (9) urethral stricture, (10) meatal stricture, or (11) rectal spasm.

It may be helpful to have the patient attempt to void while sitting in a warm bath. Bladder sedative medication may be tried. Perineal heat by way of electric or electronic pad (Aquamatic-K-Pad) or a hot water bottle (well protected) may be used. Alternatively, a rectal catheter may relieve rectal spasm and enable the patient to void. A rectal suppository containing a local anesthetic agent may relieve spasm and enable spontaneous voiding. Dibucaine hydrochloride (Nupercainal) ointment or other anesthetic ointments or suppositories may be of aid. *See below.*

Safe Insertion of Rectal Tube Following Prostate Surgery

Due to the thinness of the rectal wall following prostatectomy, by whatever method used, overzealous usage of enemata or rectal tubes is ill-advised. However, if the nurse will first insert a well-lubricated gloved finger into the rectum to feel the prostate bed anteriorly, the rectal tube may then be passed over the back side of the gloved finger. The disposable, small-volume enemas and small rectal tubes are recommended when there is specific need for an enema.

It is most surprising and gratifying to the urologist to learn of the efficacy of a colon tube, cautiously used, in relieving complete urinary retention secondary to either stool or rectal flatus.

Irradiation Therapy for Nonspecific, Resistant Post-Prostatectomy Hemostasis

Persistent mild bleeding from the prostatic fossa of a well resected or enucleated prostate may follow any type of prostatectomy. Bleeding points are not found during cystoscopy. Blood dyscrasia findings may be absent—the cause of the bleeding may remain obscure. The failure to respond to aminocaproic acid usually speaks against fibrinolysin (see section which follows). A difficult problem in management is presented.

These patients resist the use of whole fresh blood, parenteral estrogen, Vitamin C, Vitamin K, and carbazochrome salicylate (Adrenosem Salicylate).

Out of desperation, irradiation therapy to the prostatic bed has been used in some such instances with surprisingly prompt and complete remission of the bleeding after administration of only a few hundred roentgens.

Medication for Post-Transurethral-Resection Bleeding

When it is determined from the preoperative blood survey that a patient may have bleeding tendencies, complete coagulation, platelet, and vascular disorder studies must be done.

In certain instances, aminocaproic acid (Amicar) has been found helpful for bleeding following both open and transurethral prostatectomy even though no specific reason for the bleeding may have been discovered. This drug acts as an inhibitor of fibrinolysis by way of inhibition of plasminogen activator substances and also (but lesser in importance) of antiplasmin activity.

Gout Incidence Following Prostatectomy

Azotemia, acidosis, and ingestion of diuretics each account for about 20 percent of the incidence of uricemia. This must be appreciated to realize that patients with renal impairment due to prostatic obstruction will occasionally develop an attack of gout following prostatectomy.

(See also *Atrophy of the Prostatic Urethra in the Aged,* in Chapter Seven.)

Chapter Nine

THE SCROTUM AND MALE GENITALIA

THE SCROTAL CONTENTS

Differential Diagnostic Problems in the Scrotal Wall

BECAUSE OF THE TENDENCY of the scrotum to become readily edematous, this area may present problems in diagnosis. Skin lesions involving other parts of the body also frequently involve the scrotum. Extensive edema of the scrotum due to chronic cardiovascular disease may appear before signs of the disease appear in the extremities or other areas.

Edema of the scrotal wall also occurs readily as a result of trauma, chemocutaneous reactions, and venous and lymphatic obstructions. Syphilis of the scrotal skin does sometimes occur. In the presence of a scrotal ulcer, dark field examination is indicated. Carcinoma of the scrotal wall has been known to occur. Scrotal wall sebaceous cysts are most common.

Indications for Exploration

Intrascrotal Lesion Diagnosis: Torsion

Diagnosis of nonspecific orchitis, acute epididymitis, torsion of the spermatic cord, or torsion of the appendix testis and epididymis may at times pose difficult problems. When severe pain is present in the scrotum, torsion must be suspected. Torsion of the cord is for the most part confined to children and early teenagers.

Increase of pain on elevation of the scrotum is indicative of torsion of the cord, as is higher position of the testis. Swelling, discoloration, severe pain, and shortening of the cord make diagnosis fairly obvious. With the patient standing it is noted frequently that the long axis of the testis is in an anterior-posterior direction instead of the usual caudad-cephalad direction. The history of acute, sudden onset of pain is, of course, characteristic of torsion. Frequently there is a previous history of similar episodes with spontaneous regression. These signs and symptoms, however, are not always reliable.

Occasionally the patient presents himself for initial examination shortly after the torsion has spontaneously reduced. Only slight residual induration in the testis and adjacent cord may remain, with or without scrotal edema.

Torsion of the appendix epididymis and appendix testis must be differentiated from torsion of the spermatic cord. The former are generally not as totally disabling to the patient. Relieving the patient's pain will permit the examiner to palpate an indurated nodule in the expected area. Often this nodule will appear blue through the overlying scrotal skin. These conditions may frequently be treated conservatively, the pain gradually subsiding over a few days. Inflammatory hydroceles may be related to these conditions, as with torsion of the cord.

Epididymitis is usually associated with prostatitis and urethritis. The usual symptoms and signs will often be present to help in differential diagnosis. White blood cells are generally found in the urine.

The cord structures or the region of the external inguinal ring may be infiltrated with 10 ml of one percent lidocaine (Xylocaine). Pain and spasm are thereby reduced to a minimum, and more adequate examination may be made. Frequently detorsion may follow.

It must be remembered that ischemic necrosis usually occurs in two to four hours but is dependent on the severity of the torsion. There have been recent reports of viable testes preserved after delays as long as 24 hours, followed by surgery (detorsion). In a child, inability to exclude the possibility of torsion of the cord is indication enough for prompt surgical exploration.

Is the Testis Devitalized?

Having reduced the torsion of the cord at the time of surgery, it is frequently impossible to predict the viability of the testis. Superficial incision of the tunica albuginea with fresh bleeding does not necessarily indicate viable seminiferous tubules. In the past, surgeons have tended to remove the testis with poor color which has been in an avascular state beyond four to six hours.

In general, little is to be lost by preserving the testis in question when there is not associated severe inflammatory reaction of the surrounding scrotal fascial layers. Even if devitalized, pain of a severe nature quickly subsides. If the tunica albuginea has not been incised through its full thickness (or sutured through its full thickness during orchiopexy), and if the wound is not drained, drainage of sloughing seminiferous tubules through a skin sinus is rare. Healing will be *per primam*, and at worst, an atrophic testis will result, with its associated mild sensitivity to touch.

It is important to make every attempt to preserve a viable testis as the patient, who is usually a minor, may have other congenital anomalies on the contralateral side such as an absent vas deferens. The high incidence of gonorrhea among young males makes for the desirability of a "spare tire."

Orchiopexy should be performed bilaterally as the same congenital defect is usually found on the contralateral side. For this reason the midline scrotal incision is preferred. If, for some reason, drainage is desired, it should be done through a separate dependent stab wound away from the incision.

Occasionally the child with torsion of the right cord will complain only of *abdominal* pain. The hasty surgeon who does not investigate the child's scrotum may find to his embarrassment that he has performed a needless appendectomy.

(See also *Torsion of the Newborn*, under Testicle, this chapter.)

Varicocele Diagnosis and Successful Repair

The usual venous drainage of a varicocele is through the spermatic vein which within the high spermatic cord has already branched into (usually) three to four tributaries. Varicocelography has demonstrated collateral venous drainage in some individuals below the level of the internal inguinal ring. These collateral veins usually enter the spermatic cord from the abdominal wall in the region of the external inguinal ring. Failure to ligate these veins may result in an unsuccessful corrective procedure.

Ligation is accomplished by complete mobilization of the spermatic cord down to its entrance in the scrotum. During the mobilization, veins crossing to the abdominal wall may be ligated.

One may rule out preoperatively the possibility of these interconnecting veins by this simple expedient: with the patient lying in the supine position, pressure is placed over the spermatic cord (after collapse of the varicocele) in the region of the internal inguinal ring. Pressure is maintained and the patient is asked to stand. If there is rapid filling of the collapsed varicocele, collateral vessels are filling the varicocele. These collateral vessels must be located and tied off in addition to the usual high ligation of the spermatic vein tributaries.

Only in this way will repair of a varicocele be successful.

Scrotal Masses, Nodules, Indurations

Every undiagnosed mass, nodule, or induration of the spermatic cord, epididymis, testis, or its appendages should arouse sufficient suspicion to justify scrotal exploration. Little is lost in unnecessary scrotal surgery, but much can be lost by procrastination. Small indurated areas palpated in the testicle frequently turn out to be neoplasia.

A filbert-sized nodule on the upper portion of the epididymis, for instance, may remain unchanged for ten years. The nodule may then suddenly become tender, with the associated development of a hydrocele. On surgical exploration this may prove to be a leiomyosarcoma originating in the blood vessels of the epididymis, or other such unusual neoplasm.

Auto-Immune Response to Tumor

One of the authors (H.B.) did scrotal exploration on three physicians over a two-month period because of testicular nodules. The single testicular nodule measured 1 cm in two of the patients and 8 mm in the third. Two of these patients were found to have a seminoma and the third an embryonal carcinoma. All three physicians had suggestive "acute orchitis" (auto-immune reactions) for one week. Only after subsidence of the testicular swelling did the tiny nodules become apparent. All three patients are alive and free of tumor seventeen years postoperatively.

Recently Developed Hydroceles

An auto-immune response to a neoplasm may simulate an acute nonspecific orchitis. The testicular pain and swelling subsides usually within seven days. One may then palpate a small testicular tumor. As noted in the paragraph above, the tumor may be very small.

A serosal response to a tumor may also simulate a nonspecific hydrocele. For this reason recently developed hydroceles, with no history of trauma, must be viewed with suspicion. Early exploration is recommended if recent bona fide acute epididymitis, etc., has been ruled out.

Acute Hydroceles in Children

In a child with development of a relatively acute scrotal mass transillumination may occur through a solid mass. A benign teratoma may "light up." This occurs because of the relatively small size of the mass and is analogous to "lighting up" one's finger. One must remember, therefore, that transillumination in the young does not diagnose a simple hydrocele or cyst-like lesion. The examiner must be aware of the fact that a solid tumor within the cystic lesion may be present.

Epididymal Reaction Associated with Hydroceles

Following needle aspiration of a hydrocele, one frequently finds on examination an associated epididymal and vas deferens thickening suggesting chronic epididymitis. Therefore, an epididymectomy is often recommended as part of the procedure in inflammatory hydrocelectomy.

The well-known "bottle operation" has for the most part fallen into disuse. Most surgeons prefer a complete resection of the parietal tunica vaginalis close to its attachment to the testis. Hemostasis is accomplished along the incised edge of the tunica vaginalis with a running 3-0 or 4-0 chromic suture. During excision of the tunica vaginalis the epididymis is easily damaged if the operator forgets that the epididymis has been thinned out and lies some distance from the testis. This is of importance only when the epididymis is not to be removed.

In all operations involving the removal of the tunica vaginalis the testicle must be replaced within the scrotum and fixed to the scrotal wall by suture in the dependent area in at least two different locations, to prevent torsion. The spermatic cord may similarly be suture-anchored to prevent torsion.

Thrombophlebitis of the Spermatic Veins

On rare occasions, a patient may complain of scrotal or groin pain of short duration and on examination be found to have a tender indurated area within the scrotal spermatic cord. Careful examination quickly discloses a network of irregular thrombosed veins (pampiniform plexus). This may occur as an entity in itself, but has been seen associated with an ectopic ureter draining into the ipsilateral seminal vesicle.

Surgery in the Scrotum

Preparation of Penis and Scrotum

The skin of penis and scrotum is best prepared for surgical procedures by use of aqueous solutions of antiseptic or hexachlorophene soaps. Thorough rinsing with sterile water should follow, to avoid sensitivity reactions to the ingredients of the soap. The penile-scrotal skin is particularly sensitive to alcohol, acetone, ether, and iodine. Many patients show, in addition, allergic response to the quaternary ammonium compounds.

The suprapubic and scrotal hair should be removed the night before surgery. It may be easier to clip and shave this area without the use of a wetting agent initially. After the longer hairs have been removed, antiseptic soap solution may be applied to complete the shave.

At the time of surgery, it is more convenient to induce complete anesthesia before the genitalia and scrotum are prepared.

Penile Erections During Surgery

Often, under light anesthesia, erection may occur. Ice cubes within a tied sterile rubber glove applied to the penis may reduce erections. Muscle spasm relaxants such as methocarbamol (Robaxin) are of only questionable value for this purpose.

Surgical Approach

Many different incisions are used for the surgical approach to the scrotal contents. The usual incision is made in the anterolateral aspect of that side of the scrotum in which one is to operate. Some urologists will make the incision in the scrotal midline in the event they wish to also explore the opposite side. A transverse or oblique incision may also be made corresponding with the course of the scrotal skin vessels and avoiding their transection.

Inguinal incisions are favored for tumors and hydroceles with associated congenital hernia. This incision allows higher ligation of the cord in instances of tumor and eliminates intrascrotal manipulation prior to occlusion of the testicular blood supply. The spermatic cord is exposed and removed.

Using the conventional inguinal incision, large scrotal solid or hydrocele masses may be delivered into the operative area by extending the incision down toward the scrotum. Whenever possible extension downward should be avoided as the resultant inflammation in the pubic area immediately above the scrotal junction is slow to subside and suture cellulitis frequently occurs. For this reason the large hydrocele is best approached through the scrotum, reserving the inguinal approach for tumors and congenital hernia-hydroceles (patent processus vaginalis).

Eliminating Scrotum and Penis from Scrotal Field in Perineal Surgery

In performing any perineal procedure, the scrotum and the penis must frequently be held out of the field. Suturing or clipping (towel clip) the two lateral aspects of the scrotum to the abdominal wall allows complete retraction of the scrotum. The penis is held out of the way by the scrotum.

Adhesive tape used similarly is not desirable. When wet the scrotum may slip from under the tape. The close proximity of the tape to the operative area is also undesirable.

A common method of holding the scrotum out of the way is to wrap a towel underneath the scrotum and pull it on over to the abdomen. With manipulation during surgery, the scrotum usually slips out from under the towel and one then has the nuisance of attempting to get the scrotum out of the surgical field.

Scrotal Closure

Absorbable suture has the decided advantage of not requiring removal. Picking at nonabsorbable suture buried in the edematous folds of the incisional skin can be an unpleasant experience for the patient and physician. Due to the underlying dartos muscle, the incisional skin edge has a tendency to "turn in." A continuous subcuticular suture will prevent this.

Best closure of the scrotal incision is accomplished with 3-0 or 4-0 chromic interrupted catgut sutures approximating in one layer the fascia and dartos muscle of the scrotal wall. The skin is closed subcuticularly with the same suture material in a continuous fashion.

A rapid and simple method of closing the scrotum is to use a 3-0 or 4-0 catgut or chromic suture, closing all of the scrotal layers (except skin) as one in a simple continuous suture, and then continuing this same suture through the scrotal skin using alternating superficial and deep sutures to control bleeding of the superficial vessels.

We have on occasion used a subcuticular nonabsorbable suture which is removed when healing is completed.

Drainage After Scrotal Surgery

Scrotal surgical procedures invariably cause swelling of the scrotum and its contents. This can be minimized with pressure dressings and elevation of the scrotum. Most scrotal surgery, despite the best and most meticulous care, will have a collection of blood and serum for a 24-hour period. Therefore, one of us (H.B.) invariably uses Penrose drainage for 24 hours. The drain is then removed.

The fundamentals of good drainage should be followed. The drain is *led out of* the scrotum *rather than into* the scrotum to avoid the introduction of pathogens. The stab wound must be dependent in location and adequate in size to allow a loose fit of the drain through the drainage tract. Fixation of the drain to the scrotal skin is necessary to avoid premature withdrawal or "sucking" of the drain into the wound.

Hemovac drainage has been advocated by some surgeons as a satisfactory means of minimizing edema.

Postoperative Care of Scrotal Wounds

After scrotal surgery such as an operation for orchiopexy, perspiration and warm weather contribute to marked maceration and infection of the skin. Ointments inhibiting bacterial growth, such as Bacitracin®, nitrofurazone (Furacin), Aerosporin brand of Polymyxin-B Sulfate, or Polymyxin-B-Bacitracin-Neomycin (Neosporin), applied generously to a 1-inch strip of bandage doubled and placed snugly over the wound have proven very effective. Ointment is reapplied to the gauze bandage as needed. The wound will usually be found to have healed cleanly on removal of the dressing.

Prevention of Edema: Plastic Glove Contour Ice Bags

Even small ice packs applied to the genitalia have too much weight to be kept in place for long and become painful. They do not mold well over the area involved.

Disposable plastic gloves, which are filled with water and tied off at the cuff with a piece of string or suture material, make excellent contour ice bags when properly prepared. When these water-filled gloves are placed in the freezer, their thickness should best not exceed one inch. If the glove is curved slightly in the freezing process, it will permit a lightweight source of cold application which shapes itself well to the genital area involved. During the application of these cold gloves the scrotum should be kept dry to prevent maceration of the scrotal skin.

Parenzymes may also be employed to decrease edema of the scrotum postoperatively.

Scrotal Dressing

Numerous dressings have been designed for the scrotum, both for the application of pressure and for support. The "Bellevue Bridge" is most commonly used. We have found it efficacious merely to put adequate gauze dressings (fluffs) around the scrotum and to support the scrotum with a

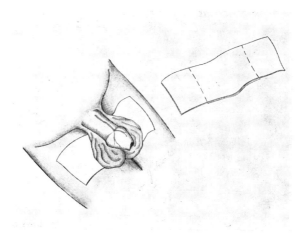

62. Bellevue bridge

large-size or extra-large-size scrotal supporter with leg straps. To better fit around the scrotum the "cup" portion of the support may be cut at its base to enlarge it. A "tight fit" is accomplished by plicating the cloth material in the midline and fixing it with a safety pin.

It may be advantageous to cover the scrotum with a thin layer of Vaseline to prevent maceration if copious drainage persists.

Scrotal Supports

BELLEVUE BRIDGE. A most helpful support may be made by pasting adhesive together back to back allowing an overlap of some of the adhesive at the outer limits. The overlapped adhesive on each side is attached to the thighs, producing a bridge. The scrotum is then placed on top of this bridge (see Fig. 62).

OTHER SCROTAL SUPPORTS. The ordinary rigid type of mask used in surgery makes a useful scrotal support. Aseptex® Surgical Mask No. 1800, manufactured by the Minnesota Mining and Manufacturing Company, Inc., or an equivalent mask, works well. The mask may be cut at one (top) edge to enlarge the size of the "cupped" area.

Another effective scrotal support can be fashioned from a foam pad sold under the trade name "Reston®" and produced by the same firm. The 8½-by 11-inch foam pad works best when cut in half longitudinally. The pad is placed under the scrotum with the legs together. It gives excellent support, with comfort, to even the most edematous inflamed scrotum. The pad is spongy in consistency, and permits the use of compresses without deteriorating.

Alternatively, 2-inch adhesive strips over scrotal dressings may be used as a bridge. The perineal area above the rectum should be previously shaved. Tincture of benzoin is applied. Two pieces of adhesive, fashioned into a "V"

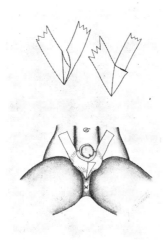

63. Adhesive cup scrotal bridge

and trimmed by scissors to a point, or one long piece folded into a V, may be applied to the midperineal area below the scrotum and led over the scrotum to the abdomen in a lateral oblique direction. Additional overlapping strips of adhesive are then applied, producing a solid adhesive cup (Fig. 63).

Intracath Needle Aspiration of Hydrocele

An intracath needle may be utilized to aspirate a hydrocele. After using one milliliter of local Xylocaine, the intracath needle with its plastic tubing is placed within the hydrocele wall. The needle is withdrawn and the plastic catheter is utilized to empty the hydrocele. The catheter is withdrawn after the hydrocele has been completely emptied. Pressure is kept on the area of puncture until bleeding is under control. A scrotal suspensory may then be worn for several days. It should be kept in mind that hydroceles, however emptied, will recur in most instances.

Injection treatment with sclerosing substance is still favored by some urologists. The intrascrotal reaction is variable and, at times, severe. Occasional slough has been reported following the treatment.

Recurrent Hydroceles

Even apparently well-executed hydrocelectomies may be followed by recurrence with reaccumulation of fluid and formation of another sac. Reoperation is difficult because of loss of fascial planes. Therefore, in performing the primary hydrocelectomy, generous excision of the sac with adjacent fascia must be accomplished. The remaining surface of the sac and visceral tunica vaginalis may be painted with phenol followed by alcohol, as is done with appendiceal stumps. Success in preventing recurrence of hydroceles has been reported with this method. Most urologists profess to extreme rarity of recurrence, so that phenol-alcohol treatment is also very infrequent.

The Epididymis

Diagnosis of Epididymitis

Epididymitis, a common disease of young and middle-aged males, may present difficult differential diagnostic signs.

Acute epididymitis is usually manifested first by pain in the groin or abdomen. On occasion, abdominal pain on the right side, before swelling of the epididymis occurs, has resulted in unnecessary appendectomy. A funiculitis first presents, and then acute swelling and pain in the region of the testicle occur. The swelling is sometimes so diffuse that the epididymis cannot be differentiated from the testis, and the accompanying pain and tenderness make it impossible at times to palpate the line of demarcation between the testis and the epididymis. Frequently orchitis accompanies epididymitis.

The differentiation between an acute torsion of the spermatic cord and an epididymitis may present. In torsion, the cord is usually foreshortened. There is a higher position of the testis within the scrotum. At times, one can palpate the cord and twisting in the cord. In a very early presentation of torsion before swelling occurs, the abnormal relationship of the epididymis to the testis may be evident. The acute and sudden onset also suggests torsion rather than epididymitis (see *Intrascrotal Lesion Diagnosis: Torsion*, at beginning of this chapter).

Exploration is sometimes required to differentiate between epididymitis and the tumor that presents as an acute problem of pain due to bleeding or necrosis within the tumor.

Causes of Epididymitis

The etiology of acute epididymitis is well defined in most standard textbooks. However, recurrent epididymitis related to straining, especially with defecation, while the bladder is distended with infected urine, has not been given enough emphasis as a possible etiological source. Once the patient has been instructed to avoid this practice, recurrent episodes of epididymitis may disappear.

Gonococcal Epididymitis

With the soaring incidence of gonorrhea in the young population group, and increased gonococcal resistance to the available antibiotics, the incidence of gonococcal epididymitis has increased.

Compensable Epididymitis

Urologists are frequently consulted in compensation cases involving epididymitis following injury while working. The usual history is that of acute pain in the scrotal area within a period of two to twelve hours after lifting or shoveling a heavy object. Most cases will be associated with a tender prostate. The most that can be said on behalf of the patient is that the epididymitis may have resulted from lifting, much as it occurs with straining to defecate, but the primary disease of prostatitis or seminal vesiculitis was preexisting.

Incidence of Epididymitis Following Prostatectomy, With or Without Vas Interruption

A recent review of the incidence of epididymitis after prostatectomy revealed the following: Less than 1 percent occurred after vasectomy. Without any type of vasoligation, the incidence of epididymitis was 6 percent. Many cases occur about the seventh postoperative day. About 18 percent of patients have epididymitis following Burdizzo clamp vas crush. This occurs usually in the fifth postoperative week.

It is the feeling of the authors that the vas deferens may recanalize following the clamp-crush procedure. An occasional funiculitis is also seen after Burdizzo clamp-crushing procedures. The judicious use of broad-spectrum antibiotics may result in a decrease in the incidence of epididymitis.

A recent series by one of us (H.B.) of patients subjected to transurethral prostatectomy may be interesting in this regard. In 200 patients subjected to transurethral prostatectomy in one year, vasectomy was performed on one side by exposing the vas, double-crushing it, and emplacing a suture ligature in between the areas of crush. Only one patient developed an epididymitis on the side in which this crush technique was used. No epididymitis developed in these same patients on the opposite side where in each instance a section of the vas was removed.

During the succeeding four years, the crush technique was done on both sides. The incidence of epididymitis did not exceed 2 percent. Follow-up examination of the ejaculate in those patients who still had ejaculation externally instead of into the bladder, revealed that many had motile sperm about three to four months following prostatectomy. It is obvious, therefore, that this crush technique is of value on a temporary basis only.

Relief of Pain in Acute Epididymitis

In patients with acute epididymitis, 10 ml of one-percent Xylocaine injected directly into the spermatic cord, high in the groin, will give immediate relief. One must be certain to aspirate to be sure the needle has not entered any of the cord vessels. This procedure must not be used if there is any evidence of a funiculitis. The relief of pain may be permanent or pain may slowly and gradually recur. Patients are grateful for the dramatic mitigation of distress. This treatment is most effective during the first 24 hours after onset of the epididymitis.

Treatment of Epididymitis

The treatment of epididymitis is well documented in most textbooks and in the literature, i.e., scrotal support, ice packs, and antibiotics or chemotherapy. The use of anti-inflammatory agents is common.

Opium suppositories with belladonna and propantheline bromide (Pro-Banthine) have been found helpful in cases with associated bladder spasm. Streptokinase, streptodornase (Varidase Buccal) tablets or bromelains (Ananase) are reported to be effective. Varidase Buccal or chymotrypsin (Chymar) in combination with a tetracycline, have been utilized. No allergic reactions to these parenzymes or proteolytic agents have been noted. Varidase, however, should not be used in patients exhibiting a deficiency in blood coagulation or depressed liver function.

Steroid preparations used in the acute phase of epididymitis shorten the clinical course of the disease. Phenylbutazone (Butazolidin) has been used successfully to accelerate the resolution of induration in instances of acute epididymitis. See additional indications and contraindications for this medication in *Phenylbutazone (Butazolidin) for Prostatitis (and Epididymitis)*, in Chapter Eight.

Tumors of the Epididymis

Tumors of the epididymis are relatively rare. Approximately 53 percent of tumors of the epididymis are thought to be adenomatoid tumors. Among the diverse epididymal tumors reported are: tuberculoma, leiomyoma of the tail of the epididymis, liposarcoma of the cord attached to the head of the epididymis, embryonal rhabdomyosarcoma of the testicular adnexa attached to the tail of the epididymis, reticulum cell sarcoma, and angiomatoid-type tumors of the epididymis. These tumors are diagnosed on exploration. The necessity for early exploration in any nonresolving, nontender mass involving the testicle or epididymis is therefore warranted.

The Testicle

Orchialgia and its Varied Indications

One occasionally sees a patient who complains of pain within the scrotum, either in the epididymis or testicle proper or along the spermatic cord. The patient will keep referring to the same specific site. Often there is no evidence of local disease on palpation, and pathological studies do not reveal the source of the pain. Surgical exploration and/or orchidectomy fail to cure the pain. One must bear in mind that search should be made for a disease process at a distant site. It is not at all unusual, for example, for a patient to have a calculus in the renal pelvis with pain only in the testis on the involved side. Prostatitis, posterior urethritis, seminal vesiculitis, hernia, deep pelvic tumor masses, pathology involving the lower ureter, diverticula or other bladder disturbances all may manifest themselves by pain only in the scrotal area.

When there is no explanation for the pain, the spermatic cord may be injected with approximately 10 ml of one percent Xylocaine. If the lesion is within the epididymis or testicle proper, or in the cord, the patient should then have relief of symptomatology. If the patient has had previous intrascrotal surgery, there is always the possibility of an area of perineurofibrosis. Therefore, repeat injection using steroids is often helpful. Bear in mind that the painful stimulus is referred to within the scrotal area from organ structures supplied by nerves originating in L1 and L2. *One must also remember that orchialgia is a leading symptom in psychoneurotic male patients with fixation to the genitalia.*

Chronic Testicular Ischemia

Spermatic cord torsion has been mentioned in indications for surgery in the scrotum. Chronic testicular ischemia should not be overlooked in those cases of hypermobile testes which have been salvaged. The testes may have suffered some permanent damage not clinically evident, and the possibility of future fertility impairment should be considered. It is therefore most important to fix the involved testicle, as well as the opposite testicle. In cases where torsion with spontaneous relief has been suspected, further recurrent attacks of partial torsion may impair the circulation and seriously damage the fertility of the testicle. Therefore, early exploration and fixation of both testes is mandatory.

Torsion of the Newborn

Torsion of the spermatic cord may occur *in utero* or in the newborn. The involved side will usually contain fluid and may appear darker than the opposite side. The testicle may feel normal or slightly enlarged. The aspirated fluid may be hemorrhagic, and the twist may be felt after aspiration.

The newborn tolerate surgery extremely well with minimum anesthesia. Cases have been reported where the scrotum has been entered one hour after birth.

Torsion of Appendix Testis

Difficulty in differential diagnosis is frequently caused by torsion of the appendix testis (see section on *Intrascrotal Lesion Diagnosis*). This may be confirmed only after exploratory surgery. Torsion of the appendix testis occurs infrequently in adults. In the young, the appendix testis is usually long and pedunculated with a well-defined stalk. In adults it is more prominent, with a less pedunculated base until older age when it becomes atrophic and sessile.

The microscopic appearance also varies with age and seems to progress through a life cycle. Microscopic findings in the various age groups are described in standard pathology and urology textbooks.

Occurrence of Cyst with Torsion of the Appendix Testis

When the diagnosis of torsion of the appendix testis is made and a small cystic structure can be palpated, aspiration of the cyst may be done. Patients usually have complete relief of symptoms. Calcification of the necrotic appendix testis also occurs after torsion. Occasionally one can palpate free-floating bodies in the hydrocele fluid surrounding the testicle. These apparently result from the appendix testis becoming necrotic, separating from the tunica albuginea and becoming calcified. Analysis of these bodies has revealed them to consist of a mass of hyalinized tissue, about 60 percent, infiltrated with microcrystalline hydroxyl apatite, about 40 percent.

Cryptorchidism: Chorionic Gonadotropins Prior to Orchiopexy

A course of chorionic gonadotropins before subjecting patients to orchiopexy will often increase the size of the undescended testis and the length of the blood vessels and vas in the spermatic cord. Testicular descent may occur in about 20 percent of instances, without surgery. It must be remembered, however, that long courses of anterior pituitary-like hormones may produce early closure of epiphyseal lines, stunting the growth of some patients. A maximum of 10 to 20,000 units of the medication preferably should not be exceeded.

Small Urethral Meatus in Patients with Cryptorchidism

A high percentage of patients with cryptorchidism have been noted to also have present a small urethral meatus. Meatotomy is therefore necessary in many patients subjected to orchiopexy. Although entirely unrelated embryologically, these two conditions are often found to coexist.

Surgery to Correct Cryptorchidism

Many articles in the literature and many textbooks adequately describe the various operations for cryptorchidism. The incision most commonly used extends from the pubic tubercle, passing diagonally upward and carried down to the peritoneum. A transverse incision may also be utilized. The peritoneum should be opened to explore for an intra-abdominal testicle if retroperitoneal search is unsuccessful. The spermatic vessels are identified and mobilized from the peritoneum to give added length to the cord. The incision, if necessary, may be extended to free the spermatic vessels almost to the renal hilus.

In right-sided cryptorchid patients, the appendix should be removed when exposed. If adequate length has not been obtained, the inferior epigastric vessels may be divided to move the whole cord medially.

The advantage of the above-described approach is that it allows adequate elongation of the cord, even in a totally intra-abdominal testis, with very little manipulation of the cord itself. It is unnecessary and undesirable to strip the cord structures, as this may impair the circulation. At times, however, this becomes necessary.

After the peritoneum is closed and the redundant hernial sac, if any, removed, the problem remains of bringing the testicle into the scrotum. If there is a tendency for the testicle to draw back from the scrotal position, it should be held down by any of the recognized methods.

Midline Approach in Cryptorchid Surgery

A midline approach for undescended testes has also been used successfully. This approach is utilized for those testicles which cannot be palpated and for testes which are high in the inguinal canal.

The anatomy is easily delineated from the inside of the pelvis. The hernia is easily repaired and the testicle is drawn up through the internal inguinal ring with little difficulty when located in the inguinal canal. Adequate cord length is usually obtained.

With a midline vertical incision the spermatic vessels may be mobilized with ease almost to the renal hilar area. The cord may then be redirected in a straight line to the scrotum. This is accomplished by first developing a space in the scrotum to accept the testis by bluntly dissecting downward into the scrotum through the lowermost point of the midline incision. It is then necessary to perforate the external abdominal fascia medial to the external inguinal ring and, with the aid of a hemostat, pull the testis down through the perforation and finally position the testis in the scrotum. A small dependent incision may be made in the scrotum to "pex" the testis.

The abdominal testis is more easily explored through this approach and must be removed if it is not feasible to bring it into the scrotum.

This operative technique is of particular value for repair of bilaterally undescended testes, doing both sides on the same day if testes have adequate length; otherwise it is best to do surgery on one side at a time.

Traction to Testis in Orchiopexy

Several methods of applying traction to the testicle are:

1) Suturing the tunica albuginea of the testicle to intrascrotal fascia and then bringing the suture through the most dependent area of scrotum. The suture is tied to one end of a rubber band. The other end of the rubber band may be held down by adhesive tape or it may be sutured to the skin of the thigh.

2) Suturing the tunica albuginea to the fascia lata of the thigh (Torek opera-

tion). This procedure is becoming unpopular because it is a two-stage operation. It is also undesirable from a spermatogenic standpoint to bury the testicle in a site in which the temperature is higher than that of the scrotum.

3) Holding the suture down to the skin of the thigh with adhesive tape.

4) Pulling the right testicle through the median septum of the scrotum and then anchoring this to the opposite left scrotal wall.

5) Taking a suture through the fascia of the cord and anchoring it to the surrounding fascia at a slightly lower level, thus placing the cord on slight tension. This serves to relieve the need of tension on the testicle *per se*. Two such well-placed sutures on the medial and lateral aspect of the spermatic cord will often fix the testicle without tension in the scrotum. The testis will remain in its dependent position. This type of anchoring allows ambulation and discharge of the patient from the hospital in a very short time.

6) Anchoring the gubernaculum to the fascia lata of the thigh with the testicle remaining within the scrotum. This seems to be a method most often assuring permanent placement of the testicle in the lower scrotal area. The gubernaculum and fascia lata may be freed three to six months later.

7) Production of a pocket in the most dependent part of the scrotal wall between the skin and dartos muscle with fixation of the testis within this pocket.

Testicular Trauma: Treatment with Steroid Therapy

In cases of well-defined testicular contusion, where the history of trauma is clear-cut, therapy with adrenocorticotropic hormones has been remarkably helpful. In some cases, symptoms have resolved within six to twelve hours following intravenous ACTH administration. The sooner the therapy is begun, the better the response. Where epididymitis or epididymo-orchitis secondary to other causes is involved, the treatment is of much less value; therefore, distinct differentiation must be made. The dosage schedule is ACTH, 40 units in 500 ml of 5% glucose in water, over four to eight hours. This may be repeated once. ACTH gel, intramuscularly, 80 units initially and 40 units every twelve hours for two doses, may then be used.

Testicular Malignancies

A definite relationship exists between cryptorchidism and testicular malignancy. Atrophy following mumps orchitis, however, has never been incriminated as a forerunner of malignancy. The incidence of malignancy in undescended or intra-abdominal testes statistically has been variously estimated as between 20 to 50 times greater than in normally descended testes. This seems to indicate that if a testicle is undescended but palpable, it can be observed for the development of a neoplasm. However, an intra-abdominal testicle which cannot be observed should be explored and prophylactic extirpation should be considered if the testicle cannot be satisfactorily brought down. Adult cryptorchid abdominal testes should be removed.

Performing an orchiopexy for cryptorchidism does not decrease the incidence of malignancy.

The reporting of a case of primary extratesticular seminoma found in the retroperitoneum points to the embryological fact that some testicular rest tissue remains retroperitoneally. Tumors in this location are readily removed.

Upper gastrointestinal bleeding and other phenomena may be signs of secondary metastatic involvement stemming from testicular primary lesions. These lesions should be suspect and thoroughly investigated whenever intra-abdominal testes are present.

Testicular Biopsy

Biopsy of the testis is a simple and rapid surgical procedure which can readily be done as an outpatient under local anesthesia, with the aid of an assistant. Biopsy should be bilateral, unless one testis is obviously atrophic.

TECHNIQUE: The scrotum is prepared and scrubbed in the usual manner. Grasping the scrotum behind the testis with the left hand (right-handed surgeon), the operator brings the anterior surface of the testis tightly against the scrotal wall. A few milliliters of one percent Xylocaine is infiltrated into all the layers of the scrotum over an area of one or two centimeters. Two fixation sutures of 2-0 chromic suture are placed parallel into the tunica albuginea and an incision (1-2 cm) is made between them down through the tunica albuginea. Allis clamps are used to grasp the edges of the skin, dartos and fascial layers.

By pressure on the testis with the left hand, the testicular tubules are forced out of the incision. Using a small iris scissors, the operator cuts off the tubules and immediately places them in the fixative—either Bouin's or Zenker's solution.

The tunica albuginea is closed with one or two interrupted 4-0 chromic sutures, and the incision in the scrotum is closed with one or two sutures of the same material. A small collodion dressing usually suffices.

VALUE OF BIOPSY. In cases of oligospermia and azoospermia, the testicular biopsy is very useful in determining whether or not therapy will benefit the patient. Seminal vesiculography and vasography should be done in conjunction with biopsy, to determine patency of the seminal tracts.

Findings of advanced tubular fibrosis, peritubular fibrosis, or germinal aplasia indicate an irreversible condition which will not respond to therapy. The patient is well advised to either adopt a child or to have his wife artificially inseminated. The finding of incomplete maturation, in the presence of patent seminal tracts, warrants therapy, even though present-day modalities are disappointing.

Mithramycin (Mithracin) for Testicular Tumors

In a combined series of 305 patients with spread of their testicular tumors treated with mithramycin (Mithracin), 33 patients (or 10.8%) showed a complete disappearance of tumor masses, and an additional 80 patients (26.2%) responded with significant partial regression of tumor masses. The longest duration of continuing complete response at the time of writing was over eight and a half years.

Since the risk of toxicity with this potent antineoplastic agent is considerable, it is recommended that Mithracin be administered only to hospitalized patients by and under the supervision of a qualified physician experienced in the use of cancer chemotherapeutic agents. All pharmacologic information and contraindications should be carefully studied before using this drug, which is administered intravenously only.

Scrotal Self-Examination Advised

Because of the frequency with which testicular tumors are seen in young adults, and because the preponderance of these tumors are seminomas, it is recommended that all male patients be instructed in self-examination of the testicles. Women are urged to palpate their own breasts for tumor. It is equally important that each young male be urged to palpate his scrotum periodically in search for any masses or tenderness. Any deviations from the normal can be brought to the attention of a physician at a much earlier stage.

It has been reported in the literature that more testicular tumors are discovered by paramours than are noted for the first time by the patient or his wife.

Hemospermia

Hemospermia is a relatively common and usually innocuous condition. When the urine itself is free from gross or microscopic blood, hemospermia probably is arising from the prostate and/or the seminal vesicles and is usually of minor significance. It should not, however, be disregarded. An occasional patient with carcinoma of the prostate may have hemospermia as the presenting symptom.

The usual etiology of hemospermia is not firmly established. It has been reported that the hemospermia accompanying dengue fever comes from the seminal vesicles.

On complete examination, including urethroscopy, very little is ordinarily found. Occasionally redness about the ejaculatory ducts can be noted, and in some cases there is evidence of a chronic hemorrhagic prostatitis. In a great majority of cases, the findings are nil.

The rare instance of carcinoma of the seminal vesicles and seminal vesiculitis must be ruled out. Nonspecific vesiculitis and granulomatous vesiculitis must also be considered. Hemospermia was the primary and single complaint in one case of carcinoma of the bladder seen in a physician patient about fifteen years ago, but was probably not related to the bladder tumor since he is living and well, having undergone only a transure-thral resection of the bladder tumor.

Hemospermia as Cause of Abnormal Vaginal Discharge in Wives

Patients may be seen with hemospermia whose wives have previously undergone dilatation and curettage because of bloody vaginal discharges. With discovery of normal findings in the females, it has been determined that this blood-stained discharge actually came from their husbands with hemospermia. This is important to bear in mind when questioning post-menopausal women who complain of vaginal bleeding.

The Vas Deferens

Vasectomy: Rationale and Elucidation

The two common indications for vasectomy are sterilization and preven-tion of epididymitis in patients subjected to prostatectomy.

Increased awareness of the importance of population limitation and of the advantages of planned parenthood, together with growing recognition of the complications of anovulatory medications and the never-ending con-troversy regarding the question of abortion, have all resulted in more and more patients demanding vasectomy for sterilization purposes.

It is essential to thoroughly explain to the husband and wife in simple language what the procedure involves. They should be informed that the purpose of the operation is to prevent any sperm from being present in the ejaculate, thus preventing conception. Emphasis should be placed on the fact that the patient is not considered sterile until it is proved that there are no sperm present, on two examinations of centrifuged ejaculate. A six-month postvasectomy ejaculate should also be examined.

The dual principal functions of the testicle—that of the production of hormones and that of the production of sperm—should be fully explained to the couple. It should be emphasized that the vasectomy will in no way interfere with either of these functions, but that it will interrupt the flow of sperm from the testicles to the ejaculatory ducts. They should be made aware of the essential permanency of the procedure. Although surgery may recanalize the vas deferens, the percentage of success is far from satisfying. The complications that may follow a vasectomy (bleeding, swelling, in-fection, and postoperative pain) should be outlined clearly to the patient.

A consent form should be signed by both husband and wife, signifying that they have both been informed as to the nature of the surgery and its possible complications. This should be witnessed. Positive identification of the spouse by having her produce a driver's license is a good idea. Women other than the legal partner have been brought to urological offices to sign consent slips for vasectomy operations.

Figures 64 and 65 have been included herein as suggested forms for consent and agreement prior to vasectomy. Also included are instructions and information regarding vasectomy which are provided for the patient and his wife.

64. Form used by authors for vasectomy consent agreement, with instruction form attached

CONSENT AND AGREEMENT   Date _____
To: _____, M.D. _____, M.D. _____, M.D.
In consideration of your performing upon me a sterilization operation (known medically as a bilateral vasectomy), I hereby consent to such operation, with the full realization and knowledge that as a result of such operation it probably will not be possible for me to ever again become the father of children, and it is doubtful if that condition can be so corrected that I can ever again become the father of children. I agree that I have requested this operation and have consented thereto and that you will not be held legally responsible for the results of this operation nor for the performance of the operation itself.
SIGNATURE _____
                    (Patient)
WITNESS _____

I, _____, wife of _____, who has signed the above Consent and Agreement, do hereby certify that I have read the above Consent and Agreement and that I have joined with my husband in requesting such sterilization with the full realization and knowledge of the consequences set forth and that my Consent and Agreement hereto is made of my own free will and desire without undue influence of any nature whasover. I agree that I will never hold _____, M.D. and/or _____, M.D., and/or _____, M.D., legally responsible for the performance of said operation or the results thereof and I do hereby release _____, M.D., and/or _____, M.D., and/or _____, M.D. from any and all claims I might have against him as a result of his performing said sterilization operation on my husband.
SIGNATURE _____
                    (Wife)

I hereby certify that I have witnessed the signing of the above document by _____, whom I know personally, and that she told me at the time of such signing that she executed the same of her own free will and desire without undue influence of any kind.
DATE _____ WITNESS _____

INSTRUCTIONS FOR VASECTOMY (STERILIZATION)
The following information has been compiled to answer those questions most frequently asked by patients who request elective sterilization (vasectomy). It is assumed that you have discussed this topic thoroughly with your wife, and that you both have some understanding of the procedure and of its consequences. Perhaps you have some questions which might be answered in the following paragraphs.

The testicles have two functions: (1) to produce the male hormone, which goes into the blood stream and is not affected by the sterilization procedure; (2) to produce sperm which are carried through small tubes (vas deferens) up the scrotum into the groin area and thence to the prostate gland, a circular gland surrounding the outlet of the bladder. The sperm are carried out at the time of intercourse, along with the prostatic fluid. Interrupting these small tubes (the vas) only interferes with transportation of sperm, and in no other way affects a man's sexual drive, attitude, or ability.

The purpose of the operation is to prevent any sperm from being present in the fluid passed at the time of intercourse, thus preventing conception. Examination of the fluid after surgery shows whether or not sperm are still present. Until we prove in our office that *not a single sperm is present, we do not consider the patient sterile.* Furthermore, *the operation has not been completed* until we have examined a satisfactory postoperative specimen which is found to be "blank," or free of sperm. Such a postoperative test is an essential part of the entire procedure.

This is essentially a permanent procedure, although there are operations to reconstruct the vas with some chance of success. Because this is a permanent, though elective, decision, one should examine the future possibilities carefully, keeping in mind the possibility of divorce, death, loss of children, remarriage, or change in attitude towards further children.

PREOPERATIVE PREPARATIONS: (1) Husband and wife, if both agree, should sign the operative permit and have this witnessed by a third party. (2) Prior to the operation, the patient should wash the area with a soap containing sterilizing solution, such as Dial or Lifebuoy. This should be done each night for about five nights before surgery. The night prior to surgery, the entire scrotum and underside of the penis should be shaved with a small safety razor; this should be done dry, before showering.

SURGERY: The procedure is performed in the office under local anesthesia, and is accompanied by minimal, if any, discomfort. The operation takes approximately one-half hour to complete. The risks of this procedure are the same as for any minor operation. The tissue of the scrotum, or sac, is much like the tissue around the eye. Any minor injury, including minor surgical procedures, may cause some degree of swelling. This can best be avoided by proper postoperative care.

POSTOPERATIVE CARE: It is important that you return home directly, after the procedure, and remain off your feet the day of surgery and the following day. This includes bedrest, or resting on a couch or sofa, or in a chair with your feet elevated. A light ice pack applied over the scrotal area for 12 to 24 hours is also helpful. All of these measures are intended to minimize any possible swelling. On the second day after surgery, light activity is allowed. Beyond this, activity is limited only by discomfort, and one may be as active as desired.

You may shower after the third postoperative day, but you are cautioned not to rub the surgical skin sites where small sutures are present (these sutures dissolve in five or six days). You may bathe after the fourth postoperative day.

You may resume sexual intercourse after one week, *but with your usual contraceptive precautions.*

We will check you in the office two or three days after the procedure, to be sure that all is well. The postoperative examination of the ejaculated material is usually done about four weeks after surgery. If this should still contain any sperm, then a further examination is required two weeks later. You will be given precise instructions as to how to present your specimen (or specimens) for analysis after the surgery. Please remember that it is your responsibility to get these specimens to us for testing, and that one of *us* must assure you personally that there are no sperm present before you can be considered sterile.

The surgical charge inculdes the consultation, the surgical procedure, and all postoperative checks until completion. The surgical fee is due and payable at the time surgery is performed.

65. Another consent and information form suggested for use by urologists doing vasectomies

INFORMATION REGARDING STERILIZATION, AND OPERATIVE PERMITS THEREFOR

The number of vas ligations requested of us lately precludes our sitting down to explain the procedure to each patient. We use, therefore, the information sheet (below) to instruct prospective vasectomy patients and their wives. The Consent and Release form shown at right is always signed before the procedure is undertaken. These forms seem to answer our needs better than any of the prepublished ones we have seen.

CONSENT TO STERILIZATION OPERATION AND RELEASE
The undersigned patient being desirous of a sterilization operation to be performed by Dr. _____, states that his reason for the same is as follows: _____
It is understood by the patient and all others that a sterilization operation, although for the purpose of preventing procreation, is not always effective in obtaining permanent results. There is no guarantee that procreation will never occur.

The undersigned patient (and spouse) represents to the doctor that he is (has) reached the age of 21 and/or has never been the subject of an application before any court alleging mental incompetency. The patient (and spouse), if any, consent to and request that a sterilization be performed by Dr. _____ and that in consideration of Dr. _____'s performing the operation, each of them discharge, relieve and release Dr. _____ of any claim, liability or cause of action whatsoever, which they have had, now have, or may ever have hereafter, by reason of Dr. _____'s services.
WITNESS WHEREOF:
WE BOTH HAVE READ AND UNDERSTAND THE BOOKLET "INSTRUCTION FOR VAS LIGATION" BY DR. _____.
WE, OF OUR FREE AND VOLUNTARY KNOWLEDGE AND ACT, AFTER HAVING FIRST READ THE ABOVE AND UNDERSTANDING THE SAME, HEREINTO SET OUR HAND, THIS _____ DAY OF _____.

Patient _____   Spouse _____
STATE OF _____
CITY OF _____
Before me, _____, a Notary Public in and for the State of _____, this _____ day of _____, 19____ appeared _____ and _____, legal age, stating that they had

read and understood the foregoing statement, and release, and that they signed the same of their own free and voluntary act.

My commission expires:

Notary Public

INFORMATION ON VAS LIGATIONS

Prior to performing a vas ligation in our office we should have a thorough discussion of the procedure with you and if possible with your wife. The indications for and the facts of the permanency of this procedure should be well understood.

The purpose of the operation is to stop sperm from leaving the testicle and prevent their being present in the ejaculate. This would prevent conception. Until we prove in the office that there are no sperm present on two examinations of the sperm specimen, we do not consider the patient to be sterile.

The testes have two functions: One is to produce the male hormone, which is released into the blood stream. This is not affected by vas ligation. The second function of the testes is to make sperm, which are carried through small tubes (vas deferens) into the groin and the prostate. The sperm are carried out in the ejaculate with the prostatic fluid at the time of intercourse. Interrupting these tubes only interferes with the transportation of the sperm and in no other way affect a man's sexual drive, attitude, or ability. There are still live sperm in and around the testicle behind the area in which the vas deferens or tube is divided.

This is essentially a permanent procedure, though there are operations which can re-construct these tubes. These operations are only fairly successful. Because it is a permanent, yet elective step, one should examine the future possibilities carefully. There is always the possibility of divorce, death, loss of present children, remarriage, or change of mind. **NOTE**—this makes the husband sterile and not the wife. The above possibility should be thoroughly discussed between the husband and the wife.

The risks of this procedure are the same as for any operative procedure, and we would like to discuss some of the complications, as we would like for you to know about these.

> Bleeding—the tissue in the scrotum is very loose tissue, it bruises easily and bleeds very easily and swells to a great size easily. (There is a definite risk of bleeding after the operation.) Because of this, we ask that you remain off your feet for about two days and limit your activities very carefully after the operation.

Both you and your wife must sign a consent form. When we agree to this procedure, we undertake to try to make you infertile or sterile. To prove that we have completed this obligation, we must have for our records, examinations of your ejaculations on at least two occasions, usually six weeks and three months after the procedure. It is possible for you to remain fertile for this length of time. This is because sperm have already traveled out beyond the area in which we interrupt the vas deferens. These sperm are stored in the seminal vesicles and in the area of the prostate gland and are only emptied out at the time of intercourse. It takes approximately eight to twelve intercourses to empty most of these out and you must use precautions for at least three months after the operation, or risk the chance of further pregnancy.

There is always the chance of some infection in any incision or cut. We will keep you on an antibiotic for several days to try to cut the chances of this down. We will give you some medication for pain, if you should have it. After the operation, you should apply an ice bag to the scrotum for the first several hours.

Do not take a tub bath for at least a week after the operation, but you may take a shower bath after about three days.

You may have sexual intercourse after about ten days, but with **precautions** until the two checks on the sperm are reported as being negative.

We will check you in two to three days after the procedure, to make sure, post-operatively, that you are getting along well. You should make an appointment at that time to be seen six weeks and three months after the surgery for the sperm checks as previously outlined. If you have any problem, please call us.

There is also the possibility that the vas deferens (tubes) can re-anastomose. In order to cut this possibility to a minimum, we remove at least a quarter inch segment and send this to the Laboratory, so that a report can be made, proving that we have removed a segment from each side. In addition, we tie off all four ends, which should give you the best chance for sterility that we are capable of.

Please wash the scrotum and penis with pHisoHex, which can be obtained at any drug store, for 2 or 3 days prior to coming in for surgery. Do not shave the scrotum, as we will do that in the office. You will be given a sleeping pill prior to the surgery, both for relaxation and also to minimize the possibility of any reaction to a local anesthetic. If you have ever had any reaction, please let us know. Because of the sleeping pill, you should not attempt to drive home. Therefore, please bring somebody with you to carry this out.

There will be three or four sutures or stitches in the incision on each side. These are catgut and should dissolve on their own within seven to ten days. If they do not, and if they give you any trouble, please let us know and we will remove them, but we very rarely have to do this, as they usually come out on their own.

Criteria to Qualify for Vasectomy

Many urologists still insist that the following criteria be met before they will perform vasectomy for sterilization purposes: (1) the husband must be 30 to 35 or more years of age; (2) the couple should have at least two or more children; (3) the marriage should be one of over ten years' duration; (4) both husband and wife must sign the consent for vasectomy after thorough discussion; (5) the urologist must be satisfied that both husband and wife are emotionally stable; and (6) the vasectomy should be scheduled three or four weeks after initial consultation to allow the couple ample time to change their mind. Medical indications, of course, take precedence over the aforementioned limitations. The criteria have been widely altered in recent years because of changing attitudes on the part of the general public.

The wife's permission for a vas reanastomosis or vasovasostomy is equally as important as it is for a vasectomy.

Functional Complaints of Vasectomized Patients

The following functional complications after vasectomy have been reported: (1) impotence, complete and partial; (2) possible acute depression; (3) pain and fullness at the operative site; (4) persistent tenderness interfering with intercourse; (5) previously faithful husband becoming a roué (wife's complaint); (6) wife becoming psychotic, wanting to become pregnant.

Many of these complications may be explained psychologically because of castration anxiety syndrome with ego loss, strong guilt complex formation in patients to whom the operation is contrary to religious principles, and loss of aggressive challenge when fear of pregnancy is abolished. The promiscuity may be explained by loss of fear of responsibility for actions.

All of these factors exemplify well the need of evaluating both the husband and wife prior to doing vasectomy.

Preparation for Vasectomy

Prior to the operation, the patient should use an antiseptic soap on the scrotum for several days. The operation is usually performed in the office (unless done in connection with prostatectomy) under local anesthesia or as an outpatient in a hospital. The patient should bring an athletic supporter or a suspensory with leg straps, and he should be driven to the office by his wife or a friend, so that he will not be required to drive home after surgery. He should be instructed to return for postoperative examination a few days after surgery and to also return to have the ejaculate examined on two occasions. (See *Proof of Sterility.*)

Technique in Vasectomy for Sterilization

There are many variations in techniques of vasectomy for sterilization purposes. These are described in standard surgical textbooks and are not touched upon in this volume.

A useful instrument for isolation of the vas under local anesthesia is the Foley vas clamp. This can be used to isolate the vas deferens after minimum local anesthetic infiltration (further anesthetic injection may be introduced if necessary after the vas has been isolated). Minimal distortion of tissue occurs when this instrument is used. It resembles a towel clamp but has ball points for grasping the vas. The ball points are per-forated to permit the insertion of a fine needle for additional anesthetic injection. Some urologists use the Allis forceps to grasp the vas in its sheath. A mosquito forceps to spread the perivasal fascias allows for easier grasping of the vas deferens with Allis forceps.

The use of a curved hypodermic needle, such as that used for ton-sillectomy, is helpful in the instillation of local anesthetic. The curved needle is passed under the vas as the anesthetic solution is injected. The needle is then advanced further and brought out through the skin on the side of the vas opposite from the starting point. This simple procedure of needle insertion and injection of the anesthetic agent anchors the vas close to the skin so that it is more easily grasped after the incision is made. The use of two ordinary towel clips is also very helpful, first to hold the vas in place in making the skin incision, and then to free the vas from its surrounding tissues by gently teasing off the blood vessels and nerves. Using this technique, one can perform vasectomy without assistance.

Some urologists routinely use antibiotics and parenzymes postopera-tively to prevent infection and speed healing.

Rapid Vasectomy: "Crush Vasectomy"

A one-centimeter incision is made in the anterolateral aspect of the scrotum. For those who prefer one incision, it may be made in the mid-line of the scrotum after one vas has been pushed over to this area with the aid of the thumb and first finger. The incision is made down to the vas, which is grasped with an Allis clamp after retraction of sur-rounding tissue by use of a Kelly hemostat. The incision need not be made through all layers covering the vas. The vas is crushed by hemostat above and below the Allis clamp. A suture ligature of 3-0 chromic is placed around one of the areas of crush as close to the vas as possible in order to avoid any of the perivasal vessels. The vas is dropped back into the scrotum.

If this is a midline incision, the opposite vas is grasped and treated in the same manner, and the scrotum then closed with the same 3-0 chromic suture. If the incision is made in the anterolateral aspect of the scrotum, the procedure is repeated on the opposite side.

In those patients in whom there is normal postoperative prostatectomy ejaculation, one may find live motile sperm again after a six- to eight-week period. This crush technique therefore holds promise as a short-term interruption of the seminal tract.

Because of the thickening and induration which occur in the spermatic cord following the Burdizzo procedure (mass crushing through skin and all fascial layers), and the possible recanalization in a blind crushing procedure, this technique is not desirable. Injury to either the internal spermatic artery or to some of the veins in the spermatic cord frequently occurs. The incidence of late epididymitis has stimulated many surgeons to abandon the Burdizzo clamp method. The above-described "crush vasectomy" technique is an improvement over the Burdizzo clamp method.

Intra-Abdominal Vasectomy

Many surgeons do intra-abdominal vasectomy while performing suprapubic or retropubic prostatectomy. The operator, by mobilizing the lateral peritoneum, can easily palpate the vas and distinguish it by its whipcord-like feel near its entrance into the internal inguinal ring. The vas is then isolated, doubly ligated, and sectioned. With the use of intra-abdominal vasectomy at the time of open surgery, no incidence of vasitis or funiculitis has been reported (to our knowledge).

Control of Bleeding During Vasectomy Prior to Transurethal Prostatectomy

If bleeding is encountered during the performance of vasectomy immediately prior to transurethral prostatectomy, one may utilize the tip of the Bovie cord to coagulate the area of bleeding.

Post-Vasectomy Bleeding

Bleeding after vasectomy may prove quite troublesome. Mild bleeding can be readily controlled with pressure and icebags. When bleeding persists, the incision is opened and a search for bleeders must be done because a small artery may have retracted. By applying pressure above and below the vasectomy site, the bleeding can be controlled and the search for the vessel accomplished. It is unwise to indiscriminately apply sutures to the area in an attempt to stop the bleeding. Because of the very nature of the scrotal wall, a very large and painful hemotoma may occur if bleeding is not controlled within a short time.

Post-Vasectomy Pain

Post-vasectomy pain is a complication which may occur years after surgery. This may be perplexing both diagnostically and therapeutically. The patient complains of sharp, stabbing, shooting pains and of aching in one or both testes. The pain may be sharply accentuated during ejaculation. The diagnosis is readily made when palpation of the vasectomy site reproduces the pain.

In these cases, excellent success in abolishing the pain may be gained by injecting hydrocortisone and Xylocaine (without epinephrine) in and around the indurated vasectomy area. Repetition of the injection for one or two times is usually sufficient for complete relief to the patient.

If perineural fibrosis is the cause of the pain, injection therapy is not too successful.

Legal Complications of Post-Vasectomy Pain

Post-vasectomy pain may also bring legal complications. Those who do elective vasectomies for sterilization are cautioned that the patient must be thoroughly informed as to the possibility of post-vasectomy pain. Intermittent pain (sometimes acute) and swelling may recur frequently over a number of years. The frequency and severity of symptoms decrease with progression of time. Examination at the end of a one- to two-year interval often reveals no abnormalities.

The proximal vas deferens lumen must dilate in most instances to accommodate the increased volume of sperm during the sexual excitement phase. In some instances, this dilation occurs slowly. Patients therefore should be told that a period of adjustment of about nine to twelve months is needed in some cases because the testis continues to form spermatozoa. It is quite common to note that the epididymis is slightly enlarged after vasectomy.

Spontaneous Vas Reanastomosis

Spontaneous recanalization of the vas has been reported in a small percentage of cases. Silk suture or other nonabsorbable ligature used by some urologists may be discharged from the wound, allowing the recanalization of the vas. Other undesirable effects such as occasional inflammatory reactions and the formation of sperm granuloma at the operative site may also result.

In the performance of vasectomy for sterilization purposes, it is important to tie back the vas on itself with removal of a large segment or to purse-string fascial layers over one end of the vas deferens to prevent its joining the opposite end. Fulguration of the lumen may also be done. Some surgeons have tied vasa to each other, overlapping the cut ends. (If this is done the overlapping sutures must be loose or recanalization may occur when the suture cuts through the adjacent vasa in the healing phase.) Hemoclips have been used by other urologists.

These and various other methods of preventing vas reanastomosis are illustrated in Figure 66.

Proof of Sterility

Some authors maintain that absence of sperm less than two months postoperatively is not conclusive, and that this state will not necessarily be permanent. Another specimen should be examined one or two months later. Several cases have been reported in which fresh semen specimens

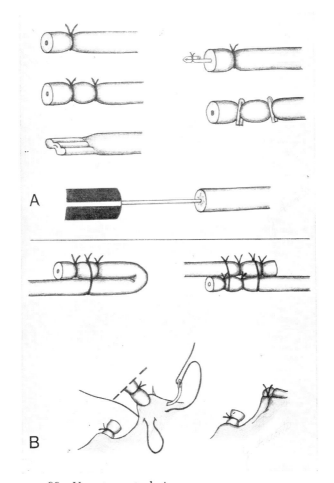

66. Vasectomy techniques
    A. Methods of obliterating lumen of vas
    B. Methods of preventing recanalization

showed an absence of sperm after two months, but six months later sperm were present. This indicates that recanalization has occurred.

It has been reported that after two negative semen specimens have been obtained approximately two months postoperatively there will be a transient reappearance of viable sperm for a short time in a few patients. This is difficult to explain, but perhaps of medical-legal value when advising patients on risks and precautionary measures.

Centrifuged Ejaculate for Post-Vasectomy Sperm Examination

Though one may find no sperm present in the ejaculates of post-vasectomy patients, when these same ejaculates are diluted with normal saline to give adequate volume in the tube, and then centrifuged, a few actively motile sperm may be seen on rare occasions. *Obviously, the centrifuged, concentrated sediment of the ejaculate should be examined as proof that no sperm are present.*

Clinical experience dictates that sperm concentration of less than 20 million per milliliter is rarely productive of conception. For medico-legal purposes, the record should show zero sperm present.

INFERTILITY

Fertility Study by X-Ray Examination

Luminal Procedures

VASO-EPIDIDYMOGRAPHY. This procedure is easily done under anesthesia in the hospital pyelographic room or in the operating room furnished with an X-ray unit. Under aseptic technique, 2 cm of each vas deferens are exposed and isolated with towel clips through a small incision in the upper part of the scrotum. A 21- to 24-gauge intradermic needle (in which the beveled tip has been cut off and filed so that the end of the needle will not have a cutting edge) is inserted into the canal of each vas, in the direction of the epididymis. A short incision is first made over the vas in a transverse or longitudinal direction, so that the lumen of the vas is exposed. This facilitates the passage of the blunt tip needle or plastic tubing. About 0.5 ml of any one of the usual X-ray contrast materials such as diatrizoate sodium (Hypaque), etc., is injected. A radiograph is made. Catgut suture, chromic 5-0, is used to approximate the cut segment of vas deferens.

Epididymography has proved valuable for the study of tumors, inflammation, malposition of the organs of the scrotum, and as a procedure for investigating the production and transportation of spermatozoa in the infertile male (see *Radiologic Aids in the Study of Male Infertility*, Chapter Three).

In the presence of white cells in the prostatic fluid or the urine the procedure is avoided, as an epididymitis may result.

VASOSEMINAL VESICULOGRAPHY. Seminal vesiculography is easily done at the same time as epididymography. The technique is the same as that for vaso-epididymography except that the direction of the needle is toward the seminal vesicle, and 2 to 3 ml of contrast material is injected. Roentgenographic exposures of the bony pelvis are made employing the usual technique. This determines continuity or obstruction of the vas and/or ejaculatory ducts and outlines the seminal vesicles.

Another method employs the insertion (after a small opening is made in the wall of the vas deferens) of a fine plastic tubing similar to that used by anesthesiologists for continuous caudal anesthesia. This is passed retrograde through the lumen of the vas to the seminal vesicle and antegrade to the epididymis, and the contrast medium is injected. Obstructions are thus easily detected.

Causes and Treatment of Infertility

The treatment of male infertility is dependent upon many factors: the presence or absence of sperm, the presence of a prostatitis, the findings on seminal vesiculography and testicular biopsy, physical findings and laboratory results.

If the urologist does not find obstructive disease, the help of a specialist in fertility should be sought. Specific therapy may be suggested by various urinary hormonal studies in conjunction with physical examination and biopsy.

The following up-to-date information was abstracted from a review article in a recently published new journal.*

Facts of Interest in Fertility

1) Sperm motility may be dependent on Leydig-cell activity. Men with hypophysectomy have loss of motility and reduction in semen volume.

2) Prostatic and seminal vesicle secretions are under the control of androgens. Both volume and contents are affected by androgens.

3) Semen absent in fructose will not coagulate immediately after ejaculation. This occurs with congenital absence of the seminal vesicles.

4) Usually the early portion of the ejaculate contains the highest number of sperm and the latter portion the highest concentration of fructose.

5) Retrograde ejaculation may occur with: a) prostatic surgery, b) surgical or chemical sympathectomy, c) spinal injury, d) deep pelvic dissection, e) diabetic neuropathy, f) abnormal anatomical position of ejaculatory ducts.

6) Low volume of semen associated with a normal sperm count may be the cause of infertility. A cervical capping treatment may result in pregnancy.

7) When there is a high volume of semen (over 4 ml), using the better half of the ejaculate may result in pregnancy.

8) Cystic fibrosis in the male is associated with congenital absence of the vas deferens.

9) Both hypothyroidism and hyperthyroidism will affect spermatogenesis.

10) Sexual habits of the couple account for 5 percent of fertility problems. Careful history-taking will uncover this.

11) Sperm agglutination with failure to liquify is sometimes corrected with ascorbic acid, 250 mg three times a day. Ascorbic acid is a potent reducing agent.

12) Husband-wife immune reaction to sperm may occur, the semen acting as an antigen. Mixing the semen with the wife's serum and incubating for 4 hours will demonstrate this reaction (agglutination occurs). The utilization of a condom for several months sometimes causes disappearance of this immune reaction long enough for a pregnancy to occur.

13) Higher-than-normal temperatures can interrupt normal spermatogenic mat-

* Richard D. Amelar and Lawrence Dubin, "Male Infertility: Current Diagnosis and Treatment," *Urology*, 1:1 (1973).

uration. Hot baths can have a definite effect. The arrest is reversible after removing the source of heat.

14) Pathogens causing prostatitis may cause agglutination of the ejaculate.

15) Certain drugs, among them busulfan (Myleran), triethylenemelamine (TEM), arsenic, colchicine, methotrexate, some amebicides, testosterone, medroxyprogesterone (Depo-Provera) and nitrofurantoin (Furadantin) may interfere with spermatogenesis.

Testicular Failure as a Cause of Infertility

Testicular failure accounts for 15 percent of fertility problems. Germinal aplasia is the commonest cause. Azoospermia with normal testis, vas deferens, and epididymis is characteristic. The follicle-stimulating hormone (FSH) may be elevated. Klinefelter's syndrome is another example of testicular failure. These patients have azoospermia, small testes, elevated FSH levels and usually a positive chromatin pattern.

With cryptorchidism, azoospermia is present if the testis has been kept out of the scrotum until puberty. If not brought down by the age of 35 to 40, androgenic activity is also lost due to total fibrosis.

Bilateral mumps orchitis and radiation are other causes of testicular failure with associated azoospermia. Radiation reaction may be reversible, spermatogenesis returning after three to four years.

Varicoceles and Infertility

The patient with a fertility problem found to have a varicocele may benefit by ligation of the spermatic veins. A good response can be expected in those patients found to have oligospermia with marked impairment of motility and increased immature forms of sperm and tapering forms. The same findings are present in adults with the adrenogenital syndrome. To differentiate the two, 17-ketosteroid determinations may be made.

With varicocele, testicular biopsy shows germinal-cell hypoplasia and premature sloughing of immature sperm similar to those seen in the ejaculate.

Contrast medium injected into the spermatic vein has demonstrated radiographically with varicocele that blood on the left mixes with blood on the right within the scrotum. It is possible that infertility in these patients is due to relatively high concentrations of toxic metabolic substances such as steroids passing directly down from the left adrenal to the testes. Increased temperature within the scrotum as a cause of infertility is not too easily explained by the mere stasis of blood secondary to the varicocele.

Endocrine Causes of Infertility

Only about 10 percent of patients will be found to have an endocrine disturbance and most of these will be due to low levels of pituitary gonadotropin. Some of these patients respond to chorionic gonadotropin.

Total urinary gonadotropin excretion is of therapeutic prognostic significance only at lower and higher extremes. At lower extremes (less than 6 M.U.U.) hypogonadotropinism is suggested. At higher extremes (more than 50 M.U.U.) primary testicular failure is suggested.

Low urinary 17-ketosteroids indicates hypoganidism or hypoadrenocorticism. Examination of the same 24-hour urine specimen for 17-hydroxy-corticoids (adrenocortical metabolite) will differentiate between these two conditions. Excretion of 3 to 10 mg per day is normal.

Elevated 17-ketosteroid excretion indicates gonadotropin suppression due to excess androgen levels. This occurs with the adrenogenital syndrome.

Nonsurgical Therapy for Infertility

The following conservative therapeutic recommendations are presented in the abstracted article (cf. previous reference to review article in *Urology*):

1) Thyroid should never be used unless specifically indicated.

2) In subfertile males with normal sperm counts and markedly depressed motility, low serum testosterone levels may indicate the usage of *very small* doses of testosterone. Suppression of the sperm count during therapy must be watched for and avoided.

3) High semen viscosity may be reduced with small doses of estrogen used for five days before the expected ovulatory phase of the female cycle. Interrupted use will not suppress spermatogenesis. Continuous use results in loss of libido, gynecomastia, and suppression of spermatogenesis.

4) Congenital adrenogenital syndrome found in boys may be treated with corticosteroids. Normal spermatogenesis and testicular development will occur.

5) Acquired adrenogenital syndrome characterized by a normal appearing male with normal or slightly small, soft testes (elevated urinary 17-ketosteroids) may be treated with glucocorticoids to reverse the gonadotropin-inhibiting effects on the excess adrenal androgens.

6) Gonadotropins may be given to stimulate germinal activity of the testes. This is of value in men with oligospermia and low urinary gonadotropin level. If a good response is to occur, it will be seen within three months.

7) Patients on testosterone rebound therapy seldom rebound and may have prolonged or permanent depression of spermatogenesis. This treatment should be reserved for patients not responding to other forms of indicated therapy who demonstrate severe oligospermia and fibrosis or sclerosis on testicular biopsy. If rebound occurs the effect is very transient, lasting only one to two months.

8) The technique of split ejaculation during the ovulatory phase of the female cycle is advised for patients with semen volume over 4 ml where motility, morphology, and liquefaction are more favorable in the first half of the ejaculum. Withdrawal midway through ejaculation has resulted in impregnation by some of these patients when other forms of therapy have failed.*

---

* End of abstract from *Urology* article.

Liquefaction of Gel-like Semen for Examination

Seminal fluids of increased viscosity are frequently seen. In most cases, sperm motility and survival *in vitro* seem to be unaffected by this condition. In others, the increased viscosity seems to be a barrier to the progressive normal motion of the sperm, and it is often difficult to obtain accurate counts in these specimens. Sometimes vigorous agitation causes liquefaction. In other cases, the addition of enzymes, such as alpha amylase, is helpful. Another method used is to aspirate and then forcefully inject with a Luer syringe and a large bone needle several times to liquefy the specimen.

Treatment with Potassium Iodide and Cervical Capping in Cases of Abnormally Thick Semen

Occasionally the semen remains very thick, with a string-like coagulum. In such cases, it is possible that the entire ejaculate can drop out of the vagina and be lost when the woman sits up or stands up. Any marked delay in liquefaction can be a cause of relative infertility.

Liquefaction often improves by treating these cases with increasing doses of saturated solution of potassium iodide. Instances have been reported where cervical capping after intercourse has resulted in pregnancy with full-term delivery. Treatment with potassium iodide is worth trying in those patients whose count and other studies have all been normal but in whom thick ejaculate prevents the passage of sperm through the cervical canal.

Spermatogenesis After Orchiopexy and Vasectomy

Not all undescended testes operated upon are defective in spermatogenesis. This has been substantiated time after time in patients subjected to vasectomy who previously had undescended testes. The vasa deferentia have been found to contain sperm. Sperm are often found in the ejaculate of patients subjected to orchiopexy after the puberty level.

Vas Reanastomosis (Vasovasostomy) and Splinting of the Vas Deferens

End-to-end and side-to-side anastomoses of the vas deferens have been advocated. Splints may consist of fine surgical wire, plastic tubing, or polyester suture material.

A splint may be inserted into the cut ends of the vas with a very fine Bunnell needle through which one has passed fine nylon suture. It is preferable to blunt the tip of the needle. The needle with suture is threaded into the lumen of the vas for a distance of about 1 to 2 cm and then makes its exit through the side of the vas. The suture is threaded in the opposite end of the vas in like manner. The sutures are usually led out through all layers of the scrotum and are tied over a bolster on the scrotal skin. Prior to tying this splint, the two cut ends of the vas deferens are sutured together with 5-0 or 6-0 silk eye sutures, one in each quadrant and only through the adventitial layer.

Proof of Nonobstruction of Distal Vas Segment at Surgery

When doing vas reanastomoses, a catheter is introduced into the patient's bladder. Several milliliters of diluted indigo carmine or methylene blue are injected into the distal vas. The dye obtained from the bladder proves the patency of the vas and ejaculatory duct.

Proof of Spermatogenesis at Surgery

In transecting the proximal vas, microscopic examination of the milky vas fluid obtained invariably shows sperm. The fact that sperm are nonmotile is of no consequence. One may obtain more fluid for examination at surgery by "milking" the epididymis.

The presence of expressed milky fluid is evidence of testicular and epididymal activity.

Subfertility After Vasovasostomy

Subfertility in patients after a vasovasostomy results from reduced motility of the spermatozoa, which is the defect accounting for 50 percent of all cases of male subfertility. Reduced motility is also seen after freezing sperm in liquid nitrogen for later use. As time progresses, the sperm become more active.

Final opinion concerning success or failure of surgical reanastomosis must await the passage of about two years of time.

THE PENIS

Penile Lesions and Their Treatment

Pathologic Significance of Pain in the Phallus

A dull aching pain in the penis is often easily overlooked. Referred pain to the penis must be explained. Examination by urethrography, cystopyelography, cystoscopy, and rectal inspection usually reveals irritation of the trigone, ureter, or urethra by a calculus or other irritant. Complete investigation for this rather benign symptom may reveal a considerable amount of silent pathology elsewhere in the urinary tract.

Condylomata Acuminata: Alternative Methods of Treatment

Condylomata acuminata are usually treated with 25 percent solution of podophyllin in mineral oil, or tincture of benzoin. A second application may be necessary in a few weeks.

With a *particularly intelligent patient* self-treatment may be tried. The patient is given silver nitrate sticks and advised to apply this morning and night for two to four days, using meticulous care. After application, the silver-nitrate-treated areas must be neutralized with an alcohol sponge. These patients should be followed at periodic intervals.

In instances where topical applications are unsuccessful, electrocautery then must be utilized. In the presence of a redundant prepuce, circumcision may be necessary.

When condylomata grow on the urethral mucosa and invade the urethra proximal to the fossa navicularis (often as far as the midportion of the anterior urethra), destruction by electrocoagulation is necessary. Stricture formation becomes a distinct possibility.

One must never overlook inspection of the sexual partner, with appropriate therapy if indicated. Often other veneral diseases will be found associated with the "venereal warts."

Multiple Recurrent Urethral Condylomata

An alternative method of treatment in severely recurrent cases of urethral condylomata consists of the surgical opening of the urethra at the coronal sulcus, the operator extending the incision even halfway to the penoscrotal junction. The urethral mucosa is sutured to the skin as in the Johanson urethroplasty for stricture. The condylomata are then individually coagulated under direct vision. The urethra is left open to heal. Recurrences then can be easily coagulated.

The urethra should be inspected every two weeks until it is certain that no recurrent lesions appear. After a period of three to six months with no recurrence, the urethra can be closed as is done in the Johanson second-stage urethroplasty.

Thrombosis of Coronal Veins

Occasionally the urologist receives a desperate call from a male patient requesting that he be seen immediately because of a lump, sometimes tender, on his penis. Inspection discloses hard coronal veins. This condition is felt to be a traumatic thrombophlebitis related to intercourse or masturbation. The condition is self-limited and will subside in two to three weeks if not aggravated by the cause.

Herpes Progenitalis

Herpes progenitalis can be very troublesome because of its frequency of recurrence. The treatment with smallpox vaccine has not proven too satisfactory. Idoxuridine, a drug used by ophthalmologists in the treatment of herpes simplex keratitis, is said to represent a pioneering achievement in antiviral chemotherapy by inhibiting the reproduction of the virus. This drug has been tried in early lesions of herpes progenitalis and appears to be effective. The 0.5 percent ointment is used three or four times a day.

It is important that the area be kept dry between treatments, and that secretions not be allowed to accumulate. Again, it is necessary occasionally to perform circumcision if there is redundant prepuce.

Paraphimosis

Paraphimosis can usually be reduced. The patient is sedated with intravenous or intramuscular opiate-like medication. Hyaluronidase, 150 N.F. to 300 N.F. units in 5 to 10 ml of saline, is injected into the edematous foreskin. Compression is done over gauze with one's fingers for three or four minutes. Reduction is attempted thus: with thumb and index finger of both hands the foreskin is pressed over the glans, while at the same time the glans is being pushed into the foreskin. Note that sometimes large doses of pain-relieving medication are required.

If there is a very tight constricting band, it may be necessary under local anesthesia to cut the constricting band in order to reduce the paraphimosis. Temporarily, one may tightly wrap Kling or any other type of elastic dressing immediately distal to the contracting band to reduce the size of the glans penis, and then pull down the foreskin. Figure 67 illustrates this method of reduction.

Another means of facilitating reduction of paraphimosis is to inject

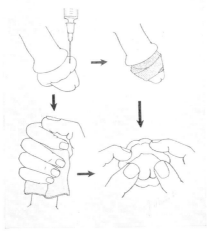

67. Method of reducing paraphimosis, showing means of wrapping elastic dressing distal to the contracting band

Xylocaine mixed with hyaluronidase into the foreskin. This will markedly reduce the inflammatory reaction, aiding reduction of the retracted foreskin. Since local anesthesia has been used, it is often wise to do a dorsal slit at this time and suture together the mucosal and skin edges with 3-0 or 4-0 catgut suture.

Urethral Meatotomy in Male Children

With the cooperative child, hospitalization for urethral meatotomy, and its attendant cost and psychological trauma, is rarely necessary. A tranquilizing medication prior to the outpatient or office visit is advised. Barbiturates alone should not be used, since they have an exciting effect on the child when pain is experienced.

A toothpick soaked with a local anesthetic agent is applied just within the meatus. After a three-minute waiting period injection of 0.5 to 1 ml of the anesthetic agent with a 25- or 27-gauge needle is made into the urethral mucosa at the frenal midline area. A mosquito hemostat applied to the area to be incised for 10 minutes before cutting the membrane assures minimal pain and bleeding for the procedure.

Continuous reassurance and diversion by the doctor before, and by the nurse during the waiting period, and separation of the meatus by the mother three times a day after the procedure, help to achieve excellent, inexpensive, and atraumatic results.

The use of ophthalmic sulfonamide ointment placed within the urethral meatus after each voiding tends to dilate and keep the meatus from healing together as well as providing excellent lubrication. The meatotomy incision should be made at least two units (French) larger than the desired size as narrowing always occurs during the healing process.

An office meatotomy is absolutely contraindicated when the child is escorted into the office by both parents (if both parents drive). This is indicative of a great deal of parental apprehension over what is about to happen. This apprehension is usually conveyed to the child, who is invariably a "spoiled little boy." If the parents and child are first interviewed in the consultation room, the problem quickly becomes apparent. After determining the need for a meatotomy, the wise physician will arrange for hospitalization.

(See also the suggestions for meatotomy and methods of maintaining patency described in Chapter Seven.)

Readily Available Penis Clamps

An ordinary laboratory wire test-tube clamp is easily sterilized and serves well as a penis clamp for adult males. For young boys ordinary adult-size penis clamps are unsatisfactory for retention of topical

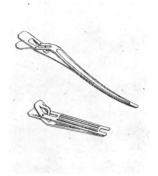

68. Penis clamps for young boys

urethral anesthetic agents. A more functional clamp may be made by using hair-curling clips found on most cosmetic counters. A small outward bend can be made in the inferior limb of the clip. This simple device is very satisfactory for the purpose stated. See Figure 68.

Stricture of Urethral Meatus—Repair and Prevention of Recurrence

In cases of marked inflammation and stricture of the urethral meatus, especially in adult males, the removal of a wedge-shaped section of skin to allow eversion of the urethral mucosa may be necessary. A sound is passed through the meatus and a section of skin is excised by means of a scalpel. Meatotomy is then performed by a vertical incision over the sound (Fig. 69).

With this method, there is redundant urethral mucosa which can be everted and sutured to the skin edge by means of interrupted 4-0 catgut suture. Recurrence of a urethral meatal stricture is rare when this technique is employed.

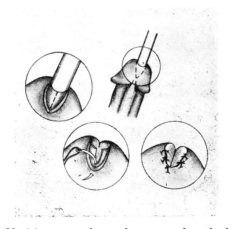

69. Meatotomy by wedge-removal method

Circumcision

The numerous operations for circumcision may be reviewed in most standard urological textbooks. A limited number of helpful procedures and instruments are herein recommended.

Loosely placed fine cotton or synthetic suture is used for circumcision by some. Others prefer 3-0 or 4-0 catgut. Catgut suture may be used for ligatures as well as for the wound approximation. Mattress suture is placed at the frenum for bleeding control. Several other sutures are also placed in adult patients subjected to circumcision due to possible wound separation resulting from frequency of erection. Interrupted sutures only are used. The continuous suture may result in contraction and paraphimosis.

The Gomco clamp has proved valuable. Some urologists use this clamp as a guide for smooth skin and mucosa edges and then separate the wound, clamp and tie off (or fulgurate) bleeding vessels, and lastly reapproximate the cut edges with catgut suture.

V-Plasty Circumcision. To allow for more circumference at the wound margin, a V-plasty on the dorsum of the penis may be done. This is accomplished by making the usual dorsal slit incision to the corona. Instead of making the circular incision at this point, the operator begins it about ¼ to ⅜ of an inch distal. This leaves a V-shaped notch in skin and mucosal edges. They are then sutured. Increased circumference at the suture line, together with nonirritating, nonabsorbable suture, makes for a more comfortable healing period. Sutures may be taken as shown in Figure 70. Added circumference of both skin and mucosa is obtained.

Circumcision by Separate Skin and Mucosal Incision. One may wish to mark the lines of incision with marking pencil or applicator stick, using methylene blue or gentian violet stain. The skin only is incised circum-

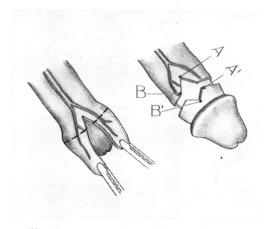

70. Circumcision by V-plasty technique

ferentially by scalpel. Following this the mucosa only is incised circumferentially. The remaining foreskin between the two circumferential incisions is then excised. After bleeding vessels are clamped and tied, or fulgurated, the skin and mucosa are sutured together with interrupted sutures. Care must be taken not to excise too much underlying fascia once the skin and mucosal incisions have been made. Excessive traction on the foreskin must be avoided.

CIRCUMCISION DRESSING. The suture at the frenal area and the one at the 12 o'clock position on the dorsum of the penis are usually left long, so that a strip of Vaseline-soaked gauze may be tied circumferentially by these sutures. The Vaseline-gauze dressing may be removed in three to four days by merely cutting these two specific sutures. Dressings soaked with Furacin, iodoform, Neomycin or Neosporin may be used in place of Vaseline. Kling or roll-gauze dressing is loosely wrapped over the moisturized dressing.

Alternatively, a sterile 4- by 4-inch gauze dressing may be cut at a folded edge, removing a V-shaped section. When the dressing is opened the penis is led through this opening. The gauze is folded back and a two-inch piece of adhesive is used to adhere this dressing to the penis at the base. See Figure 71.

Still another method is to proceed as just described. A second opened-up gauze pad is attached to the primary one with two short pieces of

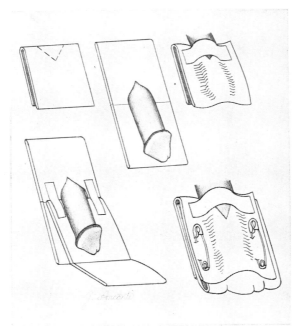

71. Dressings used after circumcision

adhesive. The second pad is folded over the top of the penis and safety-pinned to the first dressing. When the patient wishes to void, he must remove the safety pins (Fig. 71).

The dressings are changed, obviously, when soiled.

Lesions of the Glans Penis

Many penile lesions seen by the urologist fall into the category of dermatology. An edematous penis may be simply the result of a patient's habitual wearing of briefs a size too small with consequent circulatory restriction. The "sizing" used in new underwear may also cause edema.

There are instances of early carcinoma, erythroplasia of Queyrat, chronic granuloma, etc., which warrant biopsy, preferably done by the urologist. A plea is herein made for urologists to be aware of lesions of the glans penis which warrant biopsy. Wedge resection with mattress suture for bleeding control is probably the best approach. Punch biopsy with fulguration of the base for control of bleeding retards healing for a prolonged period.

Erythroplasia of Queyrat

Any persistent indurated lesion of the penis should be biopsied as early as possible. The premalignant Bowenoid skin lesions usually respond well to topical application of some antineoplastic chemotherapeutic agent such as fluorouracil (5-Fluorouracil). In the management of erythroplasia of Queyrat, confirmed by biopsy, 2 percent 5-Fluorouracil in water-soluble cream is applied once or twice daily until an inflammatory response is achieved. The treatment is then discontinued. On subsidence of the acute reaction, the lesion heals and the area looks normal. Biopsies should then be taken.

Negative biopsies have been reported after this treatment. Leukoplakias on the genitalia respond to this type of therapy but should be followed very closely by biopsy.

Priapism: Etiology

The cause of some cases of priapism remains obscure. Cavernosograms and spongiosograms have revealed that deep dorsal vein obstructions account for priapism. Infiltration of tumor, leukemia, sickle-cell disease, etc., are well-recognized causes of this condition.

Many patients on anticoagulant therapy have developed priapism. This treatment may be one cause. Consultation between cardiologist and urologist is necessary in these cases to determine whether the anticoagulation treatment should be continued or stopped.

Treatment of Priapism

Therapy for priapism has not been too satisfactory. In many cases impotence will result. This should be thoroughly explained to the patient.

The usual therapy for priapism is the aspiration of each of the corpora cavernosa, using a 16- or 18-gauge needle inserted into the base and a like needle in the distal area of each of the corpora cavernosa. Aspiration is done with a 20-ml syringe, followed by irrigation with 50 mg of heparin in 500 ml of sterile saline solution.

A recent modification of the above employs No. 14 intracaths. Two penetrations are made into each corpus cavernosum at the base and at the distal end near the coronal sulcus. The intracath placed at the base may then be connected to intravenous tubing, and the distal intracath connected to a drainage bottle. Heparinized solution may be slowly dripped into the intracath placed at the base, with drainage out of the intracath at the distal end of the penis. A pediatric blood pressure cuff may be placed around the penis between the intracaths and inflated periodically to express whole blood. Irrigation may be continued up to a maximum period of about twelve hours with this method while possible surgical correction is awaited. See Figure 72.

The saphenous-vein-to-cavernosa shunt for priapism (Fig. 73) has been reported successful if done early in the disease process. The saphenous vein is anastomosed to the corpora cavernosa first on the right side and then, if necessary, on the left side.

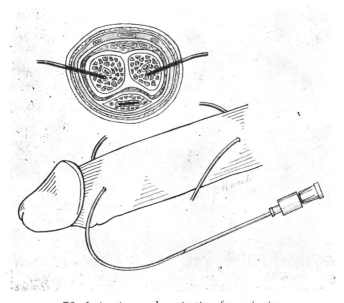

72. Irrigation and aspiration for priapism

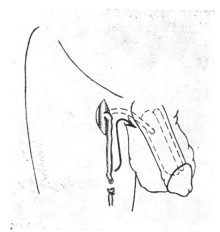

73. Anastomosis of saphenous vein to corpora cavernosa for priapism

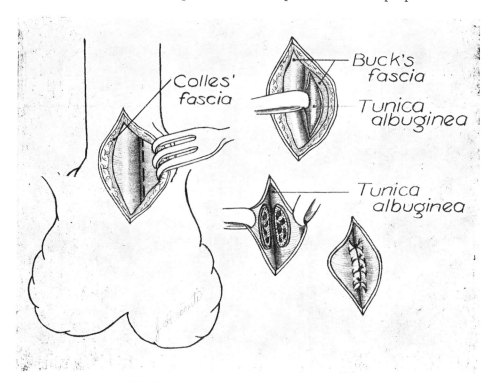

74. Cavernosa-spongiosa shunt for priapism

An alternate procedure is to cut windows (1 cm in diameter) in the corpora cavernosa and adjacent spongiosa through the tunica albuginea and suture these windows to each other (Fig. 74). This modality (cavernosa-spongiosa shunts bilaterally) is now replacing the saphenous-cavernosa shunt. More recently, multiple shunts of this type have also been done successfully. Gangrene of the penis has been reported in a case where the shunting was performed at the base of the penis.

Removal of Metal Bands Encircling the Penis

Urologists are occasionally confronted with this problem, which can produce a considerable amount of difficulty in removal. Usually the band is a ring of some sort. A considerable amount of swelling results both in front and behind the ring, so much so, that venous congestion results, calling for ingenious means of removal. The use of a file is sometimes attempted. There is considerable danger of damaging the tissues with this tool. A Gigli saw forced between a metal elevator and the ring has been used, with the ring then easily sawed in two. Occasionally, the help of hospital engineers must be elicited to remove an encircling band.

The following method for the removal of a constricting ring may be of value. A length of heavy packaging cord may be tightly wrapped around the penile shaft, and compressed for a distance of 2 to 3 cm distal to the ring. One-inch Kling dressing may also be used in like manner. By passing a curved hemostat between the ring and the wrapped penis, the operator may bring the loose proximal end of the cord through the ring. The entire area may be well lubricated with mineral oil, and the cord then slowly and completely unwrapped from the proximal end, advancing the ring along the penile shaft. The maneuver is repeated as the ring advances down the shaft. A 25-gauge needle may be used to pinprick the prepuce to allow fluid to escape during the process. This method is illustrated in Figure 75.

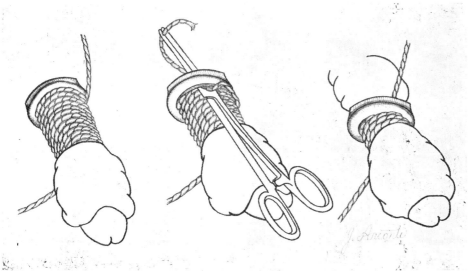

75. Suggested method for removing constricting band from penis

Tourniquet in Penile Surgery

In the performance of penile surgery a tourniquet applied at the base is most helpful in controlling bleeding. Should the skin distal to the tourniquet become cyanotic, the tourniquet should be discontinued immediately.

Various Modes of Therapy for Peyronie's Disease

In the treatment of this resistant disease, the use of local anesthesia followed by steroids and hyaluronidase injected directly into the plaques has proved helpful.

The direct injection into the plaques can be accomplished only by use of a metal syringe with screw-thread barrel, the hydrocortisone and hyaluronidase being injected under pressure into varied areas of the plaque. This therapy to five to ten injection sites once weekly may be required for as long as fifty weeks before improvement is noted in either curvature of the penis on erection, relief of pain on erection, or resolution of the plaque (or all three of the above).

The recently reported technique of incising the skin and fascial layers over the plaque and injecting hydrocortisone throughout the plaque with an air-pressure syringe (Dermajet ®) until the entire plaque shows blanching, holds excellent promise. From 50 to 100 injection sites are treated at the time of open surgical exposure of the plaque.

Dental Burr Therapy for Dense Peyronie's Disease Plaque

One of us (H.B.) has been treating the very dense plaques, not readily amenable to injection, by "shaving down" the plaques. The operating room dental drill with a diamond burr is utilized. The plaque is treated with the burr until the fine decussating fibers and the thinned-out tunica albuginea are seen. The area is thoroughly lavaged to wash away the "filings" before wound closure is done. Further trial of this modality is warranted.

Surgical Excision of Peyronie's Plaque: Sequelae; Use of Penile Prostheses

Surgical excision with closure of the incision site is almost invariably followed by impotence and recurrence of the plaques. Some authors claim success with this procedure with no erectile loss. When impotence does result, it may be amenable to treatment with the silicone prosthesis described by one of us (R.O.P.) and modified subsequently by other authors. [*]

Figure 76 is a cutaway drawing of a phallus with the implant in place.

---

[*] R. O. Pearman, "Insertion of a Silastic Penile Prosthesis for Treatment of Organic Sexual Impotence," *Journal of Urology,* 107:802 (May, 1972).

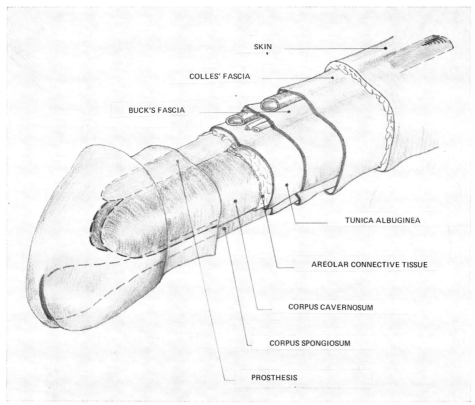

SKIN

COLLES' FASCIA

BUCK'S FASCIA

TUNICA ALBUGINEA

AREOLAR CONNECTIVE TISSUE

CORPUS CAVERNOSUM

CORPUS SPONGIOSUM

PROSTHESIS

76. Silicone prosthesis implanted in phallus

Objective Observation of Peyronie's Disease

It is difficult to assess the value of treatment in Peyronie's disease. Drawing the shape and size of the erect phallus on graph paper and following the line alongside the erect phallus at periodic intervals has proved to be a good means of evaluating the lessening of the curvature after therapy. The patient, utilizing the same graph paper, may also be able to outline the size of the plaque as he palpates it. This graphic drawing demonstrates well the progress (or lack of it) in the treatment course of the patient.

The disease is often not steadily progressive, with long periods of remission and subjective improvement.

Repair of Hypospadias

Numerous surgical procedures have been recommended over the years. The incidence of fistula formation by all methods varies from 15 to 30 percent with most urologists. It is again not the intent here to evaluate the advantages and disadvantages of the many techniques. Emphasis must be placed, however, on two factors: (1) straightening of the chordee, and (2) urinary diversion, whether it be by perineal urethrostomy or suprapubic cystostomy. Each of these diversion methods has its proponents.

Because of complications, poor results, etc., attempts to improve the surgical repair method stimulate modifications of procedures.

Penile Immobilization During Hypospadias Surgery

A simple means of penile immobilization is to place a 3-0 or 4-0 silk or polyester suture through the tip of the glans penis and tie it very loosely. This same suture is then placed into the abdominal skin in such a position in the midline below the umbilicus that the penis is placed on stretch.

Most types of surgical repair for hypospadias may be done in this manner. On completion of surgery, the suture is removed. Pressure on the needle site of the glans penis will control bleeding.

Penile Dressing Post-Hypospadias Repair

Kling dressing over Vaseline gauze is a favorite of many surgeons. Cotton batting applied wet as a cast about the penis may remain in place at least five to ten days after surgery. Vaseline, Furacin, iodoform and Polysporin dressings all have their advocates.

Battery-Operated Electrosurgical Unit for
Bleeding Control in Hypospadias Repair

A battery-operated disposable electrocautery designed for ophthalmologists which provides for minute electrocoagulation on the conjunctiva may also be useful during hypospadias repair, where meticulous hemostasis is necessary. The cautery has been found to work well for this procedure particularly around the glans penis, where it is difficult to clamp and tie. For the urethra the unit is exceedingly helpful. It is marketed under the name "OPTEMP®."

The usual electrosurgical unit with a fine wire electrode may serve the same purpose but may be exceedingly dangerous when working on a small phallus. The electrical current has to pass to the ground first through the shaft of the penis. Because of the small diameter of the penile shaft, a buildup of heat may occur, causing destruction of the penile tissue.

If the electrosurgical unit is used, the coagulating current must be set at the lowest effective current.

In hypospadias repair, the use of the loupe lens is extremely valuable in placing sutures.

IMPOTENCE

Etiology and Evaluation

Organic vs. Psychogenic Impotence

Though male sexual inadequacy is a complaint often faced by the urologist, little interest in the problem is shown by many. Less than 10 percent of the patients who complain of sexual impotency have organic basis for their complaint. The earlier in life lack of potency occurs, the more likely it is to be psychogenic. A diligent evaluation must be done, however, to rule out the presence of a Leriche syndrome, diabetes mellitus, multiple sclerosis, urological disease, cord tumors, etc. Since 50 to 60 percent of male diabetics are impotent, the urologist must be certain not to overlook this presenting complaint.

If the patient has undergone radical prostatectomy (especially perineal), orchiectomy, or is on estrogen therapy, there is no mystery as to etiology.

Other serious symptoms usually accompany impotency when an organic condition is the cause. These are more prominent or disabling to the patient, as a rule, than his sexual inadequacy. The majority of patients who complain of impotence are below the age of 40 years. In patients who complain to their physicians of this condition after the age of 40, the history reveals that the initial episode of failure generally occurred earlier in life. Such early forgotten episodes can usually be documented by careful questioning. The history of one or several episodes of sexual failure in the earlier life of the patient will constitute a strong argument in favor of a psychogenic basis for the inadequacy.

The presence of early morning erections indicates the absence of an organic disease of the reflex arc. The patient who is aware of these erections uses them as an argument against his fear of impotence. For this reason, he anticipates them, expects them, and attempts to obtain them by employing all kinds of fantasies or manipulations. The psychic inhibition can at times be so intense and persistent that the patient may notice spontaneous erections becoming progressively weaker in strength and absent for increasingly prolonged periods of time. *In most instances, psychotherapy will succeed in restoring erections.* This indicates that incomplete erections, or even the absence of spontaneous erections, do not necessarily imply an organic condition.

A superimposed psychogenic factor may frequently aggravate organic disease with resultant sexual inadequacy. The use of psychotherapy combined with testosterone (together with treatment of the organic problem if possible) has been beneficial in many such instances.

The very high increase in divorce rates among the middle aged has caused many more male patients to seek out the urologist to correct their problems with unsatisfactory erections and premature ejaculations.

These patients generally lack confidence, and time must be taken to explain to them to their satisfaction that they must relearn the act of intercourse *with one sex partner.* They may regain a very satisfying sex life with patience, but they no longer are "young bucks." The mid-life crisis (male menopause) is a very real thing, primarily emotional in origin, and must be accepted by the patient if he expects to have a satisfactory sex life.

Radical Retroperitoneal Gland Dissection Followed by Impotence

Impotency following radical retroperitoneal gland dissection is often due to the concomitant dissection of the sympathetic nerve plexus at the bifurcation of the iliac arteries. The patient must be forewarned of this possibility. Extreme caution should be used during surgery to avoid this nerve plexus, if at all possible.

Return of Function

Effect on Sexual Function of Radical Surgery and/or Estrogen Therapy for Carcinoma of the Prostate

The return of sexual function after radical surgery for carcinoma of the prostate, or after the use of estrogen therapy for same, has been reported in many instances. Sexual function may return in three to six months, or a longer period may be required. In most instances, of course, the sexual function never returns.

Stilbestrol Therapy in Cases of Impotency Due to Ejaculatory Duct Congestion

Congestion of the ejaculatory ducts often contributes to symptoms of perineal pain, tenderness in the testes, and urinary tract irritation. Stilbestrol in doses of 1 to 5 mg, three times a day for a month, causes a marked regression of the congestion; after a month, patients may gradually resume sexual activity.

UNUSUAL MANIFESTATIONS OF SEXUAL ABERRATION

The literature abounds with reports of amazing instances of sexual deviation—one is referred thereto for specific types of case reports. Almost every known object, from snakes to snails, has been reported in the urethra. The originality of man in finding substitute objects to meet his biological needs is truly incredible, and the identification and removal of such objects will continue to tax the intelligence and ingenuity of urologists—and to enhance the fascination of the most intriguing specialty in all of medicine.

APPENDIX

The following list includes the names of past and present contributors to the Weekly Urological Clinical Letter which in part inspired and formed the basis for this volume, as explained in the ACKNOWLEDGEMENTS. Note that the shared ideas have been distilled, condensed, and edited by us; we are responsible for the opinions expressed, not the contributors.

ABESHOUSE, Benjamin S., M.D.   Baltimore, Maryland
ALBERT, David J., M.D.   Buffalo, New York
ALPERN, Joshua, M.D.   Anaheim, California
ARCONTI, John S., Jr., M.D.   Reseda, California
ATKINS, Dale M., M.D.   Denver, Colorado

BAIRD, John M., M.D.   Bryan, Texas
BAIRD, Sydney S., M.D.   Dallas, Texas
BANALAPH, Thongchai, M.D.   Buffalo, New York
BANDELL, Herbert, M.D.   Fontana, California
BECK, Sidney H., M.D.   Bridgeport, Connecticut
BELT, Elmer, M.D.   Los Angeles, California
BENJAMIN, Victor A., M.D.   Jaffna, Ceylon
BERLIN, Bert B., M.D.   Hartford, Connecticut
BERRY, John L., M.D.   Loudonville, New York
BIEL, Leonard, Jr., M.D.   New York, New York
BIORN, Carl L., M.D.   Palo Alto, California
BLUM, John A., M.D.   San Diego, California
BOATWRIGHT, Donald C., M.D.   Scottsdale, Arizona
BODNER, Henry, M.D.   Van Nuys, California
BOSWORTH, N. Lewis, M.D.   Lexington, Kentucky
BOYLAN, Richard N., M.D.   Riverside, California
BRADHAM, Allen C., M.D.   Anderson, South Carolina
BRADY, Edward A., M.D.   New Brunswick, New Jersey
BRENNER, M. A., M.D.   Newport Beach, California
BRIDGE, Robert A. C., M.D.   San Diego, California
BRODNY, M. Leopold, M.D.   Chicago, Illinois
BROWN, Richard J., M.D.   Richmond, Indiana
BURNHAM, John P., M.D.   Ventura, California

CONROY, Frederick D., M.D.   Edmonton, Alberta, Canada
COONER, William H., M.D.   Mobile, Alabama

COOPER, John F., M.D. — Los Angeles, California
CRENSHAW, W. B., M.D. — Seattle, Washington
CROWELL, Bruce, M.D. — Tampa, Florida
CURD, Howard H., M.D. — St. Petersburg, Florida
CUTLER, Harry, M.D. — St. Louis, Missouri

DANIEL, William R., M.D. — Orlando, Florida
DAVIS, Phillip, M.D. — Beverly Hills, California
DEDDENS, Lloyd E., M.D. — Jackson, Mississippi
DeKOVESSEY, Charles A., M.D. — Olney, Illinois
deKERNION, Jean B., M.D. — Los Angeles, California
DESAI, Priyakant K., M.D. — Erie, Pennsylvania
DICK, Arthur L., M.D. — Los Angeles, California
DILLON, James R., Jr., M.D. — San Diego, California
DORMAN, Parker S., M.D. — Washington, D.C.
DOVEY, E. G., M.D. — Elkhart, Indiana
DUCOTE, Martin J., M.D. — Lafayette, Louisiana

ELIASON, Orland D., M.D. — Redwood City, California
EWELL, George H., M.D. — Madison, Wisconsin

FALK, David, M.D. — Bakersfield, California
FEENEY, Michael J., M.D. — San Diego, California
FIEDLER, George A., M.D. — Columbia, Tennessee
FINE, Myron G., M.D. — Dallas, Texas
FINE, Stuart W., M.D. — Milwaukee, Wisconsin
FINK, Aaron J., M.D. — Mountain View, California
FISCHMAN, J. L., M.D. — New Orleans, Louisiana
FISHER, Harry E., Jr., M.D. — Salt Lake City, Utah
FITE, Edward H., Jr., M.D. — Muskogee, Oklahoma
FITZPATRICK, Terence J., M.D. — Los Angeles, California
*FREED, Ezekiel, M.D. — Northridge, California
FREED, Selwyn Z., M.D. — Bronx, New York
FRUMKIN, Jacob, M.D. — Schenectady, New York

GARRETT, Jerry S., M.D. — Mission Hills, California
GARRETT, Robert A., M.D. — Indianapolis, Indiana
GENS, John Paul, M.D. — Norwalk, Connecticut
GERRIE, Wallace A., M.D. — Newport Beach, California
GERSH, Isadore, M.D. — Denver, Colorado

*Chief Radiologist Northridge Hospital, Northridge, California (contributor to information on Table IV, Pages 52, 53—not a W.U.C.L. member)

GERSON, Stanley, M.D.	Paterson, New Jersey
GHORMLEY, Kenneth O., M.D.	Redlands, California
GITTES, Ruben F., M.D.	San Diego, California
GOLDFARB, Morton, M.D.	Massapequa Park, New York
GOLDSTEIN, Abraham M. B., M.D.	Los Angeles, California
GOODWIN, Willard E., M.D.	Los Angeles, California
GRAY, Cary P., M.D.	Palo Alto, California
GREY, David N., M.D.	Ventura, California
GRIFFITH, Thomas L., M.D.	San Leandro, California
GROBERT, Marshall J., M.D.	Long Beach, California
°GUMAS, Thomas, M.D.	Sherman Oaks, California
HARP, Grady E., M.D.	Los Angeles, California
HARRISON, Richard H., III, M.D.	Bryan, Texas
HARROLD, Jesse F., M.D.	Lansing, Michigan
HART, Joseph B., M.D.	Newport Beach, California
HEINEMANN, S., M.D.	Carlsbad, New Mexico
HOLLAND, Harold, M.D.	Beverly Hills, California
HORSLEY, T.A., M.D.	Norwalk, California
HOWARD, Allan H., M.D.	Laguna Hills, California
HOWE, Gerald E., M.D.	San Diego, California
HUDSON, Henry C., M.D.	Birmingham, Alabama
HYMAN, Jack, M.D.	Mobile, Alabama
IMMERGUT, Sidney, M.D.	Brooklyn, New York
ISAAC, Charles A., M.D.	Newton, Kansas
JEPPESEN, F. B., M.D.	Boise, Idaho
JEROME, Shepard, M.D.	Mobile, Alabama
KAMINSKY, Anthony F., M.D.	Erie, Pennsylvania
KAPLAN, Joseph H., M.D.	Los Angeles, California
KAPLAN, Ronald J., M.D.	Sherman Oaks, California
KAY, Harold, M.D.	Oakland, California
KELLY, Timothy L., M.D.	Arlington, Virginia
KESHIN, Jesse G., M.D.	Mount Vernon, New York
KIES, Norman A., M.D.	Grass Valley, California
KOPP, Jules, M.D.	St. Louis, Missouri
KROLL, Kenneth M., M.D.	Anacortes, Washington
KUHN, Mark A. R., M.D.	Fort Lauderdale, Florida

°Dept. of Anesthesiology, Sherman Oaks Community Hospital, Sherman Oaks, California (contributor to information on Brevital amnesia, Pages 16-18—not a W. U. C. L. member)

LANDA, Eastwood, M.D. — Vancouver, B.C., Canada
LANDES, Ralph R., M.D. — Danville, Virginia
LAVELLE, Patrick J., M.D. — Los Angeles, California
LEADER, Abel J., M.D. — Houston, Texas
LEIFER, William W., M.D. — Kansas City, Missouri
LIPSHUTZ, Harold, M.D. — Philadelphia, Pennsylvania
LUBIN, E. N., M.D. — Tulsa, Oklahoma
LYONS, Richard C., M.D. — Erie, Pennsylvania

McGAVRAN, Harry G., M.D. — Quincy, Illinois
McKENZIE, Kenneth R., M.D. — Redlands, California
McLAREN, H. J., Jr., M.D. — Erie, Pennsylvania
McLIN, Patrick, M.D. — San Rafael, California
McROBERTS, J. William, M.D. — Lexington, Kentucky

MAGID, Moreton A., M.D. — Waco, Texas
MALIS, Irving, M.D. — Van Nuys, California
MARCONIS, Joseph T., M.D. — Pottsville, Pennsylvania
MAYERS, Morton, M.D. — Los Angeles, California
MILLER, J. Bernard, M.D. — Santa Ana, California
MINER, W. R., M.D. — Covington, Kentucky
MOOS, Mitchell A., M.D. — Grants Pass, Oregon
MORROW, James, M.D. — Los Angeles, California
MURPHY, Gerald P., M.D. — Buffalo, New York

NATION, Earl F., M.D. — Pasadena, California
NEWMAN, Harry R., M.D. — New Haven, Connecticut
NICELY, Park, M.D. — Knoxville, Tennessee
NEEDELL, Mervin H., M.D. — North Miami, Florida

O'HEERON, Michael K., M.D. — Houston, Texas
OHMAN, Albert C., M.D. — Seattle, Washington
OPPENHEIMER, Gordon D., M.D. — New York, New York
ORTEGA, Eduardo M., M.D. — Guayaquil, Ecuador
OZAR, Milton B., M.D. — Kansas City, Missouri

PALMER, James K., M.D. — Salt Lake City, Utah
PATTERSON, Joseph H., M.D. — Denver, Colorado
PEARLMAN, Carl K., M.D. — Santa Ana, California
PEARMAN, Robert O., M.D. — Encino, California
PECK, Sam, M.D. — San Diego, California
PIERCE, W. Vinson, M.D. — Covington, Kentucky

PINARD, Carl J., Jr., M.D.	Seattle, Washington
PLUMB, Robert T., M.D.	San Diego, California
POLSE, Sanford, M.D.	Encino, California
POWELL, Platt, M.D.	Burlington, Vermont
PRESMAN, David, M.D.	Chicago, Illinois
PRINS, Leo R., Jr., M.D.	Albert Lea, Minnesota
RAWLING, John C., M.D.	St. Petersburg, Florida
REED, Josiah F., Jr., M.D.	Montgomery, Alabama
*RIESER, Charles, M.D.	Atlanta, Georgia
RIOS, Jacinto B., M.D.	Canoga Park, California
RITTER, Henry, Jr., M.D.	Redwood City, California
ROLL, William A., M.D.	Kettering, Ohio
ROTH, Russell B., M.D.	Erie, Pennsylvania
ROTHFELD, Samuel H., M.D.	Great Neck, New York
RUBIN, Seymour W., M.D.	Miami Beach, Florida
RUSSO, C. Paul, M.D.	Ithaca, New York
SAMPSON, D., M.D.	Buffalo, New York
SCANLAN, David B., M.D.	Atlantic City, New Jersey
SCARDINO, Peter L., M.D.	Savannah, Georgia
SCHLOSS, Walter A., M.D.	Hartford, Connecticut
SCHMIESING, Clifford A., M.D.	Santa Ana, California
SCHNEIDERMAN, Clarence, M.D.	Montreal, Canada
SEARS, Bernard R., M.D.	Brookline, Massachusetts
SHAPIRO, Irving J., M.D.	Chicago, Illinois
SHARGEL, George M., M.D.	Huntingdon, Pennsylvania
SHASKY, Florian J., M.D.	Medford, Oregon
SHIELDS, John R., M.D.	Renton, Washington
SILBAR, John D., M.D.	Milwaukee, Wisconsin
SILBAR, Sidney J., M.D.	Milwaukee, Wisconsin
SILBER, Igal, M.D.	Tustin, California
SIMON, Samuel, M.D.	Poughkeepsie, New York
SINGER, Paul L., M.D.	Phoenix, Arizona
SLATER, Gregory S., M.D.	New Britain, Connecticut
SMART, William R., M.D.	San Rafael, California
SMITH, Baxter A., Jr., M.D.	Minneapolis, Minnesota
SPAULDING, Robert W., M.D.	Fresno, California
SPILLANE, Richard J., M.D.	Hartford, Connecticut
SPITALNY, August, M.D.	San Francisco, California
STEWART, B. G., M.D.	Bakersfield, California

---

*Contributor to information on Page 187—not a W.U.C.L. member

STEWART, B. Lyman, M.D.   Los Angeles, California
STITT, Ronald W., M.D.   Kansas City, Kansas
STOUTZ, Henry L., M.D.   Ventura, California
STRAUSS, Bernard, M.D.   Beverly Hills, California
SU, Shaw C. T., M.D.   Savannah, Georgia
SUTHERLAND, James W., M.D.   Quincy, Illinois

TEHAN, Timothy J., M.D.   Bethesda, Maryland
THOMPSON, Ian M., M.D.   Columbia, Missouri
TURNER, A. Fred, Jr., M.D.   Orlando, Florida
TYVAND, Raymond E., M.D.   Seattle, Washington

ULLMAN, Arthur, M.D.   Santa Ana, California

VARKARAKIS, Michael J., M.D.   Buffalo, New York
VILDIBILL, J. W., M.D.   Lafayette, Louisiana

WARRES, Herbert L., M.D.   Springfield, Missouri
WERSHUB, Leonard P., M.D.   New York, New York
WINER, Julius H., M.D.   Beverly Hills, California
WISE, M. F., M.D.   Kansas City, Missouri
WOOD, Lorne G., M.D.   Vancouver, B. C., Canada

ZANGRILLI, James G., M.D.   Pittsburgh, Pennsylvania

INDEX

309